Assessments for Sport and Athletic Performance

■ ■ ■

David H. Fukuda, PhD, CSCS,*D, CISSN

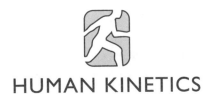

HUMAN KINETICS

Library of Congress Cataloging-in-Publication Data

Names: Fukuda, David H., 1980- author.
Title: Assessments for sport and athletic performance / David H. Fukuda.
Description: Champaign, IL : Human Kinetics, [2019] | Includes bibliographical references and index.
Identifiers: LCCN 2018036040 (print) | LCCN 2018054826 (ebook) | ISBN 9781492586876 (epub) | ISBN 9781492559894 (PDF) | ISBN 9781492559887 (print)
Subjects: LCSH: Athletic ability--Testing. | Physical fitness--Testing.
Classification: LCC GV436.5 (ebook) | LCC GV436.5 .F84 2019 (print) | DDC 796--dc23
LC record available at https://lccn.loc.gov/2018036040

ISBN: 978-1-4925-5988-7 (print)

The web addresses cited in this text were current as of September 2018, unless otherwise noted.

Senior Acquisitions Editor: Roger W. Earle; **Developmental Editor:** Laura Pulliam; **Managing Editor:** Miranda K. Baur; **Copyeditor:** Marissa Wold Uhrina; **Indexer:** Andrea J. Hepner; **Permissions Manager:** Martha Gullo; **Senior Graphic Designer:** Joe Buck; **Cover Designer:** Keri Evans; **Cover Design Associate:** Susan Rothermel Allen; **Photograph (cover):** Laszlo Szirtesi/Getty Images; **Photographs (interior):** © Human Kinetics; **Photo Asset Manager:** Laura Fitch; **Photo Production Coordinator:** Amy M. Rose; **Photo Production Manager:** Jason Allen; **Senior Art Manager:** Kelly Hendren; **Illustrations:** © Human Kinetics, unless otherwise noted; **Printer:** Sheridan Books

Human Kinetics books are available at special discounts for bulk purchase. Special editions or book excerpts can also be created to specification. For details, contact the Special Sales Manager at Human Kinetics.

Printed in the United States of America

10 9 8 7 6 5 4 3 2 1

The paper in this book is certified under a sustainable forestry program.

Human Kinetics

P.O. Box 5076
Champaign, IL 61825-5076
Website: www.HumanKinetics.com

In the United States, email info@hkusa.com or call 800-747-4457.
In Canada, email info@hkcanada.com.
In the United Kingdom/Europe, email hk@hkeurope.com.

For information about Human Kinetics' coverage in other areas of the world,
please visit our website: **www.HumanKinetics.com**

To Tamiko, for all of the revisions and ramblings you've endured over the years without receiving the credit you deserve. Without your love and unconditional support, this project would not have been possible and my days would certainly be incomplete.

To Brogan and Josette, I can only hope to add as much meaning to your lives as you have to mine. When we find ourselves at the bottom of a valley, we always dig in, support each other, and go for broke, so that we can enjoy the view from the top of the next peak together.

Contents

ASSESSMENT FINDER

Chapter 7   Power

Chapter 8   Muscular Strength and Endurance

(continued)

ASSESSMENT FINDER *(CONTINUED)*

Preface

The content of this book was developed to provide coaching and fitness professionals an accessible, comprehensive overview of assessments that was different from the information typically packaged in academic textbooks. The opportunity to serve as author for this project was especially appealing because I was a coach long before I received a PhD in exercise physiology and began my career teaching at the university level and conducting research studies.

Normative data tables with columns containing more percentile values than anyone would ever need are commonly included in books focused on assessments for sport and exercise. This book takes a different approach while simply dividing normative data into a few categories and presenting the information in a uniform, easily interpreted manner. Also unique to this book, assessments are described in a script format in order to clearly convey the protocols and assist in the standardization process between testing sessions.

Most of my early experiences as a coach fell within sports where success could not simply be measured by changes in distance or height, weight, or time, and improvements in performance in these activities tended to be based on my own potentially biased perception. The inclusion of even just a few assessments would have put my mind at ease when faced with the difficult task of evaluating the progress of my athletes. Additionally, for all of the grassroots coaches and others volunteering their time to allow others to engage in sport and fitness-based activities, it is important to provide resources to ensure everyone involved has a positive experience while achieving their full potential.

The National Library of Medicine defines athletic performance as the "carrying out of specific physical routines or procedures by one who is trained or skilled in physical activity," which is influenced "by a combination of physiological, psychological, and socio-cultural factors." It is important to note that this definition does not limit athletic performance to only the elite and that coaching and fitness professionals play a major role in each of the listed influential factors. Furthermore, athletic performance exists on a spectrum, and advancement along this spectrum of training and skill development signifies a very personalized journey. From the weekend warrior or the recent retiree to the up-and-coming prodigy, everyone involved may benefit from assessments along the road to accomplishing their goals.

Acknowledgments

I am very fortunate to have had so many great colleagues help me throughout my career as well as a wide variety of coaches and mentors who pushed me to succeed. There are certainly too many to mention here, so a generic "thank you" will have to suffice until I can attempt to return my debts of gratitude.

Roger Earle from Human Kinetics was a source of steady encouragement and guidance throughout the development of this book. His wealth of experience and creativity certainly made a positive impact on the final product. I would like to thank Justin Klug and Jeff Mathis for their contributions early on in this project, and Laura Pulliam for her feedback and direction during the editing process.

My entire family has always provided a steady mix of unfettered wisdom and enthusiasm, and I cannot begin to describe how important that has been amid all of my endeavors. Thanks!

PART I

BASICS OF ASSESSMENT

The first section of this book begins by providing support for the inclusion of assessment within the basic set of skills for coaching and fitness professionals as well as considerations for decision-making and implementation. This introduction is followed by a description of the various pieces of equipment that may be used to successfully conduct assessments. Finally, the basic fitness attributes are discussed, and a general outline of the assessment selection process is described.

CHAPTER 1

Assessment 101: Who, Why, and How?

> *"Carefully observe oneself and one's situation, carefully observe others, and carefully observe one's environment. Consider fully, act decisively."*
>
> Jigoro Kano, Founder of Judo

Coaches and fitness professionals are focused on optimizing health, physical fitness, and athletic performance. Assessments are part of the specialized toolbox they use to provide a clearer view of the current state of their client, athlete, or team. However, assessments should be used for more than just evaluation and can be used as key indicators of the effectiveness of decisions related to athlete or client management, general demographic information, personnel selection, talent development, and standardized training programs.

Oftentimes, we as coaches and fitness professionals get dialed in on our own system or personalized approach to improving the lives of our athletes or clients and the day-to-day support required to maintain positive development throughout this process. While this is certainly a trait of a successful professional, continuous improvement and unique situations likely dictate the need to answer the questions, "Is what I'm currently doing effective?" and "Can I be better serving my athlete or client?"

When you bring your car to a service center, a technician likely runs a series of diagnostic tests in order to recommend adjustments or to identify the cause of an existing issue. In the same manner, a client or athlete seeks out coaches and fitness professionals to provide feedback and guidance while working to achieve their individual goals. Following a general health evaluation and establishing the goals and needs of the client or athlete, the natural next step is to perform baseline assessments to answer the question, "What are we working with?" This process of identifying strengths and weaknesses allows for a clearer path to success to be laid out. For clients or athletes, an ongoing evaluation helps to identify progress or to determine the need for potential changes to be made.

INPUT FOR THE DECISION-MAKING PROCESS

While the phrase "garbage in, garbage out" illustrates that an informed decision requires accurate information, decision making without any, or with limited, input is simply guessing. The appropriate use of assessments by coaches and fitness professionals provides quality data that can inform the decision-making process. For example, a coach or fitness professional might notice that the client or athlete is noticeably slower toward the end of a soccer match and assume that this fatigued state is caused by a lack of aerobic conditioning. With this snap judgement, and without knowledge gleaned from a general fitness profile, the coach may select a course of action involving additional aerobic exercise that would take up valuable technical training time or extend the duration of an existing training session. However, periodic assessments, including those related to aerobic capacity or self-reported exertion/fatigue measures, might indicate that the individual was slower due to accumulated or residual fatigue and actually needed decreased training time or extended recovery.

While aerobic capacity measures evaluated at this point might be influenced by the fatigued state of the individual, preseason aerobic capacity measures and subsequent training focused on addressing any identified issues would allow the coaching staff to be confident that the athlete was properly prepared and not likely out of shape. Daily (or even weekly) assessments of perceived exertion or fatigue would then help to identify when training sessions could be adjusted to address these types of issues.

Whether the focus is on general management, performance, education, or health, the aim of most coaches and fitness professionals is to see progression in the individuals who put their aspirations or development in our hands. The intersection between these areas of focus and the use of the scientific method is complicated and sometimes problematic. This is made clear by the collective groans produced during coaches' meetings when a new evaluative approach is mentioned. Coaching can and should be viewed as an art form; however, without periodic quantitative feedback, the aforementioned progression may become stagnant. Particularly, in activities that have a storied history (think martial arts), change does not come easily, and there is an inherent "stick to what we've always done" mind-set. However, just as we would expect reflection on the part of our clients or athletes during periods of change, we should aim to evaluate our practices and be flexible with our approach.

As many programs face dwindling resources, coaches and fitness professionals are often tasked with a broad range of responsibilities outside their typical areas of focus. While it may be ideal for specialists to conduct separate assessments in a well-equipped laboratory, most programs are limited by both time and resources. Due to these limitations, assessments are often included as part of sport-specific practices or fitness/conditioning sessions and conducted by the sport-specific coaching staff, trainers, or fitness professionals.

USEFULNESS OF ASSESSMENTS

Typically, the outcomes of assessments are used to characterize skill sets to determine the appropriate playing positions or event specialties of an athlete. Fitness professionals may be interested in these results to compile comparison or normative data to evaluate clients, while the potential to predict performance might be particularly appealing to coaches. Assessments can also be used for educational purposes to inform athletes, parents, and coaches regarding the particular skill sets that may be of importance for a given sporting activity. More recently, results of these assessments have been used to aid in injury prevention via prehabilitation or to identify muscular imbalances. The usefulness of assessments within each of these areas is explained in more detail in the following sections.

NORMATIVE DATA COMPARISON

One of the difficulties of working with individuals or small groups of clients or athletes is the pitfall of potentially viewing their abilities in a vacuum without comparison to others. This can lead to complacency or a lack of focus on fundamental skills and physical capacities. A great example of this conundrum is when an athlete classified as a big fish in a small pond transitions from junior to senior levels of competition or from high school to college varsity athletics. For example, the fastest athlete on the team may struggle when suddenly surrounded by a group of equally strong runners, and a state champion high school wrestler might be overwhelmed in a college wrestling room filled with state champions touting several years of collegiate experience. In the first case, the fast athlete could have engaged in additional preparatory training with the goal of being competitive. In the second case, the wrestler might undergo assessments to identify potential deficiencies compared to more senior counterparts. Regardless of the situation, access to normative assessment data on similar individuals or the accumulation of previous assessment data provides a clearer perspective on where the clients or athletes currently stand or how far they have progressed toward their intended goals.

RELATIONSHIPS WITH PERFORMANCE

A wide variety of research in the field of exercise science is dedicated to determining the relationship between specific physical attributes and the potential for performance (18, 23). Prediction might come in the form of the ability to differentiate between individuals of higher and lower competitive or skill levels or to classify individuals as having specific groups of skills similar to successful athletes. However, it should be noted that most of the time, these predictions are really based on the determination that two specific outcomes are highly related rather than one specifically causing the other, or vice versa. Perhaps the most explored assessments in this regard are the determination of aerobic capacity to predict endurance performance or the determination of maximal power output to predict success in activities involving explosiveness. Assessments that can be easily executed outside of the laboratory (termed *field-based tests* or simply *field tests*) have also been explored for their usefulness in quickly evaluating large groups of athletes on their potential to excel in a given sport. For example, elite youth soccer players have lower body fat percentages and higher aerobic capacities while tending to score higher on agility and speed

assessments compared to non-elite players (19). Many experienced coaches also develop their own personal approach by which they identify individuals who they believe have the capacity to be successful. In this case, assessment data could play a key supplemental role to reinforce or fact-check qualitative evaluations.

In statistics, the term *parsimonious* is used to describe the desire to maximize predictive power while minimizing the number of inputs. This concept is sometimes referred to as the "law of briefness" and should be at the forefront of the planning and implementation process with respect to both complexity of the procedures and the time available to complete them. Parsimony in the context of assessments refers to the ability to compile as much useful information as possible with just a few assessments.

EDUCATIONAL AND INFORMATIVE DATA

Assessment data is particularly useful when working to educate or provide feedback to clients or athletes and other relevant stakeholders (family members, teammates, other coaches or fitness professionals) on a particular topic. Early on in our lives, our parents or guardians are exposed to crucial assessment data in the form of basic anthropometric measurements (height, weight, body mass index, etc.), which is compared to normative data presented as growth charts. This information is meticulously tracked by health care providers and family members to make sure that normal development is occurring. Ask most parents or guardians about statistics and you will get a blank look, but they will most likely be able to tell you what percentile of height and weight their child was and how big their child was supposed to get. In a similar manner, we can use assessments, including anthropometric data, to illustrate progress and to support the decision-making process. This is particularly helpful when working with those same stakeholders (parents or guardians) and educating them on why we train the way we do and what the next step might be.

In the case of clients or athletes, results from assessments help promote commitment to the training program or buy-in or support for an intervention. For example, in hot and humid environments, many clients or athletes show up to training sessions dehydrated and fail to properly rehydrate following training (20). A simple self-reported urine color assessment might illustrate this issue with athletes (1, 2), and a brief educational session highlighting the relationship between hydration and fatigue as well as performance (13), such as sprinting and dribbling performance in soccer players, might provide incentive to drink fluids throughout the day and following training sessions.

TRAINING PROGRAM DESIGN AND REVISION

Assessments can be used when designing new training programs or to introduce modifications to existing programs. The determination of baseline values allows for personalized programming and provides the basis for setting appropriate training goals. For example, a new coaching staff that puts a premium on speed may inherit athletes from a previous coach who focused primarily on size or strength, and initial assessments may be required to determine specific training emphases. The development of training groups based on strength versus speed or explosiveness versus aerobic capacity could also be considered. This might be an option for off-season training in which specific training programs and goals are provided to groups of clients or athletes with opportunities for improvement identified through the assessment process.

When the initial targets have been surpassed, progression can be built within the training program. With respect to strength, when an individual who was initially identified as weaker than the peer group has achieved comparable maximal strength or muscular endurance values, that individual's program may be adjusted to focus on another desirable physical fitness quality or to further develop strength. Consistent assessment may also be used to monitor fatigue and manage rest and recovery. Methods for evaluating fatigue might include routine evaluation of a variety of measures (6, 22), including, but not limited to, perception of effort, explosiveness (e.g., jump height or distance), or velocity of movement (e.g., bar speed). For example, a simple vertical jump test conducted prior to a training session resulting in a jump height less than usual for a particular client or athlete might indicate the need for reduced training intensities for the day or other modified programming options.

INJURY AND PREHABILITATION

Prehabilitation refers to engaging in specifically selected exercise programs in an effort to minimize the potential for injury (14). Muscular imbalances identified through various testing methodologies (between-limb, upper/lower body, push/pull comparisons, etc.) could be related to injury or performance deficits from individual anatomical features or induced by training. Some athletes are susceptible to knee injuries, particularly with respect to anterior cruciate ligament (ACL) tears during landing or quick deceleration. This issue could potentially be due to differences in limb alignment and muscle development that are more common in females than males (8, 26). Deficits in strength and flexibility between muscle groups (quadriceps dominance), between legs (leg dominance), and between body segments (trunk dominance) related to the increased risk of ACL injury may be identified using assessments (7). For example, single-leg hop tests that are indicative of lower-body strength and power could be used to identify muscular imbalances as well as the need to engage in unilateral (e.g., primarily using one leg) exercise (21). Subsequently, preventative training programs can be enlisted to minimize the potential for this type of injury.

PERFORMANCE-BASED CONTINUOUS IMPROVEMENT

The process of client or athlete management should be viewed as a process of continuous improvement. With this in mind, and with an emphasis on quality feedback via the scientific method, a model stemming from the field of quality management (9), termed the Plan-Do-Check-Act (PDCA) cycle (see figure 1.1), may be used to illustrate the importance of assessments.

The Plan, Do, and Act portions of this cycle represent the traditional qualitative strengths of coaches and fitness professionals. The Plan portion entails the initial strategic analysis and goal-setting procedure, Do is the execution of the plan, and Act is the summative response

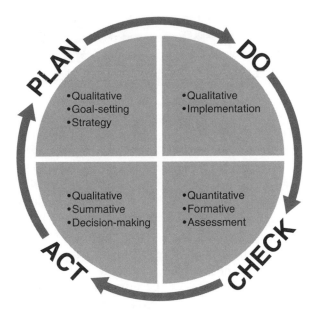

Figure 1.1 PDCA cycle.

(i.e., evaluating or making sense of the available information) and adjustment to this implementation. The Check portion of the PDCA cycle represents formative feedback (i.e., bringing together or monitoring of the available information) from knowledge-based quantitative data collection via appropriate assessments that inform the decision-making process. This cyclical approach with integrated qualitative (via observation) and quantitative (via data) components allows for the management of both individual client or athlete needs as well as reflection on the strategic approach. For example, through use of the PDCA cycle, coaches and fitness professionals might determine if specific adjustments need to be made on an individual basis from a single cycle or, as a result of several cycles, if a change to the process employed by the training staff should be considered.

Assessments should allow for a properly informed decision-making process. The results of well-designed and appropriately selected assessments can be used by the coaching or training staff and other stakeholders to design and modify training programs, and they can be used in the identification of proficiencies or deficiencies from both the individual and team perspectives. A common pitfall of many well-intended assessment initiatives is the one-and-done approach—

represented by a failure to conduct follow-up sessions. This is unfortunate because regularly planned assessments allow for benchmarking against previous performance, goal setting, and recognition opportunities.

USING THE PDCA CYCLE: CLIENT OR ATHLETE PERSPECTIVE

From a client or athlete perspective, the PDCA cycle allows for a clear, process-oriented, results-based approach to training and fitness preparation. It provides the opportunity for the client or athlete to provide input on specific goals and to either be actively engaged in the development plan or to gain a greater level of understanding of the decision-making process. The initial consultation or meeting constitutes the Plan portion of the cycle, where the goals and perceived strengths and weaknesses of the client or athlete are identified and a strategy for the initial assessment can be outlined. When first implementing the PDCA approach, the Do and Check portions are combined and consist of implementation of a series of assessments (the testing battery) to verify the perceived strengths and weaknesses of the individual as well as the potential to achieve the previously outlined goals.

The Act portion provides an opportunity for coaches and fitness professionals to evaluate and interpret the quantitative data through their own qualitative lens or perspective. If needed, the Plan portion can be revisited with feedback from the client or athlete prior to engaging in the first iteration of the training program or intervention as part of the full-blown Do portion of the cycle. Thereafter, periodic Checks can be performed to demonstrate progress toward the client's or athlete's goals and to inform changes to the training program or intervention. As the PDCA cycle continues, opportunities and threats, which require additional changes, might be identified. For example, if performance data from one of the assessments does not change over time, its relevance to the client or athlete should be questioned.

USING THE PDCA CYCLE: COACH AND FITNESS PROFESSIONAL PERSPECTIVE

In addition to designing and modifying training programs or interventions, coaches and fitness professionals can leverage the PDCA cycle to assist in their evaluation of clients or athletes and to optimize the assessments used in this process. Namely, coaches and fitness professionals can use their existing knowledge and experience of the sport or intended activity to select an initial series of assessments designed to identify important strengths and weaknesses of clients or athletes. Moving forward with the PDCA allows the coach or fitness professional to methodically adjust this set of assessments to account for the relevance of the recorded measurements to the activity of interest. The potential inclusion of new or alternative assessments that may shed some additional light on the fitness profile of the client can also be evaluated. Eventually, this set of assessments will become the customized assessment battery used by the coach or fitness professional while allowing the option to fine-tune the included assessments. This iterative process helps coaches and fitness professionals avoid making wholesale changes to their overall approach, which is a common pitfall for many programs.

CLIENT OR ATHLETE DEMOGRAPHICS

We can think about any group of clients or athletes as representing a bell-shaped curve, with the majority possessing the most similar athletic or fitness traits (typical) and relatively fewer possessing either advanced (outstanding) or underdeveloped (suboptimal) capacities (see figure 1.2). The assessment approach and evaluation process, or the coach's or fitness professional's perspective, may limit the pool of clients or athletes who would be considered for inclusion on a team or within a specific training program. Our tendencies as coaches, and oftentimes former competitors, is to gravitate toward those outstanding individuals with the most highly developed skill sets or physical abilities. Certainly, the assessment process may magnify this potential issue because these athletes are the easiest to recognize. However, it also allows us to determine how most of our athletes are performing and, combined with knowledge from previous measurement sessions, enables documentation of recently improved individuals. Furthermore, for the educator in all of us, it provides the opportunity to identify individuals in need of our assistance or those who have suffered recent setbacks with respect to the fitness measure being evaluated. This is a chance to truly demonstrate our own coaching abilities and promote our own growth and development through the implementation of a new or unique intervention.

So what exactly does this bell curve actually represent? When we first start coaching or working with clients, our knowledge base may be very limited. Each additional client or athlete with whom we work adds new information to that base, and our definition of outstanding athletes constantly changes. As we gain experience, our knowledge base grows and eventually we can clearly differentiate between the outstanding and suboptimal athletes and the large number of typical athletes. This knowledge base becomes our own bell curve upon which each new set of athletes can be compared. The beauty of normative data is that they provide us with similar information

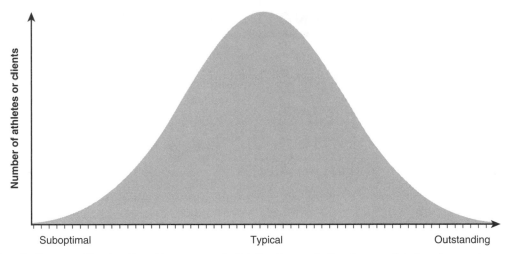

Figure 1.2   Bell curve illustrating the general distribution of clients or athletes for a given outcome.

and allow us to make more informed evaluations.

Occasionally, we are presented with a group of athletes who primarily fall within the suboptimal area of the bell curve. When this occurs, we might be inclined to lose hope; however, because most of the physical fitness characteristics determined via assessments can be changed, we have the ability to improve specific attributes through coaching or training interventions. In fact, it could be argued that changes may be more easily attained in the suboptimal or typical individuals as compared to the outstanding individuals, who have little room to improve. In this sense, it would be prudent to consider working with a larger group of athletes who have potential to improve rather than only those who currently possess the most developed attributes. This brings us to several interesting questions with regard to the evaluation and preparation of athletes. Do we have a tendency to consider primarily above-average individuals? Do all of the athletes need the same type of preparation? These questions may be most problematic when working with youth athletes, in whom physical (and mental) capacities and the ability to improve differs dramatically both between and within age groups. This issue lends credence to the notion that the coaches or trainers with strong teaching or skill-based backgrounds, as opposed to amateurs or volunteers, should be working with youth athletes, whereas those coaches or trainers with strong management backgrounds should be working with more advanced athletes.

TALENT EVALUATION AND MANAGEMENT

This approach is particularly important with respect to the processes of talent identification, selection, development, and transfer (15, 27). During talent identification, assessments may be used to evaluate individuals uninitiated to a particular sporting activity in an effort to gauge their potential for success. After athletes have been identified and introduced to the sport, additional assessment procedures more specific to the sport are valuable for placement in developmental and competitive situations. For those athletes for whom a particularly developed physical capacity is identified through this process but who do not continue with the originally intended sporting activity, transfer or referral to another sporting activity might be an option. These concepts have direct application to youth development. Longitudinal data collected at specific intervals may be used by coaches and other stakeholders to make decisions that will likely have long-term consequences for the athletes.

TALENT IDENTIFICATION AND SELECTION

Talent identification tends to involve the use of assessments aimed at evaluating generic fitness attributes and physical capacities in large groups of individuals (23). Because these individuals have yet to engage in the sport or physical activity, the results of these assessments may be predictors of, or more appropriately described as "highly related to," success or attainment of a particular goal or outcome. This process is conducted to more rapidly align the interests and abilities of individuals with competitive opportunities. Talent selection might include more specific assessments with consideration for known indicators of successful athletes or sport-specific skills that can aid in directing individuals into the appropriate developmental pipelines (11). Taken together, assessments provide crucial information during talent identification and selection that likely has an impact on the long-term decision-making process as well as the future experiences of the client or athlete within the sport or activity.

TALENT DEVELOPMENT

Talent development can include the use of assessments for monitoring youth athletes throughout the maturation process (10, 12). The comparison of individual athletes to age-specific normative data potentially allows for the identification of early, average, and late maturers with respect to various physical capacities. When dealing with youth athletes, coaches and fitness professionals must recognize that physical fitness attributes will undergo major changes but that the specific age at which this occurs and how quickly this occurs vary drastically between individuals. A common phrase among pediatric exercise physiologists is that "children are not mini-adults"; however, an argument could be made that two randomly selected youth athletes between the ages of 11 and 14 may exhibit physical and physiological differences in a similar manner. These distinctions are crucial in encouraging coaches and trainers to manage the training and assessment process with respect to the needs of the athletes and to minimize dropout from the sporting activity. In particular, some developing athletes may experience adolescent awkwardness, which might require revisiting some basic motor skills (or movement patterns) prior to focusing on strength and power improvements (10, 17). In adults, assessments can provide input to the talent development process specific to the competitive level or across the span of individual careers.

TALENT TRANSFER

The concepts of talent identification and selection can also be applied to a more diverse talent pool of experienced athletes who may not have made progress toward their originally defined goals through a talent transfer evaluation. An interesting example of talent transfer was the Sports Draft conducted by the Australian Institute of Sport (3). The Sports Draft focused on several combat sports as well as paddling sports in which specific physical skills, including speed, power, and agility, might be exploited when combined with focused coaching and technical preparation. While this approach might be viewed as overly ambitious, more common examples of talent transfer include sprinters finding success in the sport of bobsledding and gymnasts excelling in aerial sports. The knowledge of coaches and fitness professionals may be of particular importance when determining the assessments used for the purpose of talent transfer decisions.

IMPLEMENTATION OF ASSESSMENTS

The process of assessment can and should be viewed from both the coach or fitness professional and client or athlete management perspectives. It may be particularly useful to first apply approaches used to determine the needs of a client or athlete to the coach or fitness professional.

Coaches and fitness professionals should avoid the introduction of assessments simply for the sake of implementation. However, the following questions must be addressed: What does the coach or fitness professional hope to gain from the assessments? Can the identified data be used to help the client or athlete progress toward goals? This needs-based approach will ensure that unnecessary assessments and the impact on resources associated with them are limited. Furthermore, with this type of

> ## Motivating With Assessment Outcomes
>
> Assessments may be used to provide motivation through the process of setting and achieving tangible goals. For resistance training, athletes may be incentivized by the potential inclusion in groups with elite status, such as a 500- or 1000-pound club for weightlifters representing the total amount of weight lifted from several different lifting techniques. Similar groups can be outlined for speed (<4.6-second 40-meter times) or endurance (<5- or 6-minute mile times). However, recognition in this manner may have the unintended consequence of setting unattainable goals for some individuals. Therefore, a more appropriate approach for a varied group of individuals (with both high-level performers and beginners or lower performing clients or athletes) may be individualized goal setting based on realistic percentage or incremental improvements. With respect to the team-based environment, the motivation of attaining specific results from assessments may assist in either establishing or identifying group, team, or clubhouse leaders.

approach, the focus of those involved will remain on continuous improvement driven by value-added decision making rather than on the process of data collection. Therefore, for the purpose of this section of the chapter, considerations will be presented from the view of a coach or fitness professional who, despite a strong foundational knowledge, might be hesitant to engage in the assessment process due to unfamiliarity, the desire to keep things simple, fear of commitment, or deviating from standard operating procedures.

RESOURCES AND POTENTIAL BARRIERS

To determine the resources needed, we must first determine how many clients or athletes need to be evaluated. Drastically different resources are required if only a handful of clients or athletes will be assessed on a sporadic basis versus an entire team (or teams) on a specific timeline. For example, vertical jump tests for a group of keepers or tight ends could simply be conducted prior to the beginning of a training session using minimal facilities, whereas aerobic capacity or maximal strength tests for an entire team may require the use of an entire field, pitch, gymnasium, or weight room. Many barriers exist to the implementation of assessment by coaches and athlete stakeholders. Chief concerns include financial resources, expertise, and time; however, a wide variety

of assessments have been developed, ranging from inexpensive and simple to complex and time-consuming. The process of implementing the appropriate system of evaluation can be streamlined by identifying the needs and capabilities of both the clients or athletes and coaches or fitness professionals as well as any limitations that could be encountered.

DEPTH AND BREADTH OF AVAILABLE ASSESSMENTS

Generally, assessments are geared toward evaluating physical measures, such as body size and composition, flexibility, and balance, as well as performance measures, such as speed, agility, and strength, but they also include functional capacities related to the cardiovascular system or power output. Within each of these functional areas, specific assessments may be used to focus on the activity of interest or for a particular movement pattern. Assessments may be applied to client or athlete monitoring through periodic personal evaluation (perceived exertion, fatigue, soreness, etc.) or other health-related measures (heart rate, body composition, etc.). The decision to focus on a variety of assessments spanning several physical fitness attributes, functional capacities, and health measures, or to drill down into specific subareas is up to the discretion of the coach or fitness professional according to the needs of the client or athlete.

OVEREMPHASIS ON SPECIFICITY

The previously mentioned benefits of testing in an environment similar to competition or training have led to the suggestion that sport-specific testing modalities may also be ideal. However, the balance between useful data collection and specificity tends to result in highly engineered testing environments that are not conducive or readily available to most fitness professionals. Some examples include skating treadmills featuring the ability to control speed, incline, and direction for hockey athletes wearing skates or immersive virtual or augmented reality simulators for evaluating visuomotor capabilities. While both of these opportunities for testing athletes provide unique sport-specific features in controlled laboratory-type situations, coaches and fitness professionals with their own unique experiences and knowledge may select from a wide variety of assessments such as those covered within this text that present fewer barriers to implementation.

FOUNDATIONAL KNOWLEDGE OF COACHES AND FITNESS PROFESSIONALS

One of the cornerstones of successful implementation with respect to assessments is the input and guidance from coaches and fitness professionals. Knowledge of the needs of clients or athletes, the demands of the sport or activity, and potential constraints to implementation must all be considered through the lenses of these individuals. These areas are where the wisdom gained through personal and professional experience can truly amplify both the planning and eventual effectiveness of the selected assessments. In this regard, when properly implemented, assessments should be considered an extension of the coach's or fitness professional's skill set.

CONSTRAINTS TO IMPLEMENTATION

Newell's model of constraints is commonly used to describe the "optimal coordination and control of an activity" (16, 24). While traditionally applied to instruction through identification of individual, task, and environmental constraints related to human movement and decision making, this approach can also be used to develop a framework and outline factors associated with the implementation of assessment programs, potentially through a SWOT analysis, as outlined in the final section of this chapter. Individual constraints reflective of the coach's or fitness professional's personal influence on this process might include expertise related to assessment, desire for personal development, ingenuity, flexibility, and level of commitment. Task constraints reflecting the nature of assessments would include the activity or sport of interest, the use of laboratory- or field-based measures, and the desire to examine sport-specific or general fitness qualities. Environmental constraints that could influence

Paralysis by Analysis

Comprehensive analyses provided by testing device software and the desire to please a large group of constituents (coaches, trainers, administrators, parents or guardians, athletes, etc.) often yield excessive amounts of data that could be overwhelming to a coach or fitness professional, leading to the dreaded condition termed *paralysis by analysis*. Anyone who has ever been presented with a readout of heart rate or global position system (GPS) data for the first time understands that we can easily get lost in the weeds or lose the forest for the trees by delving into the specifics of the numbers rather than focusing on what happened during the evaluation or training session. This situation could easily be avoided by implementing assessments that have a simple outcome, such as average heart rate or peak running speed, and perhaps an estimated value for some physiologically relevant variable, such as aerobic capacity or rate of perceived exertion.

implementation are related to the availability of resources, including personnel or staff, external support (administrators, family, boosters), athlete buy-in, funding, and time.

SUSTAINABILITY

In order to ensure long-term success, a clear timeline must be determined. After accounting for the number of clients or athletes needing to be evaluated and the amount of time needed to accomplish the selected assessments, the dates for multiple assessment sessions should be identified. Logical points to begin this process might include prior to beginning a specific training program or before the start of a season. As mentioned earlier in this chapter, completing a single round of assessments might provide important information; however, the true benefits of this process will not be realized until several iterations have been completed. Therefore, follow-up assessment sessions, such as after sufficient time has elapsed in a given training program or at the midseason and postseason periods, should be planned and consistent in order to evaluate progress or aid in decision making.

BUDGETARY CONSIDERATIONS

Budgetary considerations could be a limiting factor for the implementation of assessment procedures by coaches or fitness professionals, including the lack of financial resources or limited access to the appropriate facilities and equipment. However, athlete assessments do not necessarily need to be conducted in a research laboratory or even in a strength training facility. In fact, some would argue that evaluating athletes in an environment as similar to competition or practice may be ideal. Financial concerns may also be tied to the wide variety of available testing devices that are aggressively marketed and tend to be associated with unanticipated expense or commitments. These common barriers may be exacerbated by the real or perceived use of technologically advanced hardware and software, the sensational nature of sport science programming in the popular media, and the potential overcomplication of results. For example, while a wearable metabolic analyzer with built-in GPS and environmental sensor capabilities could be used to determine aerobic capacity for an individual athlete, an intermitting shuttle run test with a simple timing system and the local weather report would provide similar information, with the added bonus that multiple athletes could be tested at once.

SWOT ANALYSIS

In order to ascertain if incorporating assessments into a coach's or fitness professional's toolbox would be a worthwhile pursuit, we first might need to engage in some reflection and information gathering. Therefore, the SWOT (strengths, weaknesses, opportunities, threats) analysis framework (4, 5, 25) may help determine the feasibility of implementing assessments.

A SWOT analysis involves identifying internal factors at which an individual is particularly skilled (strengths) or where deficiencies may be present (weaknesses), which are then paired with an appraisal of the coach's or fitness professional's current situation including identification of those external factors that may be benefits (opportunities) and barriers (threats) to implementation. The following generic analysis, which uses some of the SWOT factors discussed throughout this text, helps to identify how a typical coach or fitness professional might move forward with the implementation of an assessment program.

INTERNAL AND EXTERNAL FACTORS RELEVANT TO SWOT

When considering the inclusion of assessments, a coach or fitness professional may be hesitant to commit to this endeavor due to the additional time burden or the potential of taking time and focus away from training. They may also fear the unknown in that their lack of prior knowledge of assessments could stymie the potential benefits. These weaknesses should then be compared to the strengths of a high level of familiarity with the clients or athletes and a wealth of sport- or activity-specific knowledge.

Consideration should be given to potential threats, such as the availability of resources, including the coaching or training staff as well as technical expertise, that may be needed to implement assessments. Furthermore, depending on the selected assessments, there may be costs related to equipment, consumables, training, and access to the appropriate training or testing facilities. These threats can be weighed against the opportunities associated with implementation—for example, the wealth of information related to the fitness profiles and potential for improved performance of clients or athletes, and the prospect for growth for the coach or fitness professional.

SWOT MATRIX

The intersection of opportunities and strengths (OS) yields potential for increased client or athlete performance or goal achievement through optimized decision making and planning by the coach or fitness professional. This offers the best-case scenario by leveraging the clearly positive aspects of the SWOT analysis. Considering the relevant opportunities and weaknesses (OW) together provides the prospect of overcoming weaknesses through personal and professional growth by expanding knowledge of assessment procedures and gaining experience that benefits the clients or athletes. Perhaps the most intriguing situation lies with the connection of threats and strengths (TS) in that coaches or fitness professionals might leverage their individual knowledge and skill sets to produce an assessment battery that minimizes the perceived need for excess resources. Finally, in the worst-case scenario, where the coach or fitness professional ultimately decides that the assessment program is not feasible, the intersection of potential threats and weaknesses (TW) might produce a strategy for future implementation. See table 1.1 for an example SWOT analysis aimed at examining the implementation of an assessment program considering the factors relevant to coaches or fitness professionals.

SUMMARY

Assessments allow coaches and fitness professionals to refine the decision-making and goal-setting processes while enhancing the development of the client or athlete. Several factors, including the availability of resources and the specified outcomes, likely play a role in determining the feasibility of engaging in these endeavors. A variety of compelling reasons exist for the inclusion and implementation of assessments within a given strategic framework. Subsequent chapters will provide additional insight to aid in successfully accomplishing this task through an examination of the equipment needed and the process of selecting the appropriate assessments.

Table 1.1 Generic SWOT Analysis for Implementation of an Assessment Program From the Coach or Fitness Professional Perspective

	Strengths Sport- or activity-specific expertise, familiarity with clients or athletes	**Weaknesses** Limited knowledge of assessment procedures, fear of compromising training environment
Opportunities Expanded knowledge of clients or athletes	**OS:** Advances in client or athlete performance and improved decision making by coach or fitness professional	**OW:** Personal and professional growth; continuous improvement
Threats Exhaustion of resources (human, financial, technical)	**TS:** Development of unique situation-specific assessment procedures; creative leverage of resources	**TW:** Identification of specific needs that can be addressed when resources or personal development opportunities arise

CHAPTER 2

Assessment 201: What Equipment?

"I learned quickly, as I tell my graduate students now, there are no answers in the back of the book when the equipment doesn't work or the measurements look strange."

Martin Lewis Perl, Nobel Prize for Physics, 1995

The types of equipment used for assessments are a function of the specific procedures selected and the allotted budget but likely include both measurement devices (stopwatches, scales, meter sticks, cameras, personal computers, etc.) and implements (weights, benches, markers, cones, etc.). While there is often a desire by those involved with assessment to adopt the most innovative, and often complex, technological devices, consideration should be given to the generalizability of the data collected and the potential for overcomplicating a given testing session. The means by which the coach or fitness professional will conduct and record the results of the assessments must be considered, while a properly outfitted assessment space with amenities such as a semi-controlled environment, safe testing surfaces, adequate room to maneuver, and support facilities is necessary.

PERFORMANCE MEASUREMENT

The primary measurement of most assessments is the ability to complete work over a certain amount of time, more specifically defined as power, in one form or another. As such, the equipment used generally helps determine the factors associated with power output, including force/resistance, distance/displacement, and time. While the relationship with performance is very clear for some of these measures (strength, speed, etc.), others may not be as straightforward. For example, body mass is not necessarily a performance measure; however, when we gain an understanding of body composition (i.e., the relative amounts of muscle, fat, etc. that make up body mass), its influence on the ability to sprint or jump comes to the forefront with a potential trade-off between the positive effects of force production specifically coming from muscle mass and the negative effects of body mass in general due to the impact of gravity (1). Because performance is a relatively ambiguous term that can be described in many different ways, assessment equipment is equally diverse and can be used to quantify many different measures.

COST-BENEFIT

The equipment available for assessments varies considerably with respect to both cost and complexity. While the basis of traditional strength testing simply requires a heavy implement to lift up and down or, for conditioning assessments, a stopwatch, recent technological advancements and a growing consumer market for monitoring devices have caused the depth and breadth of equipment accessible to coaches and fitness professionals to become overwhelming. Devices offering research-grade capabilities with precise measurements and a variety of control features as well as specialized software may be exceedingly expensive and unnecessary in most applied settings. However, a greater demand for consumer products and the use of standardized mobile technology allow many assessments that were previously confined to a laboratory to be conducted in the gym, on the field, or in the weight room. Increased computing power has also decreased the price of these types of assessments while providing the opportunity to integrate several simultaneous streams of data collected during a single test. Therefore, how complex an assessment session becomes ultimately is a function of the needs of the coach or fitness professional and the client or athlete, the available budget, and the amount of technological know-how and support.

GENERALIZABILITY

Normative data is developed from a group of standard values or norms from either a large number of different individuals or a large group of people who share some similarities. Therefore, it is important to understand the type of equipment used during the assessments to create the normative data. While it is tempting to use the latest and greatest assessment technology, if a coach or fitness professional plans to compare client or athlete data with others, they must determine if there is enough comparative data available, specifically, comparative data of similarly trained individuals. Furthermore, the standards of a particular sport or profession may dictate that a particular type of equipment be used rather than the most appropriate or recently developed. This could be the case in events such as scouting combines or team selection, particularly if years of normative data have been compiled.

The ability to compare and contrast the results from assessments may be dictated by the equipment used. When large-scale normative data are collected, the researchers select specific equipment that is standardized across all of the study participants, which allows for the results to be standardized. In terms of body composition, the devices and technology used to evaluate body fat percentage can drastically change the final estimated value (8). While both skinfold calipers and bioelectrical impedance devices can be used to estimate body fat percentage, the technical approach is very different (as outlined briefly later in this chapter) and may result in different results. Certainly, a debate can be had over which is most correct, but for the case of comparing the values of clients or athletes, it is more important to select normative data that used similar equipment or to select equipment that aligns with the most relevant normative data. Examples from a performance perspective include the type of barbell used (9), the use of lifting straps (2) or belts for strength and endurance assessments (12), or the type of timing device used for speed and agility assessments (3). Therefore, coaches and fitness professionals must understand how the normative data was collected and the type of equipment at their disposal.

Occasionally, scientists who develop the normative data or evaluation procedures miss the mark. For example, a research team (one of which may or may not have been the author of this text) was excited to develop a standardized assessment procedure to enhance training prescriptions for older adults (4). They selected several simple assessments (height, weight, and handgrip strength) to categorize clients according to their estimated body composition characteristics as compared to a highly clinical (and expensive) procedure. Great idea, right? Height, weight, and handgrip strength are simple enough; however, the researchers decided to use a digital handgrip strength testing device as opposed to a more commonly used hydraulic device. While a case could be made that the digital version allowed for more precise measurements, most practitioners already owned the hydraulic version of the handgrip testing device. Ultimately, the usefulness of the published results to practitioners was limited due to this discrepancy.

ADJUSTABILITY

When selecting equipment, a coach or fitness professional should ask themselves, "Who will I be testing?" and "Are all of my clients or athletes built the same?" The answer to the second question in most cases will be no. As such, individual requirements with respect to the size and perhaps even the design of equipment may affect performance.

DOES ONE SIZE FIT ALL?

The design of most consumer products, including equipment used during assessments, poses an interesting predicament with respect to adjustability because they are typically built for the average body size and type and are meant to quantify average values. However, the nature of sport and human performance in general dictates that coaches and fitness professionals constantly try to push clients or athletes to the extremes. Furthermore, standout athletes and extreme performers tend to have unique body sizes and shapes (think jockeys, gymnasts, professional basketball players, sumo wrestlers), or large variations may exist on a single team (think American football players). Whenever possible, simple differences in size between men and women, or adults and children, or women and pregnant women should be accounted for with respect to equipment.

DOES DESIGN AFFECT PERFORMANCE?

A simple example of this potential issue is a handgrip strength device, which was one of my first purchases as a new exercise science researcher. This particular model allowed me to record force production over time, and with my background in combat sports, particularly judo, I was excited to set it up in the lab. I had not considered the potential need for adjustability, and the design of the device (shaped sort of like the handle of a baseball bat) did not allow for it. What if I wanted to test youth athletes with small hands or elite basketball players with much larger hands? In the context of judo, the question I had to ask myself was, "Do the athletes get to pick and choose the size of their opponents and the specific design of their uniforms?" Ultimately, we decided that, for the purpose of assessment, we did not want hand size to dictate our results. Interest-

Training Evaluators Before Going Live

While this chapter primarily focuses on equipment used for the purpose of assessment, the requirements of the support personnel and coaches cannot be overlooked. In order to successfully conduct the assessments, these individuals must be familiarized with the equipment and how it is to be used for potentially specialized purposes. All of the coaching staff and support personnel who will be participating in the assessment process should be appropriately informed of the standardized protocols as well as common mistakes or issues that may arise during testing. This type of training will assist in the consistent delivery of the assessments and increase the quality of the data by limiting the amount of factors unrelated to performance that might affect the results.

The development of standard operating procedures should be considered; however, at a minimum, a basic script with simplified language to explain the assessment to all clients or athletes should be prepared. This simplified language should be selected to ensure a basic understanding of tasks. The script can then be practiced and presented in a uniform manner to everyone being tested. Furthermore, variations in the amount of enthusiasm and encouragement or intensity in the delivery of the instructions between assessments could influence performance. Prior to going live, a practice round of assessments should be conducted in an environment as similar to the actual testing environment as possible to identify any unforeseen issues and to give the personnel and coaches some additional experience.

ingly, the available options for handgrip devices with the specific capabilities that I was looking for at the time were somewhat limited. Luckily, most of the standard handgrip strength devices that would be used in the field are adjustable… but they still might be too large for children! Coaches and fitness professionals must determine if a one-size-fits-all device is appropriate or if any alternatives, either individual sizes or adjustable options, are available.

DATA COLLECTION AND ORGANIZATION

Perhaps the most inexpensive instrument used during assessment is the data collection form (see figure 2.1), which contains important information, such as client or athlete identification, date and time of testing, environmental conditions, and, last but not least, the results! Throughout the assessment process, particularly in the case of comprehensive testing of large numbers of clients or athletes, a standardized method of recording and organizing the data collected is crucial. Whenever possible, it is important to document inconsistencies during testing or relevant information that may affect performance. While many assessment devices come with their own software and many people are now skilled at using mobile recording devices, hard copies of the most important data collected in a given testing session should be kept to guard against any technological difficulties or the potential loss of crucial information. Regardless, accurate record keeping is important in order to fully evaluate changes over time and to ensure the proper communication of collected data among coaching and training staff when needed.

TYPES OF EQUIPMENT

The wide range of physical fitness attributes, from body composition to strength to aerobic capacity, dictates that the equipment used be equally diverse. Some of the equipment is designed for a

Figure 2.1   Sample data collection form

Location: _____   Testing Surface:_____   Assessment Date: _____

Temperature: _____ °C   Relative Humidity: _____ %   Time of Day: _____

_____ °F   Barometric Pressure: _____ mmHg   Evaluator: _____

Athlete/Client ID#: _____   Age: _____ yr   Clothing/Footwear: _____

Sex: ❑ Male   Height: _____ cm   Weight: _____ kg

❑ Female   _____ in.   _____ lb

Assessment: Countermovement Jump

	Total jump height (cm or in.)		Standing reach Height (cm or in.)		Vertical jump Height (cm or in.)
		-		=	
Trial 1		-		=	
Trial 2		-		=	
Trial 3		-		=	
			Average	=	
			Best	=	

From D. Fukuda, *Assessments for Sport and Athletic Performance* (Champaign, IL: Human Kinetics, 2019).

very specific purpose, such as skinfold calipers to determine body fat percentage, while some is more generic and intended for a variety of assessments, such as barbells and dumbbells. Due to this variety and the potential use within multiple types of assessments, the equipment will be presented in the following categories: anthropometric equipment, resistance equipment, gravity-based equipment and other implements, distance or length measuring equipment, timing equipment, heart rate and GPS monitors, treadmills and rowing ergometers, instruments and questionnaires, and clothing and performance apparel.

ANTHROPOMETRIC EQUIPMENT

The most basic anthropometric measurements involve standing height and body mass or weight. Standing height is usually measured manually with a stadiometer using a vertical measurement column that may be free-standing, wall-mounted, or part of a physician's scale (see figure 2.2). Sitting height to approximate trunk/leg length can generally be measured using the same device with the person being tested in the seated position on a chair or platform. The most commonly used device for body mass or weight assessment is the balance beam scale, typically known as a physician's scale. Specific benefits of this type of device include the ability to use it without a power supply and a clear calibration procedure (verifying that it reads zero when unloaded), but the manual nature of the measurement does introduce some drawbacks, including lack of precision and extended testing duration. Digital scales offer greater precision with no need for technical expertise; however, these devices require a power supply, and the user relies on electronic features for calibration. The difference in cost between balance beam and digital scales is minimal, but the overall cost of scales in general can increase exponentially with expanded features as well as the need for high levels of precision.

Measuring tapes are used to determine the lengths and circumferences of specific body parts, such as the waist, hips, biceps, etc. While a standard flexible measuring tape may be used for these types of assessments, an anthropometric measuring tape made of woven fabric or fiberglass material featuring a push-button retracting mechanism and Gulick attachment is preferred. Woven fabric or fiberglass material allows the

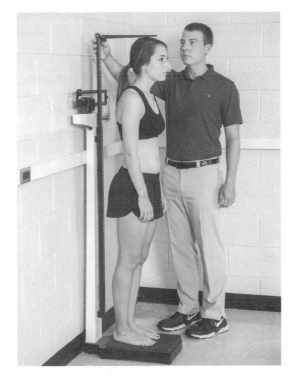

Figure 2.2 Stadiometer.

measuring tape to adjust to the contours of the body and being retractable limits the device from becoming tangled or damaged over time. The Gulick attachment is a spring-loaded mechanism on the end of the measuring tape that provides a precise method for standardizing measurements based on the application of uniform tension between assessments.

A variety of body composition methods are currently used but tend to focus on the assessment of body fat percentage or fat-free mass. Skinfold thickness measurements, which can be input into equations to estimate body fat percentage, are generally conducted with skinfold calipers (see figure 2.3). Skinfold calipers vary in price due to differences in precision, reliability, and durability. The least expensive options simply rely on plastic molding and tension provided by the evaluator but may have a limited lifespan and calibration options. More durable and precise devices feature metal casing with spring-loaded mechanisms that allow for consistent tension and calibration procedures. It must be noted that the equations used to estimate body fat percentage from skinfold thickness are developed using a specific type of skinfold caliper, and the use of different calipers likely results in estimation errors. When there might be a concern that the available equations

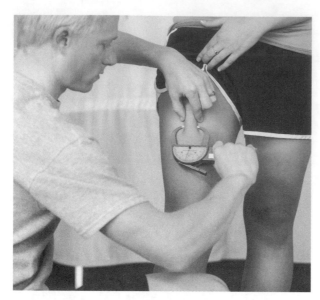

Figure 2.3   Skinfold calipers.

do not cover the types of people being tested, the actual skinfold thicknesses can be used. If fact, this method may be preferred when the actual body fat percentage is not crucial as is often the case in lean athletes or young people.

Bioelectrical impedance analysis (BIA) devices offer an alternative method of determining body fat percentage through the estimation of total body water (from the measurement of resistance). The most commonly available and user-friendly BIA devices feature leg-to-leg analysis via foot electrodes embedded in a body mass scale. While all body composition methods require standardized diet and physical activity in order to provide valid estimates, body fat percentages from BIA are particularly influenced by hydration (5). As a result, many weight monitoring programs such as those used in the sport of wrestling, require urine-specific gravity evaluation to verify appropriate levels of hydration in conjunction with BIA assessments.

RESISTANCE EQUIPMENT

Strength and power assessments rely on the ability to quantify force production during resistance training exercises. Thus, resistance training equipment, including free weights (i.e., barbells and dumbbells) or weight machines, is needed to conduct these types of assessments. While many

types of barbells exist, standard weightlifting bars are straight and made of steel, are approximately 7 feet (2.2 m) long, with a 1.1-inch (28 mm) grip diameter, and weigh 45 pounds (20 kg) with the sleeves, which are used to load weight plates (see figure 2.4a). Powerlifting barbells, such as the Texas Power Bar, are more rigid in order to withstand greater resistive capacities, while Olympic weightlifting barbells contain bearings that allow them to spin during dynamic lifts. Knurling/crosshatch patterns (the rougher portion of the bar intended to increase friction for gripping) vary between models. More recently, hybrid barbells with overlapping Olympic and powerlifting features have been developed and smaller barbells (33 lbs [15 kg], 6.6 ft [2 m] long, 0.98 in. [25 mm] grip diameter) are also available for smaller individuals or adolescents. Lightweight training bars made of aluminum are also used but should not be loaded in the same manner as other barbells because they may permanently bend due to having lower weight capacities. The use of chalk to enhance handgrip strength during a variety of lifts or lifting straps to minimize the influence of handgrip strength, specifically during deadlifts, may also be considered. Finally, safety clips or collars should be used at all times to secure the weights to the barbell (see figure 2.4b). Spring-loaded and clamp-style collars add minimal weight to a loaded barbell, while metal competition-style collars weigh 5.5 pounds (2.5 kg) each.

Depending on the nature of the assessment, standard cast iron weight plates ranging from 2.5 to 45 pounds (1.25-20kg) should be sufficient. If the assessments include dynamic movements where the weights might be dropped or swiftly set to the floor, rubberized bumper plates within a similar weight range are recommended. Similarly, cast iron and rubber-coated dumbbells and kettlebells, normally purchased in pairs, are available; however, larger weights may be needed to provide enough resistance for certain individuals. Other types of implements that may be used to provide resistance during muscular strength and endurance assessments include medicine balls, sandbags, sleds, and weight vests. In particular, medicine balls come in a number of forms, including hard, rubberized versions that are capable of bouncing and softer vinyl or leather versions that give upon impact. Depending on

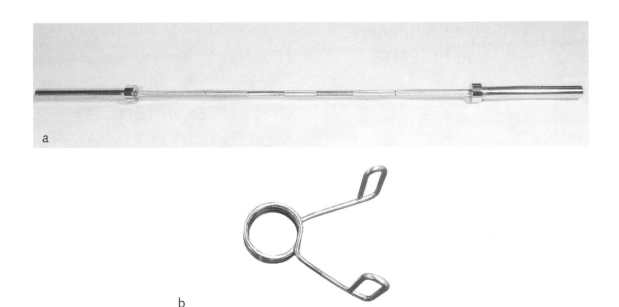

Figure 2.4   *(a)* Barbell and *(b)* collars.

the size of the person using them or the intended activity, coaches or fitness professionals might select medicine balls that increase in diameter with increasing weight or ones that have a uniform diameter regardless of the weight.

Weightlifting racks or stands and benches are likely needed when conducting strength assessments and must be of sufficient quality and construction to withstand the weights being used. Flat utility benches and adjustable angled benches may be used for specific assessments, primarily those focused on evaluating the upper body musculature. Commonly, power racks (see figure 2.5), which are freestanding structures featuring four upright columns and adjustable-height J-hooks that hold a barbell and safety bars which prevent the barbell from dropping past a certain point, are used to allow for many different lifts to be safely performed. Wall-mounted racks, freestanding squat stands, and combination racks with integrated benches are also common devices used for testing purposes.

Weight machines with selectorized weight stacks and pulley systems or modified bars used to load standard weight plates provide an alternative to free weights when conducting assessments. These devices usually mimic movements similar to those expected while lifting free weights; however, they are generally limited to a single

plane of motion. Because of this, weight machines may provide an additional level of safety or at least comfort for those individuals unaccustomed to lifting free weights. However, it should be noted that these devices vary greatly with respect to quality and adaptability.

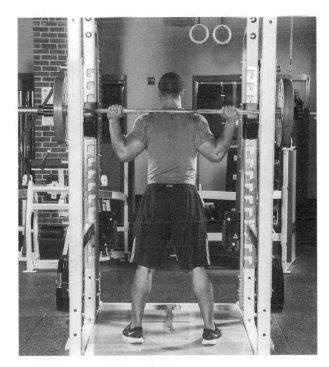

Figure 2.5   Power rack with J hooks.

GRAVITY-BASED EQUIPMENT AND OTHER IMPLEMENTS

Specific equipment may be useful even when body weight is the primary form of resistance during assessments. Implements such as plyometric boxes, step benches, stairs, or overhead mounted ropes require clients or athletes to displace their body weight to perform work that can be quantified and evaluated. With respect to safety during dynamic high-intensity activities, nonslip surfaces should be present when using plyometric boxes, step benches, and stairs, and cushioned mats may be needed when using overhead mounted ropes. Freestanding or rack- or wall-mounted pull-up bar or dip stations provide similar resistive capabilities when assessing muscular endurance. Furthermore, these implements should be stable and sturdy so that it is difficult to tip them over.

As mentioned several times earlier in this chapter, handgrip strength devices, otherwise known as handgrip dynamometers (see figure 2.6), are commonplace in field-based settings to estimate overall strength without the influence of movement-based technical prowess. Additionally, implements used to test balance (e.g., balance beams and foam stability pads) or to aid in attaining a specific body position (custom pads or benches) may also be needed to conduct a thorough assessment.

DISTANCE OR LENGTH MEASURING EQUIPMENT

Maximizing distance or length is the primary goal for a large majority of assessments. Measuring length or distance is also a key component for the determination of total work done and power output. For shorter length measurements, a meter- or yardstick may be sufficient, while longer distances may require the use of an extended-length measuring tape. These measuring tapes commonly feature a utility handle and a reel system in order to quickly and easily retract the tape after marking the desired distance. In order to clearly identify specified lengths, the use of cones, markers, or other indicators will likely be required. Speed- or agility-based assessments over commonly evaluated distances may be conducted using standardized, premarked surfaces such as a track, field turf, or basketball court. Large-scale custom measurements may need to be made using a combination of commercially available items, such as a measuring wheel, field string, and field paint.

While custom devices are available for certain assessments, alternative methods are available that do not require additional equipment. For example, flexibility testing can be conducted using a sit-and-reach box with a built-in measurement system (see figure 2.7), and vertical jump testing can be conducted using a device outfitted with uniformly spaced vanes extending from a vertical beam (see figure 2.8). Alternatives to these devices include taking appropriate measurements on the floor (flexibility) or wall (vertical jump) with some sort of marker or visual verification.

TIMING EQUIPMENT

The most basic piece of equipment to record time is the stopwatch (or chronometer), and due to its cost, ease of use, and relative utility, it is perhaps the most common. However, when greater levels of precision are required, and in order to control for human error, various timing systems have been developed. Timing gates featuring infrared

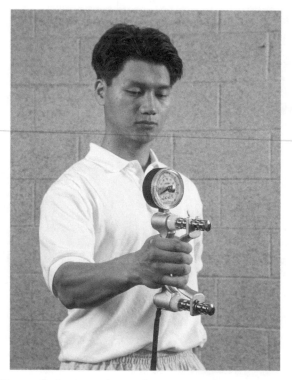

Figure 2.6 Handgrip dynamometer.

photocells are available for sprint and agility assessments. These wired or wireless devices are connected to a computer or receiver that records when the infrared beam (or beams) are broken to indicate the start and stop of a specific test. Optical timing systems or contact mats (see figure 2.9) that are triggered with pressure work in a similar fashion to record flight and contact time during jumping. Several desktop computer and mobile apps have also been developed that

examine the accumulated time between specific events within recorded video of sprinting, weightlifting, and jumping activities.

While many assessments rely on start and stop or directional signals given directly by the evaluator, the recent integration of technology allows for coordinated visual or auditory signals to be conveyed and staged within a given protocol. Furthermore, metronomes designed to make sounds set to a specific beat may be used to standardize movement velocities during weightlifting (repetitions per minute), jumping (cycles per second), or cycling (revolutions per minute) assessments.

HEART RATE AND GPS MONITORS

Some assessments may require the measurement of the client's or athlete's heart rate during exercise. This can easily be accomplished by manually counting the number of heartbeats over a designated amount of time using a watch or clock; however, there is skill involved with this type of assessment, and access to a pulse during some activities may be difficult. Heart rate monitors (see figure 2.10) are a relatively

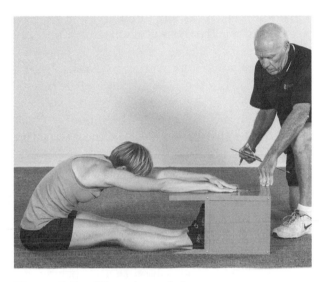

Figure 2.7   Sit-and-reach box.

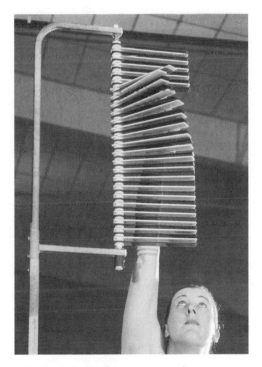

Figure 2.8   Vertical jump test device.

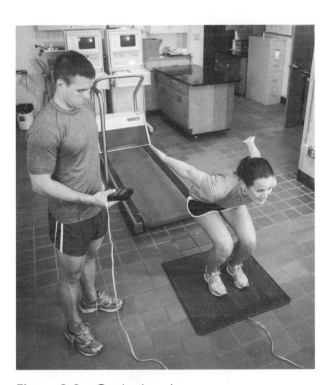

Figure 2.9   Contact mat.

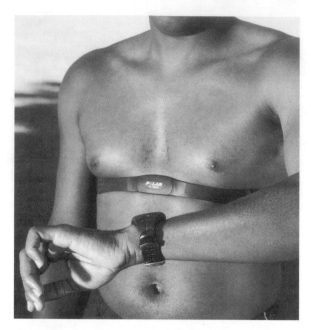

Figure 2.10   Heart rate monitor.

inexpensive option that are now commonplace on the athletic field and in the gym. Chest straps that transmit to watches or a mobile app as well as watches with integrated wrist pulse monitors are available and provide real-time display of heart rate during physical activity. To take it a step further, many watches now also feature global positioning system (GPS) capabilities that allow for the determination of speed and acceleration in addition to time and distance.

Privacy and placement, particularly with respect to chest straps, may need to be taken into consideration when using heart rate monitors. A clear explanation of how the monitor is to be worn and a private area, such as a locker room, in which the client or athlete can put the device on, are needed.

TREADMILLS AND ROWING ERGOMETERS

While most assessments can be conducted without the use of treadmills and ergometers, a few special cases may lend themselves to using this type of equipment. In cases where inclement weather or difficulty in determining controlled conditions (e.g., geography), treadmills may be ideal. When selecting a treadmill, considerations should be given to the maximal potential speed (many devices

are limited in this regard), the width and length of the running belt and deck, and the space required to maintain safe conditions. The running surface should be clean and not overly worn in order to deliver the appropriate amount of friction while running. Furthermore, some amount of treadmill incline may be needed to simulate outdoor or overground running or to allow for reasonable comparison with existing normative data.

While a variety of rowing ergometers (see figure 2.11) are available, large amounts of normative data and the recent development of several specific tests make those available from Concept 2 a popular option. These ergometers use fan-based air resistance while providing a wealth of useful data from their integrated display and are housed in many gyms. Coaches and fitness professionals should be aware that while the intensity or air resistance delivered by these rowing ergometers are dependent on how hard a person pulls, there are adjustable damper settings (similar to gears on a bicycle) that affect how much air is allowed to interact with the fan on a given pull, which may also influence performance. Therefore, in most cases, damper settings should be recorded and standardized between assessment sessions. It should also be understood that proper rowing technique greatly affects performance, and adequate familiarization is likely needed. As with all of the previously described equipment, regular maintenance and periodic calibration are essential for proper operation and longevity of treadmills and rowing ergometers.

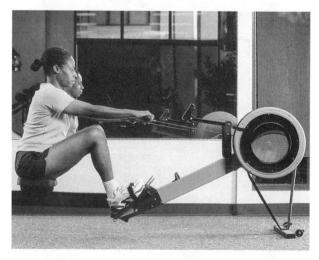

Figure 2.11   Rowing ergometer.

INSTRUMENTS AND QUESTIONNAIRES

Some assessments may be delivered as either paper or electronic instruments or questionnaires. These assessments generally require the client or athlete to self-report how they feel with respect to a particular topic at a given point in time according to a predefined rating scale or comparative value. The questions should be written such that they are understood by most clients or athletes and standardized in order to be compared between assessments. Preferably, the instrument or questionnaire has been produced and evaluated by knowledgeable professionals who have verified its usefulness in a similar setting. When a specific rating system is to be used, such as a number-based scale (from 1 to 10, for example, as shown in figure 2.12) or a visual scale, anchors should be provided that clearly define specific values within the scale for the client or athlete to consider. An example anchor for a number-based scale might include values and terms such as "6 = no exertion at all" being equivalent to sitting on the couch and "17 = very hard" exertion being just prior to exhaustion. An anchor for a visual scale might include the left side of a straight line being equivalent to "no fatigue/soreness" and the right side of the same line being equivalent to "very severe fatigue/soreness." The description of these anchors as well as the ability of the client or athlete to understand the rating scale is of utmost importance to the applicability of the results.

A great example of this issue comes from peer review during group presentations in an academic setting. Students are asked to rate each group using a scale of 1 to 5 on several criteria, with 1 considered "poor" and 5 considered "excellent." As students know that the instructor will be reviewing their responses and that it may affect the final grade of the group members, values of 4 and 5 are most commonly reported. However, one student gives across-the-board values of 1 for all groups, leaving the instructor to wonder if the student had extremely high standards (or some personal vendetta against the entire class), if the directions were poorly conveyed, or if the student simply misunderstood the anchors and the rating scale. This situation also highlights the potential influence of the person conducting the assessment and how the client or athlete might respond if they assume some specific outcome will result from their responses.

CLOTHING AND PERFORMANCE APPAREL

Even though it seems that the question of what to wear would seem obvious, this topic should be explicitly addressed as it could alter the process of conducting assessments. Think about a client or athlete (outside of a military setting) trying to complete a sprint or agility test in combat boots or someone attempting a jump test in sandals or flip-flops. Therefore, footwear recommendations should generally include closed-toe, surface-specific, properly fitted shoes designed for the intended activity. For example, flat-soled shoes may be most appropriate during assessments related to muscular strength and cushioned shoes may be most appropriate for assessments involving running, whereas cleats would be best for agility assessments conducted on turf or grass. However, the latter recommendation might be dictated by whether the assessments used to compile the available normative data were conducted with cleats on a similar surface. With respect to other pieces of clothing, breathable garments that allow full range of motion but are not overly loose fitting should be recommended in order to address the ability to move freely and to ensure safety. In the case of sport- or activity-specific testing, standard uniforms or clothing typically worn during

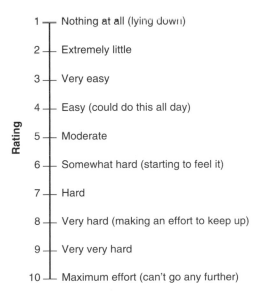

Rating	
1	Nothing at all (lying down)
2	Extremely little
3	Very easy
4	Easy (could do this all day)
5	Moderate
6	Somewhat hard (starting to feel it)
7	Hard
8	Very hard (making an effort to keep up)
9	Very very hard
10	Maximum effort (can't go any further)

Figure 2.12   Rating of perceived exertion scale.

practice or competition would also be appropriate. Finally, any accessories used, such as lifting belts, straps, etc., should be checked to be in proper working order and to determine if anything else worn (watches, jewelry, hair ties, etc.) may be causing some undue influence on performance.

MATHEMATICAL FORMULAS AND NOMOGRAMS

The results of many assessments can be used to estimate other values that may be difficult to measure without expensive equipment or by invasive means. These estimated values are determined through research studies and subsequent statistical analyses to develop prediction equations. Prediction equations require the use of formulas that may range from simple and straightforward algebra to highly complex with the need for advanced mathematical knowledge. One way of simplifying the use of prediction equations is through nomograms that provide for quick graphical calculations (7). An example of a nomogram is given here using midparental height, which allows for a rough

estimation of a child's potential adult height with consideration for the average 13-centimeter difference in height between men and women (13). Midparental height can be calculated for boys by adding 13 centimeters to the mother's height and averaging that with the father's height, and for girls by subtracting 13 centimeters from the father's height and averaging that with the mother's height. In this rudimentary example, if the parents' heights are known for a given boy or girl, they can be located on the outer vertical lines and a straightedge can be used to connect the appropriate height markers. The intersection of the straightedge and the middle vertical line give the estimated midparental height. For a boy whose father's height is 180 centimeters and whose mother's height is 160 centimeters, the following manual calculation can be completed:

$$\text{Midparental height} = \frac{(160\,\text{cm} + 13\,\text{cm}) + 180\,\text{cm}}{2} = 176.5\,\text{cm}$$

This result can be verified using the graphical calculation provided in figure 2.13. While the calculation of midparental may not require this

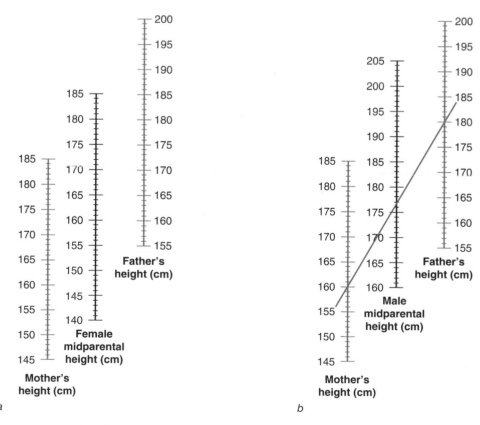

Figure 2.13 Nomograms depicting graphical calculation of midparental height for (a) girls and (b) boys.

Formula from (13)

Calibration and Maintenance of Equipment

An often forgotten but crucial component to selecting equipment for the purpose of assessment is the notion that a particular device consistently provides accurate performance data. If the equipment used during assessments provides inaccurate information or is greatly affected by factors not related to performance, the gathered results are of little use to coaches and fitness professionals. Even if we assume that the equipment comes in proper working order, if it is used on a regular basis then there will likely be the need for periodic calibration. Furthermore, the facility and equipment being used to conduct the assessments should be clean and well-maintained in order to ensure safety to the client or athlete and coaches or fitness professionals (6). Figure 2.14 provides a basic facility and equipment safety checklist.

While most of our assessment procedures do not require the level of precision required to maintain the international standards for measurement, we do want to be as accurate as possible and to identify when our clients or athletes have improved or declined. Thus, consideration should be given to the need for regular maintenance and calibration procedures, including how often they should be performed, the level of technical knowledge needed to complete the procedures, and any potential costs associated with performing them. Many commonly used pieces of equipment (e.g., treadmills, bodyweight scales, etc.) will likely require professional assistance to maintain accuracy and consistency. Even if calibration procedures are deemed inappropriate for a particular piece of equipment, regular maintenance and cleaning should be conducted in order to prolong its lifespan. Furthermore, properly functioning and maintained equipment will help to ensure the safety of the evaluators and the individuals being tested. A checklist that includes necessary cleaning and maintenance procedures and a running list of the dates they are completed may be needed.

Figure 2.14   Basic facility and equipment safety checklist

❏ Inspect all flooring for damage or wear

❏ Clean (sweep, vacuum, or mop and disinfect) all flooring

❏ Clean and disinfect drinking fountain

❏ Inspect fixed equipment's connection with the floor

❏ Clean and disinfect equipment surfaces that contact the skin

❏ Inspect all equipment for damage; wear; loose or protruding belts, screws, cables, or chains; insecure or nonfunctioning foot and body straps; improper functioning or improper use of attachments, pins, or other devices

❏ Clean and lubricate moving parts of equipment

❏ Inspect all padding for cracks and tears

❏ Inspect nonslip mats for proper placement, damage, and wear

❏ Inspect measurement devices for proper tension, time, and revolutions per minute

❏ Ensure adequate lighting and airflow

❏ Ensure that equipment is returned and stored properly after use

From D. Fukuda, *Assessments for Sport and Athletic Performance.* (Champaign, IL: Human Kinetics, 2019). Adapted from A. Hudy, "Facility Design, Layout, and Organization." In *Essentials of Strength Training and Conditioning,* 4th ed., edited for the National Strength and Conditioning Association by G. G. Haff and N.T. Triplett (Champaign, IL: Human Kinetics, 2016), 637.

approach, when more complex formulas are used nomograms are particularly valuable and will be provided throughout the text.

ASSESSMENT SPACE AND AMENITIES

Particular attention should be given to the space in which the assessment procedures will be conducted and the equipment will be housed. Dedicated assessment space is usually available in traditional laboratory settings (and some weight rooms); however, space for assessments in the field tends to be temporary, and both the portability and storage of equipment must be addressed. In both cases, the availability of electrical outlets and potentially an internet connection may require consideration. While technology tends be a large part of our day-to-day activities, we must remember that simpler solutions may be ideal. In a recent sport science planning session, a five-minute conversation about how to get Wi-Fi access on the training pitch to record posttraining perceived exertion was stopped immediately after a suggestion to "clipboard it" and simply record the numbers (1-10) by hand.

Regardless of the space being dedicated or temporary, safety should be of the utmost importance and adequate room should be given for the assessments and the number of evaluators and individuals being tested. If the assessment requires a distraction-free environment or a limited audience during testing, a staging area or a private room may be needed. Similarly, the ability to manipulate the environment, including temperature, humidity, noise, and lighting, would be ideal in order to re-create similar conditions between testing sessions or to simulate the competitive environment. The preferred or available testing surface (court, turf, grass, mat, etc.) must also be determined with specific consideration for the trade-off between transferability to the sport or activity and limiting injury or the ability to complete the outlined assessment procedures. Furthermore, the testing surface affects the client's or athlete's potential performance and should be similar to that used to collect the normative data.

Adequate room to move during assessments and spacing between testing stations should be maintained. Additionally, there should be minimal exposure of electrical cords or other potential hazards. Appropriate consideration should also be given to proper storage of equipment to decrease the likelihood of damage or inappropriate usage. Fortunately, most coaches and fitness professionals are also required to be certified in first aid and cardiopulmonary resuscitation (CPR); however, a well-stocked first-aid kit and access to an automated external defibrillator (AED) will allow for them to fully use these skills in the case of an emergency. Finally, a written plan to alert proper medical support when needed should be instituted.

Environmental conditions, such as the heat, cold, humidity, and wind, may not only adversely affect the performance of the client or athlete but also that of the equipment being used during the assessments (10, 11). Certainly, any time electronic devices are being used there is potential for malfunction due to environmental extremes, but even the simple interaction of the athlete and the ground, turf, or implements could be affected by changes in frictional forces. Another case might be the influence of headwinds or tailwinds on a variety of field-based performance measures. Therefore, coaches and fitness professionals should have a clear understanding of the daily forecast or indoor climate during assessments and the limitations of the equipment being used.

SUMMARY

General considerations for the use of equipment during assessments include the potential costs and benefits of specific devices or instruments, adjustability, maintenance, and safety. Additionally, issues related to the data collection process, availability of technology, and eventual generalizability of the results to other athletes or normative data should be addressed prior to beginning the assessment procedures. Appropriate training and experience with respect to the equipment used during assessment by the coaches and training staff as well as the ability to standardize the testing environment are factors that may affect the ability of the client or athlete to perform optimally. Lastly, different types of equipment are available that may be used to measure or support assessments related to anthropometrics, physical performance (force or resistance, distance or length, speed, etc.), and other key areas.

CHAPTER 3

Assessment 301: Which Tests?

"A common mistake among those who work in sport is spending a dispro-portional amount of time on X's and O's as compared to time spent learning about people."

Mike Krzyzewski, Duke University Men's Basketball Coach

While the multitude of assessments available may be daunting, the selection process can be simplified through the determination of the activity-specific needs of the athletes or clients being evaluated and the information deemed crucial by the coach or fitness professional. Furthermore, the identified protocols should be easily implemented from the perspective of both the clients or athletes and the coach or fitness professional to allow for repeatability. Once the assessments are complete, the athletes or clients and coach or fitness professional must be able to compare the results with benchmark data from either baseline testing or the general population. Therefore, the needs of the client or athlete and the coach or fitness professional should be balanced with selecting and implementing relevant assessments that lead to informative feedback.

NEEDS OF THE CLIENT OR ATHLETE

The selection of assessments should be made through the lens of either the self-identified needs of the client or athlete or the knowledge and experience of the coach or fitness professional. These needs are likely to be in the form of specific goals or performance outcomes. It is important to consider that the available assessments may not directly address the goal or outcome but may be used to provide additional information about the physical fitness attributes or the current situation of the client or athlete. A cross-country runner may want to improve performance times, which may be directly related to aerobic capacity, but they may also have a tendency to lose at the end of races where sprinting ability could be relevant.

A wide receiver may want to earn the starting spot on the football team, which requires sprint speed, strength, and power. A client simply may want to get stronger or gain muscle while losing body fat, but the simple process of identifying baseline levels of strength of various muscle groups and body composition would still need to be conducted.

NEEDS OF THE COACH OR FITNESS PROFESSIONAL

Coaches and fitness professionals can use their knowledge, expertise, and experience to focus and expand the goals or performance outcomes of the client or athlete prior to engaging in the actual selection of assessments. Furthermore, the selected assessments will aid in the decision-making process with respect to training or competition. Perhaps the goal or performance outcome will be tied directly to a specific decision aided by the results of the selected assessment. However, more typically, several decisions from a variety of assessments covering many physical fitness attributes result in incremental improvements, termed *marginal gains*, ultimately leading to the eventual attainment of the client's or athlete's needs. This approach really gets to the core of the benefits provided by the combined perspectives of coaches or fitness professionals and exercise or sport scientists through the selection and implementation of assessments.

RELEVANCE OF THE ASSESSMENT

While the terms *validity* and *reliability* (to be described shortly) are key indicators of the soundness of a particular assessment, the term *relevance* may be more useful when initiating the process of assessment selection. More specifically, the questions that must be asked are, "How relevant is the assessment for the individual or situation?" or perhaps, "How well does the assessment help me address my client's or athlete's needs?" The first piece of this puzzle is to determine which physical fitness attributes are relevant. For a general fitness assessment, a broad testing battery would make sense. If clients or athletes have specific goals or easily

identified deficiencies, this process is relatively straightforward. Many sports also have commonly used assessments that may provide the basis for developing your own set of testing procedures.

As indicated in chapter 1, the intention of assessments is to shed light on the identified goals of the client or athlete or coach or fitness professional. These goals or performance outcomes may not be easily quantified with a single physical fitness attribute. In this case, assessments representing the potentially relevant physical fitness attributes should be thoughtfully selected in an effort to explain as much of the goal or performance outcome as possible. For example, if the client's or athlete's goal or performance outcome is related to endurance performance, the first selected assessment would likely be related to cardiorespiratory fitness (represented by the dark inner circle labeled "Assessment 1" in figure 3.1). Perhaps a client or athlete is smaller and potentially weaker than peers, so assessments related to body composition and muscular strength would also be selected (represented by the dark inner circles labeled "Assessment 2" and "Assessment 3" in figure 3.1). This process of including additional assessments (represented by the dark inner circles labeled "Assessment 4" and "Assessment 5" in figure 3.1) would continue until the client or athlete and coach or fitness professional are confident that implementing this assessment battery will sufficiently increase their knowledge of the agreed-upon goal or outcome. Using our simplified theoretical example, the assessment battery consisting of individual assessments (represented by the dark inner circles in figure 3.1, sized to represent their relevance) would help to explain or "predict" as much of the intended goal or performance outcome (represented by the light outer circle in figure 3.1) as possible.

EASE OF IMPLEMENTATION

The selection of assessments must be made while keeping in mind the available resources and any barriers to implementation. To this end, any specific equipment or facilities that may be needed should be identified and a determination should be made if they are currently available or if there are any costs associated with them. For example, some muscular strength assessments may require the use of resistance training equipment. If access to a resistance training facility is easily attained, the assessment may be easily implemented; however, if this is not an option, gaining access to or purchasing the equipment may be prohibitive. If the assessment is new to either the client or athlete or the coach or fitness professional, the potential for a learning curve must be considered. If the inclusion of the selected assessments will be useful in the long run, a learning curve typically would not be an issue because the benefits outweigh the upfront investment (namely, time).

ISSUES WITH REDUNDANT ASSESSMENT

If one assessment is so incredibly useful, why not conduct as many as possible? A typical scenario occurs when a coach or fitness professional, who wants to get to know a bit more about their athletes and has a specific physical fitness attribute in mind (e.g., agility), meets with an exercise or sport scientist. The coach or fitness professional leaves the meeting with a list of too many assessments

to keep straight (and a headache!). This also consistently occurs when designing research studies until someone points out that there is a budget and a timeline for completion.

While implementing a comprehensive and exhaustive battery of assessments is ideal, presumably all clients or athletes and coaches or fitness professionals are limited by time and budget constraints. Therefore, the aim should be the selection of a sufficient number of assessments to address the identified needs while minimizing overlap among those assessments associated with specific physical fitness attributes. Returning to our simplified theoretical example, we want to avoid the situation where an additional assessment (represented by the dark inner circle labeled "Assessment 3" in figure 3.2) is included and significantly overlaps an existing assessment (represented by the dark inner circle labeled "Assessment 2" in figure 3.2) while not adding enough insight into the intended goal or performance outcome (represented by the light outer circle). In this case, the time or financial burden may not justify the use of the third, potentially redundant, assessment.

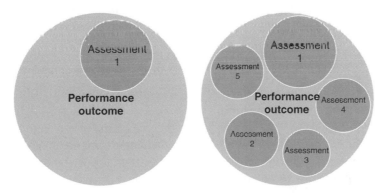

Figure 3.1   Example 1 of determining the relevance of assessments based on a performance outcome.

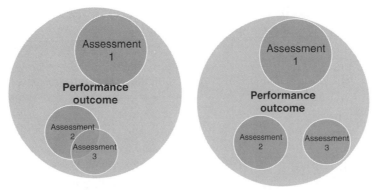

Figure 3.2   Example 2 of determining the relevance of assessments based on a performance outcome.

ASSESSMENT OF BASIC FITNESS ATTRIBUTES

The assessments included in this text are generally focused on basic physical fitness attributes (14, 19), including anthropometrics and body composition, flexibility and balance, speed and agility, power and explosiveness, muscular strength and endurance, cardiovascular fitness, and client or athlete monitoring. While these physical fitness attributes will become much clearer throughout the proceeding chapters, which contain specific assessments and suggested evaluation procedures, an overview of each is provided here.

ANTHROPOMETRICS AND BODY COMPOSITION

Anthropometrics are values that quantify the size and proportions of an individual. Body weight and height are typical anthropometric assessments that can also be used to calculate body mass index. The relative size of specific segments of the body measured as lengths or circumferences and the comparison of these segments as ratios provide insight into the individual shape or physique of the client or athlete. The waist-to-hip circumference ratio is a common anthropometric value that is used to quickly evaluate potential health risks, but distinct values can be seen in specific types of athletes as well as between men and women.

Body composition provides an overview of the separate components (fat, muscle, water, bone, etc.) that make up the total body mass of an individual. The term *body weight* (measured as force in Newtons by scientists or, more generally, in pounds) is distinguished from body mass (measured in kilograms by scientists) due to the variable influence of gravity. Because all of our assessments will presumably be conducted on Earth under relatively stable gravitational conditions and the results will not end up in scientific journals, we will stick with the term *body weight* (measured in pounds or kilograms) for the purpose of this book. Skinfold assessments and bioelectrical impedance analysis are two commonly used field-based methods of assessing fat mass, as body fat percentage, and fat-free mass, which is represented by the rest of the body including muscle mass. Any idea on which athletes

have been reported to possess the largest fat-free mass values? Sumo wrestlers! One athlete had a fat-free mass of more than 265 pounds (120 kg) with 33 percent body fat, equaling a total body mass of approximately 397 pounds (180 kg) (9). This information provides unique insight into the training status of the athlete that may not have be otherwise evident. These types of values are crucial components of a physical fitness profile and influence the decision to engage in various weight management and exercise training strategies. The selection process for determining the most appropriate method of estimating anthropometrics and body composition will likely be influenced by the equipment available, the costs associated with the assessments, and the expertise of the individual conducting the testing.

FLEXIBILITY AND BALANCE

Flexibility describes the ability to move segments of the body (arms, legs, torso, head, etc.) around joints (elbows, knees, hips, neck, etc.). Similar to body composition assessments, flexibility assessments tend to affect performance indirectly. A minimum level of flexibility may be desired to allow the appropriate mobility for a given activity, but an excess of this attribute, termed *hypermobility*, may result in injury. Therefore, flexibility assessments tend to be used to verify the requisite mobility needed or to identify deficits in specific joints or muscle groups in order to develop stretching programs or manage the training process.

Balance is made up of several separate attributes but can generally be defined as the ability to hold the body in a desired position or to maintain stability during both static (limited movement) and dynamic (with movement) situations. Balance assessments can be conducted in a variety of ways while examining how well clients or athletes can keep their body (more specifically, their center of gravity or mass) within the contact area of their feet (their base of support).

These assessments range from measuring the amount of time clients or athletes can hold a specific position or orientation, to the distance that can be reached while extending their body to the edge of its base of support, or the distance traveled while moving within a limited base of support. Further levels of complexity can be added to these balance assessments with alterations to the environment, such as having the eyes closed, changing the base of support, or making the surface unstable. For example, balance measures that were reportedly similar between ballet dancers and judo athletes under stable conditions with their eyes open changed in favor of the judo athletes when they closed their eyes and were exposed to unstable conditions, presumably because the ballet dancers relied heavily on visual feedback during their training and performances (17). As with flexibility, balance deficits may be related to injury risk, but the implications of this attribute could also be expanded to include relationships with body composition, motor control, and sport performance.

SPEED AND AGILITY

Speed is simply defined as the distance covered over a specific duration of time; however, it can be described further by the ability to gain speed, termed *acceleration*, and the ability to achieve as high of a speed as possible, termed *maximal speed*. As the equipment used to determine acceleration and maximal speed is not commonly available, the time needed to cover a predefined distance is usually measured as an indicator of these values. The selected distance is chosen to provide meaningful information based on the sport or activity of interest. Furthermore, repeated sprint ability based on several (<10) short-distance sprints (5-6 sec or 20-40 m) separated by brief rest periods (<30 sec) may also be evaluated if the activity is intermittent in nature.

Agility is defined as the ability to change direction while incorporating speed, balance, and coordination. Furthermore, acceleration (speeding up) and deceleration (slowing down) are key factors that affect agility performance. Assessments of agility vary depending on the number of directional changes, the distance between changes in direction, the total distance covered, and the patterns of movement. Most agility assessments include preplanned movement patterns; however, an additional level of complexity can be included by having the client or athlete react to signals indicating the appropriate directional change. For example, while limited differences in preplanned agility were reported between elite and non-elite rugby players, the scores for reactive agility (with randomized changes in direction) were clearly superior for the more accomplished athletes (20).

POWER AND EXPLOSIVENESS

Power is formally defined as the amount of work completed over a specified time period or, alternatively, as the product of force and velocity. In practice, power, or explosiveness, is dictated by the ability to produce extremely high levels of force very quickly (termed *rate of force development*). As such, there is a trade-off between force production and speed that must be balanced to optimize power output. For example, let's compare powerlifting, where the specific lifts are conducted at slower speeds with a limited range of motion, versus Olympic weightlifting, where the specific lifts require rapid movements and thus would result in less weight (relatively speaking!) being lifted. In support, Olympic weightlifters have been shown to perform better in countermovement jump tests, a common assessment for power output, compared to powerlifters (13). Sometimes power assessments are labeled "anaerobic" due to their use of the energy system that supports short-term, high-intensity activities. This also explains why assessments used to determine power are very short in nature, generally completed in just a few seconds. Field-based measurements of power usually quantify this physical fitness attribute by determining the displacement of the client's or athlete's body or an implement, or the time needed to displace the body or implement over a specified distance.

MUSCULAR STRENGTH AND ENDURANCE

Muscular strength is the result of force production by specific muscles or muscle groups that is potentially affected by the muscle fiber composition, muscle size and architecture, and the neuromuscular system. For the purpose of assessments, muscular strength is typically defined as estimated maximal voluntary strength and measured as the highest amount of weight an individual can lift during just a few (1-5) repetitions. Regardless of the number of repetitions completed, these assessments require that clients or athletes load additional weight onto their body. Thus, proper technique and safe movement patterns are extremely important to minimize the potential for injury. While muscular strength assessments are usually measured as the actual amount of the weight lifted or force produced (termed *absolute strength*), some coaches and fitness professionals may elect to divide the results by the client's or athlete's body mass or weight (a measurement termed *relative strength*) for the purpose of comparison.

Alternatively, muscular endurance can be defined by the ability to repeatedly produce voluntary strength or to maintain voluntary force production by a specific muscle or muscle group at submaximal levels for an extended period of time. Most muscular endurance assessments use a predefined load (e.g., body weight, percentage of body weight, or a percentage of maximal strength values) and count the number of repetitions a client or athlete can complete of a specific movement. For example, the Scouting Combine conducted annually by the National Football League features a bench press test where athletes are instructed to complete as many repetitions as possible of 225 pounds (102 kg) (12), while the National Hockey League's Scouting Combine features a similar test with a weight equivalent to 70 to 80 percent of the player's' body weight with the additional caveat that they must keep up with a pace of 25 repetitions per minute (3). Due to the relationship between muscular strength and endurance, the number of repetitions from muscular endurance assessments are sometimes used to estimate the maximal strength values. Another method of evaluating muscular endurance involves timing how long clients or athletes can hold themselves in a particular body position without moving (termed *isometric strength*).

CARDIORESPIRATORY FITNESS

Cardiorespiratory fitness is a function of the body's aerobic capacity or its ability to take in and use oxygen through the lungs, heart, and muscles during exercise. Sometimes cardiorespiratory fitness assessments are labeled "aerobic" due to their use of the energy system that supports longer duration activities with athletes specializing in distance events possessing higher values than those specializing in shorter events. In this regard,

these assessments feature testing protocols that quantify the time needed to complete a given amount of work (i.e., a specific distance covered) or the amount of work completed (i.e., distance covered) in a given amount of time. Depending on the training status of the client or athlete or the needs of the coach or fitness professional, maximal or submaximal assessments with or without increasing intensities (i.e., increasing speeds) can be conducted. While maximal assessments require that the client or athlete exercise until exhaustion, submaximal assessments might be terminated at a predefined intensity level as indicated by perception of effort or heart rate.

CLIENT OR ATHLETE MONITORING

Another beneficial avenue of assessment is through the process of client or athlete monitoring. The monitoring process includes a variety of different assessments focused on day-to-day or week-to-week measures of physiological or psychological strain, training load or volume, and recovery. Some of these assessments are used to quantify external training load, defined as work completed by the client or athlete, whereas others are used to quantify internal training load, defined as either physiological or psychological stress related to training. Additional measures include the monitoring of recovery, soreness, and hydration status. The bulk of the monitoring assessments can be completed by the client or athlete on their own through self-reporting, making them ideal to be recorded on more of a recurring basis than the previously discussed assessments. Due to the highly individualized nature of these monitoring assessments, changes from the client's or athlete's typical values, rather than comparisons to normative data, may be used as inputs to aid in the adjustment of training programs or other lifestyle factors (e.g., sleep, diet, etc.).

ASSESSMENT SELECTION USING SWOT ANALYSIS

One approach to evaluating assessments for a single client or athlete or a group of individuals at a given point in time is to use a SWOT (strengths, weaknesses, opportunities, threats) analysis (2, 4, 22). In a slightly different approach from that described in chapter 1, this process involves a selection of assessments to identify internal factors or areas in which a client or athlete is particularly skilled (strengths) or to identify particular physical fitness attributes where improvement may be needed (weaknesses). This determination would be paired with an appraisal of the client's or athlete's current situation and environment, including identification of those external factors that may be benefits (opportunities) and barriers (threats) to attaining the intended goal or performance outcome. Let's take a look.

INTERNAL FACTORS

For this comparison, strengths and weaknesses can be interpreted much more literally, with the perceived physical fitness attributes of the client or athlete serving as the internal factors. For example, perhaps a coach or fitness professional has identified that a basketball player may be particularly gifted at jumping for rebounds (supported by power or explosiveness and lower-body strength) but is limited by poor cardiorespiratory fitness (consistently fatigues during the second half of games) and upper-body strength (struggles when being guarded by average defenders). During baseline testing, assessments can be used to verify these perceived strengths and weaknesses. In follow-up testing sessions, previously identified strengths and weaknesses can be checked to see if any improvements have been achieved.

EXTERNAL FACTORS

Consideration should be given to potential threats, such as the availability of resources, which includes the time commitment of the client or athlete and the coaching or training staff needed to conduct the selected assessments. Furthermore, depending on the selected assessments, costs related to equipment, consumables, training, and access to the appropriate training or testing facilities may be factors. These threats can be weighed against the opportunities associated with either clear improvements or marginal gains made in the identified physical fitness attributes and any influence on the intended goal or performance outcome of a client or athlete.

Table 3.1 shows how a generic analysis using some of the SWOT factors discussed throughout this text helps to identify how the selection of assessments might influence progress toward the intended goal or performance outcome of a client or athlete.

The intersection of opportunities and weaknesses (OW) yields the best case for clear improvements in deficient or suboptimal physical fitness attributes, which will likely result in progression toward the client's or athlete's goal or performance outcome. This offers support for the appropriate selection of assessments and uses the positive aspects of the SWOT analysis. Considering the relevant opportunities and strengths (OS) together poses the potential for incremental improvements (or marginal gains) in the physical fitness attributes classified as typical or outstanding that could yield progress toward the client's or athlete's goal or performance outcome. Perhaps

Table 3.1   Generic SWOT Analysis for Assessment Selection From the Client's or Athlete's Perspective

	Strengths Perceived or verified physical fitness attributes	**Weaknesses** Perceived or verified physical fitness attributes
Opportunities Clear improvements OR marginal gains	*OS:* Marginal gains in existing strengths with potential to benefit performance outcome	*OW:* Clear improvements in existing weaknesses with benefit to intended performance outcome
Threats No improvements AND depletion of resources (human, financial, technical)	*TS:* Wasted resources and inappropriate focus on existing strengths	*TW:* Justified use of resources through identification of alternative interventions

the most informative situation for the coach or fitness professional lies with the connection of threats and weakness (TW), where minimal progression in the deficient or suboptimal physical fitness attributes occur, resulting in modifications to the training program or other interventions. Finally, in the worst-case scenario, where the use of resources to continue evaluation of the typical or outstanding physical fitness attributes are not justified, the intersection of potential threats and strengths (TS) might result in a discontinuation of the assessments or the intervention.

It should be noted that this generic SWOT analysis relies on the assumption that identified physical fitness attributes can be improved, which may not always be true. Nonetheless, we will rely on the coach's or fitness professional's knowledge and experience to take care of this issue.

ASSESSMENT PRINCIPLES

Adherence to the concepts of validity and reliability will help ensure the effectiveness of assessments. Furthermore, appropriate management of the clients or athletes as well as the sequencing and timing of the selected assessments must be considered.

SPECIFICITY

After the appropriate physical fitness attributes have been identified, coaches and fitness professionals must select relevant assessments. This step of the process necessitates that clients or athletes rely on a key principle, namely specificity to the sport or activity of interest. A number of factors may be used to determine how specificity affects the selection of assessments. These factors include, but are not limited to, the general movement patterns of the activity, the speed and duration of the activity, the muscles used, and how these muscles are used (6, 15). However, as noted with respect to the initial evaluation steps, specificity must be considered with some degree of common sense.

General Demands of the Sport or Activity

The movement patterns within the context of the sport or activity of interest must be considered during the assessment selection process. This process entails determining the types of exercise required (or exercise mode) during the sport or activity (e.g., running, jumping, throwing, cycling) and if they can be classified as being completed in a single (discrete) movement, a series of a few interconnected (serial) movements, or a repeated pattern of the same movements (cyclical). Within discrete and serial movements, the physical actions are usually easily identified; however, they may need to be broken down into phases in order to home in on the specific demands. When considering cyclical movements, the repeated physical actions are the primary focus and how long they need to be repeated becomes a major indicator of the types of assessments that need to be conducted. Brief, simplified examples of this process are provided throughout this section for the sport of tennis (5, 10).

Tennis is made up of several serial movements, such as service, forehand and backhand strokes, and net play, that are separated by short-duration sprints. Each stroke consists of unique initial preparation, backswing, impact, and follow-through phases.

From this point, the physical actions of the body and the motors, or muscles, used to accomplish these actions are identified. A description of the physical actions of the body includes whether the sport or activity primarily uses the arms (upper-body dominant), legs (lower-body dominant), or both (full-body), as well as whether it requires mostly pushing, pulling, rotating, stabilizing, or, more than likely, a combination of these actions. Furthermore, it may be relevant to determine if the use of a dominant limb (arm/leg) influences these actions or if the limbs are engaged simultaneously (bilaterally) or independently (unilaterally). This information can then be used to determine the specific joints and muscle groups used, which are of particular interest in selecting relevant assessments.

Lower-body strength and power, along with general balance and stability, help support the upper-body power or explosiveness needed to complete the tennis stroke.

The overall duration and intensity of the movements, which reflect the use of metabolic energy, associated with the sport or activity of interest must also be considered. The anaerobic energy system is made up of two components: the phosphagen and glycolytic systems. Very short-duration, explosive activities lasting just a few seconds are primarily governed by the phosphagen system, whereas high-intensity activities lasting >10 seconds to several minutes are primarily governed by the glycolytic system. Because they have a clear beginning and end and last for just a few moments, discrete and serial movements are generally supported by the phosphagen system. Cyclical movements conducted at very high intensities may be supported by the glycolytic system. However, when the cyclical movements continue on for long periods of time at lower intensities or when the high-intensity (serial or cyclical) actions are interspersed with rest or recovery periods (think sprint intervals or high-intensity intermittent training), the aerobic energy system, with its responsibility for extended duration activities, takes over the support duties.

A tennis match consists of repeated serial actions (<10 sec each) interspersed with brief rest periods (approximately 20-40 sec) between points. The entire match varies in duration, potentially lasting several hours.

Don't worry, there's no quiz after this section, but general knowledge of the energy systems used during the sport or activity of interest and the physical fitness attributes to be evaluated will aid in the appropriate selection of assessments. For example, a testing battery consisting of the following assessments may be appropriate for the sport of tennis (5):

- Reactive agility test to evaluate speed, balance, and coordination
- Repeated sprint ability test to evaluate speed
- Vertical jump to evaluate lower-body power or explosiveness
- Medicine ball throw to evaluate upper-body power or explosiveness
- Three-repetition maximum squat test to evaluate lower-body strength
- Intermittent shuttle run test to evaluate cardiorespiratory fitness

Predominance Versus Influence

Some situations might warrant a more thorough evaluation of the goals of the client or intended activities of the athlete. These evaluations can become very complex, spanning from knowledge gleaned from time motion analysis to energy system contributions—perhaps without reason or to the detriment (or at least confusion) of the evaluator. Examples from two separate sports can be used to illustrate this issue. Time motion analyses of soccer matches reveal that the greatest portion of the game is spent walking (23), and during combat sports, research shows that the aerobic energy system is primarily used (8). In both cases, an evaluation conducted without knowledge of the activity might lead the uninitiated to determine that the most important assessments would fall within the realm of cardiorespiratory fitness. However, coaches and trainers would be quick to tell you that speed and agility for soccer players and power for combat sports athletes should be the primary focus. That is not to say that cardiorespiratory fitness is irrelevant in either case, but it does help us understand that we must consider both the predominant attributes for a given activity as well as the decisive attributes that lead to success.

Client or Athlete Constraints

As mentioned previously, Newell's model of constraints is commonly used to describe the "optimal coordination and control of an activity (16, 21)." In this regard, the identification of the potential individual, task, and environmental constraints to movement or human performance may assist in the appropriate selection of assessments.

Individual   Individual constraints reflective of the client's or athlete's physical and psychological state will likely affect which assessments are selected. In particular, body composition may dictate if an individual can successfully complete an assessment or if the results need to be interpreted with respect to key anthropometric factors, such as body weight, height, arm and leg length, etc. The nature of certain protocols may limit their applicability to all individuals, and special consideration should be given to children and older adults to ensure safety. Advanced maturity (both physical and psychological), fitness level, and training experience of the client or athlete may allow for more complex and physically demanding assessments to be conducted. Depending on the severity or location, preexisting injury or the potential for injury may preclude some individuals from completing specific assessments. The availability of sex/gender-specific normative data (and a variety of other individual factors) may also pose a limitation.

Task Task constraints reflecting the nature or demands of the sport or activity of interest and the corresponding physical fitness attributes strongly influence which assessments are appropriate for a specific client or athlete. This is where the concept of specificity is particularly important, and agreement between the task constraints, the physical fitness attribute, and the selected assessment is crucial. The work-to-rest ratio of specific sports may dictate the types of physical fitness attributes and corresponding assessments that should be used. Considering the previous example from soccer, where a typical work-to-rest ratio is greater than 1:4 (11), the relevant work represents short-duration sprints and changes in direction whereas the extended-duration rest periods represent walking and standing. In this case, short-distance speed and agility assessments may be selected. For some athletes, the requirements of specific playing positions will likely dictate which assessments are relevant. For example, in American football, vertical jump tests may be more appropriate for wide receivers, who are expected to catch the ball at as high of a point as possible, than for offensive linemen, who are expected to defend opposing linemen by pushing them away and for whom tests of maximal upper strength and endurance may be more appropriate. The competitive level or level of participation, and potentially the rule set, of the sport or activity of interest may also have an impact on the assessment selection.

Environmental Several environmental constraints could have an effect on the assessment selection, including the policies of the training facility or sporting organization, such as limitations on the type of information that can be measured or interpreted, and the physical environment, such as indoor or outdoor facilities, noise, privacy, etc. Furthermore, social norms as well as expectations from coaches or fitness professionals and other individuals in the client or athlete support group (administrators, family, friends, boosters) with respect to the type of assessments conducted and the information made available must also be considered. In general, environmental or organizational support for change and continuous improvement will aid in the selection and implementation of assessments.

VALIDITY

The concept of validity is different than usefulness, as mentioned previously, and can be applied to assessments in a variety of ways (7, 15, 18). In general, validity—or, more specifically, logical or face validity—refers to the ability of an assessment to measure what it is intended to measure, but it can be expanded to include the notion of ecological validity where the results of the assessment make sense in the real world outside of the testing environment. From a research perspective, a valid assessment means that it provides values similar to the best available methods to evaluate a particular physical fitness attribute. For example, an assessment aimed at estimating aerobic capacity might be considered valid if it provides values similar to maximal oxygen uptake determined using gas exchange analysis with a metabolic cart.

Due to some limitations with the direct comparison of field-based measures used during assessments and gold-standard laboratory-based measures, coaches or fitness professionals often rely on a strong correlation between these two types of measures, which is referred to as concurrent validity. Ecological validity is one of these issues where discrepancies between clinical-type outcomes measured in a more controlled setting (e.g., a laboratory) and performance outcomes measured in a setting more likely to be encountered by clients or athletes could lead to the inability to generalize the results. Another form of validity, discriminant validity, occurs when the results of a specific assessment can effectively differentiate between individuals who would be expected to possess different physical fitness attributes (e.g., athletes versus nonathletes, endurance athletes versus strength or power athletes, etc.). The assessments included in this text have been selected with these types of validity considerations in mind. However, coaches or fitness professionals should be sure to consider how valid a specific assessment is for their particular situation.

RELIABILITY

The concept of reliability, which refers to the consistency of obtaining a specific value (7), has been addressed previously with respect to the implementation of assessments and the equipment used to conduct the assessments. A reliable assessment that is highly correlated to the gold standard, but that may not provide the exact same outcome, can still be used to verify changes in a particular physical fitness attribute. The term *precision* can be considered a subcategory of both reliability and validity, describing how confident one can be about a given data point (7). More specifically, precision gives us an approximate range in which a specific result might fall. For example, we can be confident that a body mass of 220 pounds (99.8 kg) measured on a scale with a precision 0.1 pounds (0.05 kg) is between 219.9 and 220.1 pounds (99.74 and 99.84 kg). This confidence in the measurement of a particular physical fitness attribute allows us to appropriately compare changes between assessment sessions. Because one of the primary purposes of assessment is to determine if improvements in the athlete's or client's performance have been made, the coach or fitness professional must consider the reliability of the selected assessments with respect to the actual protocol, the testing environment, and the equipment.

ATHLETE OR CLIENT STAGING

The number of athletes or clients that need to be evaluated and the time available to complete the assessments are primary questions that need to be addressed. This information will dictate the types of assessments selected, the amount of equipment needed, and the number of personnel or staff required. Depending on the assessments and available resources, athletes or clients may need to be evaluated individually, such as reactive agility testing during which external distractions may compromise performance, or in manageably sized groups, such as endurance tests or shuttle runs. The final determination relies heavily on the coach's or fitness professional's knowledge of requirements of the activity or sport, the athletes or clients, and the testing environment.

SEQUENCING

Because several assessments are usually conducted in the form of a testing battery, coaches or fitness professionals must consider the time needed for each assessment (including rest or recovery time), how many assessment sessions will be needed, the number of clients or athletes to be tested, and the order in which the assessments are completed. Generally, assessments should be arranged in such a manner that the previous assessment does not result in decreased performance on the next assessment (24). With this in mind, nonfatiguing assessments should be conducted first, followed by speed or agility, power, muscular strength or endurance, and cardiorespiratory fitness assessments. These general guidelines may need to be modified depending on the specific assessments selected, with an attempt to perform tasks requiring more skill before physically exhausting tasks, and those relying on strength prior to those relying on endurance (15, 18). If the total time needed to complete the selected assessments is longer than the time available, multiple sessions must be scheduled within the given time constraints. In this case, separating the assessments with consideration for the previously mentioned guidelines is recommended.

The time between assessment sessions should be sufficient to allow recovery from the first session (hours to days depending on intensity of the assessments) but not so long that the general fitness of the clients or athletes might be susceptible to change. Furthermore, if a large number of clients or athletes need to be tested, they may need to be separated into different sessions. Depending on the number of testing stations, assessments that may not cause limited residual fatigue for each other could be grouped and completed before moving on to more physically taxing assessments. This approach might expedite the assessment session by minimizing the rest time between assessments.

TIMING

Timing is another consideration when implementing assessments. Time limitations may stem from decisions related to sport- or activity-specific requirements (will the assessment adversely affect training time or progression?), client or athlete availability (will the assessment adversely affect the client's or athlete's other personal or professional commitments?), and coordinating with facilities and other staff or personnel (are any special accommodations required?).

It is recommended that baseline assessments be conducted during times of relative training stability prior to engaging in planned training progression. The preseason timeframe or the transition between training cycles are commonly selected for baseline evaluation; however, results from a single baseline assessment may be limited due to difficulties associated with identifying relative training stability in a large group of clients or athletes. Therefore, assessments conducted at regular intervals should be considered. The duration of regular intervals will vary by situation, but periods of transition, such as pre- to postseason or between training phases, provide great opportunities for assessment that aid in future planning. Adequate time between assessments should be given to allow for intervention-related adaptations. For youth athletes, assessment every three months is recommended to account for maturity-related growth and development (25).

AVAILABILITY OF NORMATIVE DATA

The selection of specific assessments may be dictated by the availability of normative data against which the results of the client or athlete can be compared. This normative data is developed from a group of standard values or norms from either a large number of different individuals (providing a comparison to the general population) or from a large group of people who share some similarities (providing a comparison to specific populations of interest). The specific populations of interest are useful and become much more relevant when they match the demographics of the client or athlete being evaluated (similar age, gender/sex, sport or activity, skill level, etc.). While some coaches or fitness professionals will have accumulated enough assessment results from their own clients or athletes to allow for comparison, existing normative data will be provided for the included assessments in subsequent chapters.

Taken together, the previously outlined physical fitness attributes (or subsets of the attributes deemed relevant for a particular situation) and the assessments selected to represent them can be used to represent the fitness profile (or strengths and weaknesses) of the client or athlete. The values measured for each attribute can be compared to normative data, and using the previously described terminology, the client or athlete can be evaluated as suboptimal, typical, or outstanding for each physical fitness attribute. An example spider plot (also called a *radar chart*), depicted in figure 3.3, includes the physical fitness attributes described in this chapter. To illustrate how to interpret the spider plot, bell-shaped curves, as explained in chapter 1, have been included along with the shaded regions representing suboptimal, typical, and outstanding values.

This information can enhance the decision-making process by providing a visual representation of the relevant assessments. For example, deviations from typical values for specific physical fitness attributes may be used to determine if specific interventions should be selected or if the client or athlete is more developed, at the same level as, or behind their peers. The spider plot in figure 3.4 depicts an athlete who appears to have particularly developed flexibility, balance, power, and explosiveness but lacks cardiorespiratory fitness. Conversely, figure 3.5 depicts an athlete who appears to have particularly developed cardiorespiratory fitness but lacks muscular strength and endurance.

Following a review of the client's or athlete's fitness profile or the profiles of an entire team or group of clients, the coach or fitness professional can make decisions, including the modification of training programs or adoption of some intervention, to address these findings. Follow-up assessment can then be used to see if the selected response was successful by comparing the previous (black line and markers) and current results (white line and markers) as depicted in this spider plot (see figure 3.6). In this case, muscular strength and endurance appears to have improved from suboptimal to typical along with small changes in several other physical fitness attributes.

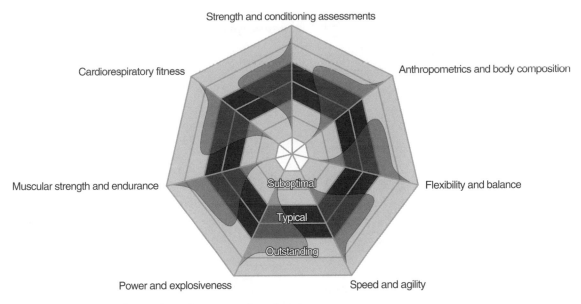

Figure 3.3 An example spider plot (or radar chart).

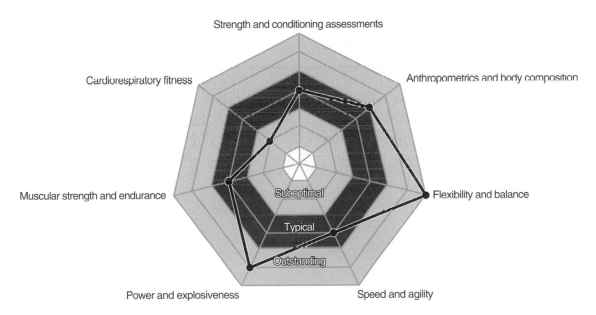

Figure 3.4 A spider plot showing developed flexibility, balance, power, and explosiveness but deficient cardiorespiratory fitness.

GENERAL RECOMMENDATIONS

Prior to outlining specific assessments related to the previously mentioned physical fitness attributes, a number of general recommendations for supporting these procedures should be reviewed. These include procedures related to client or athlete screening, familiarization, pretesting guidelines, warm-up, and delivery of the assessments.

PREPARTICIPATION SCREENING AND PHYSICAL EXAMINATION

The general health and ability to participate in exercise of the client or athlete must be verified prior to engaging in assessments. For the purpose of this text, it is generally assumed that the client or athlete is currently involved with the sport or activity of interest and has already been cleared to participate by means of a physician or some

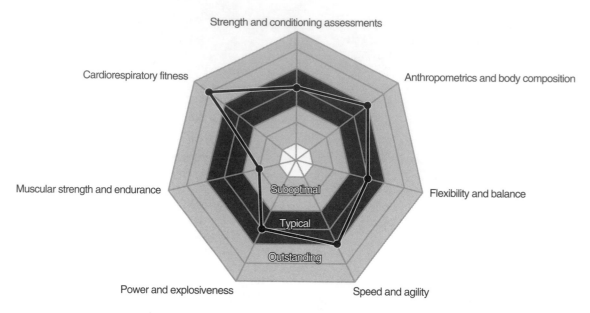

Figure 3.5 A spider plot showing particularly developed cardiorespiratory fitness but deficient muscular strength or endurance.

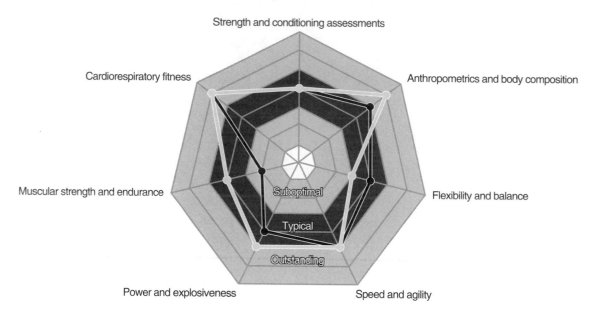

Figure 3.6 A spider plot showing comparative improvements.

other manner. The self-guided Physical Activity Readiness Questionnaire for Everyone (PAR-Q+), provided in figure 3.7 (starting on page 44),, starting on page 44 may be an option to help identify when physician clearance is warranted. It should also be noted that some preexisting conditions, such as lingering injuries or impaired movement patterns, may warrant special considerations by the coach or fitness professional when selecting assessments.

FAMILIARIZATION

Conducting several familiarization (or practice) assessments prior to the official data collection allows both the client or athlete and coach or fitness professional to become acquainted with the procedures and equipment. This run-through session will help identify any procedural issues or external influences that might affect the ability to achieve the most useful and relevant results.

The ability to quickly pick up novel tasks, termed the *learning effect*, through rapid improvements related to motor learning or tactical strategy may need to be considered. Thus, the use of familiarization assessments may allow the client or athlete to move along the learning curve in order to clearly identify changes related to training programs or other interventions.

PRETESTING GUIDELINES

Just as relative training stability is desired, daily homeostatic conditions (defined as equilibrium within the surrounding environment) are also recommended. This includes factors related to hydration, diet, residual fatigue from previous physical activity, and sleep that can be addressed through communicating specific pretesting guidelines (18). Due to these recommendations and to account for daily variations in biological activity, assessment sessions are normally conducted during a specified time of day. In order to minimize drastic alterations in eating and drinking habits, the morning hours are the most common time to complete body composition testing. Clients or athletes should avoid engaging in high-intensity physical activity for a period of approximately 24 hours before the assessment and to avoid large meals for a period of 2 to 4 hours (4-6 for weight testing) prior to testing depending on requirements of the assessments. If a novel intervention has recently been completed, particularly with respect to resistance training, performance improvements may be delayed and additional de-loading and de-training time may be needed to capture changes adequately. When the assessment results are used as indicators of competitive readiness, coaches and clients or athletes might consider minimally fatiguing assessments prior to real competition or more demanding assessment procedures prior to simulated competition. This approach would allow clients or athletes to engage in their standard preparation, which does not always represent stable day-to-day conditions.

WARM-UP

Prior to engaging in assessments, some form of general and activity-specific warm-ups should be completed (15). It is recommended that the client or athlete avoid extended duration static stretching prior to most assessments because this may result in potentially negative effects on performance. Thus, dynamic movements of progressively increasing intensity should be employed. An example of a general warm-up is outlined in table 3.2 (starting on page 48). For the purpose of this text, activity-specific warm-ups will be communicated within the assessment protocols in subsequent chapters.

CLEAR AND CONCISE ASSESSMENT PROTOCOLS

In order to trust the data and effectively compare the results between individuals and time points, standardization of procedures through consistent delivery and execution of assessments is of paramount importance. Therefore, effective communication should be used both when describing and conducting assessments so that the client or athlete has a clear understanding of the expectations. As mentioned previously, instructional delivery may be enhanced by using a written script that has been practiced and adapted by the coaches or fitness professionals for the specific situation. This approach lends itself to the ability to identify and minimize deviations from the protocol between testing sessions. However, when deviations do occur (such as clients or athletes altering their movement patterns or arriving in a compromised state, such as little to no sleep or wearing less than desirable clothing or footwear), the coach or fitness professional should record these potential issues in the testing notes for consideration with the assessment results.

Standardization will be aided by having the same coach or fitness professional conduct a given assessment for all of the clients or athletes to be tested. This practice will minimize differences in instructional delivery and increase the comfort level of the client or athlete while tempering the influence of personality, encouragement, and feedback given on performance. Whenever possible, positive feedback should be provided with the intention of maintaining high levels of engagement and motivation in the assessment environment. With this in mind, it is particularly important that the coaches or fitness professionals verify that the necessary levels of effort are achieved during testing and that, when applicable, clients or athletes do not enlist any pacing strategies (withholding effort for specific moments during the test). In both cases, the results may not be valid and

2018 PAR-Q+

The Physical Activity Readiness Questionnaire for Everyone

The health benefits of regular physical activity are clear; more people should engage in physical activity every day of the week. Participating in physical activity is very safe for MOST people. This questionnaire will tell you whether it is necessary for you to seek further advice from your doctor OR a qualified exercise professional before becoming more physically active.

GENERAL HEALTH QUESTIONS

Please read the 7 questions below carefully and answer each one honestly: check YES or NO.	YES	NO
1) Has your doctor ever said that you have a heart condition ☐ OR high blood pressure ☐?	☐	☐
2) Do you feel pain in your chest at rest, during your daily activities of living, **OR** when you do physical activity?	☐	☐
3) Do you lose balance because of dizziness **OR** have you lost consciousness in the last 12 months? Please answer **NO** if your dizziness was associated with over-breathing (including during vigorous exercise).	☐	☐
4) Have you ever been diagnosed with another chronic medical condition (other than heart disease or high blood pressure)? **PLEASE LIST CONDITION(S) HERE:** _____	☐	☐
5) Are you currently taking prescribed medications for a chronic medical condition? **PLEASE LIST CONDITION(S) AND MEDICATIONS HERE:** _____	☐	☐
6) Do you currently have (or have had within the past 12 months) a bone, joint, or soft tissue (muscle, ligament, or tendon) problem that could be made worse by becoming more physically active? Please answer **NO** if you had a problem in the past, but it *does not limit your current ability* to be physically active. **PLEASE LIST CONDITION(S) HERE:** _____	☐	☐
7) Has your doctor ever said that you should only do medically supervised physical activity?	☐	☐

☑ **If you answered NO to all of the questions above, you are cleared for physical activity.**
Please sign the PARTICIPANT DECLARATION. You do not need to complete Pages 2 and 3.

- ▶ Start becoming much more physically active – start slowly and build up gradually.
- ▶ Follow International Physical Activity Guidelines for your age (www.who.int/dietphysicalactivity/en/).
- ▶ You may take part in a health and fitness appraisal.
- ▶ If you are over the age of 45 yr and NOT accustomed to regular vigorous to maximal effort exercise, consult a qualified exercise professional before engaging in this intensity of exercise.
- ▶ If you have any further questions, contact a qualified exercise professional.

PARTICIPANT DECLARATION
If you are less than the legal age required for consent or require the assent of a care provider, your parent, guardian or care provider must also sign this form.

I, the undersigned, have read, understood to my full satisfaction and completed this questionnaire. I acknowledge that this physical activity clearance is valid for a maximum of 12 months from the date it is completed and becomes invalid if my condition changes. I also acknowledge that the community/fitness centre may retain a copy of this form for records. In these instances, it will maintain the confidentiality of the same, complying with applicable law.

NAME _____ DATE _____

SIGNATURE _____ WITNESS _____

SIGNATURE OF PARENT/GUARDIAN/CARE PROVIDER _____

⬤ **If you answered YES to one or more of the questions above, COMPLETE PAGES 2 AND 3.**

⚠ **Delay becoming more active if:**

- ✓ You have a temporary illness such as a cold or fever; it is best to wait until you feel better.
- ✓ You are pregnant - talk to your health care practitioner, your physician, a qualified exercise professional, and/or complete the ePARmed-X+ at **www.eparmedx.com** before becoming more physically active.
- ✓ Your health changes - answer the questions on Pages 2 and 3 of this document and/or talk to your doctor or a qualified exercise professional before continuing with any physical activity program.

Copyright © 2018 PAR-Q+ Collaboration   1 / 4
01-11-2017

Figure 3.7   Physical Activity Readiness Questionnaire.

Reprinted with permission from the PAR-Q+ Collaboration and the authors of the PAR-Q+ (Dr. Darren Warburton, Dr. Norman Gledhill, Dr. Veronica Jamnik, and Dr. Shannon Bredin).

2018 PAR-Q+

FOLLOW-UP QUESTIONS ABOUT YOUR MEDICAL CONDITION(S)

1. **Do you have Arthritis, Osteoporosis, or Back Problems?**

If the above condition(s) is/are present, answer questions 1a-1c   If **NO** ☐ go to question 2

1a.   Do you have difficulty controlling your condition with medications or other physician-prescribed therapies? **YES** ☐ **NO** ☐
(Answer **NO** if you are not currently taking medications or other treatments)

1b.   Do you have joint problems causing pain, a recent fracture or fracture caused by osteoporosis or cancer, **YES** ☐ **NO** ☐
displaced vertebra (e.g., spondylolisthesis), and/or spondylolysis/pars defect (a crack in the bony ring on the
back of the spinal column)?

1c.   Have you had steroid injections or taken steroid tablets regularly for more than 3 months? **YES** ☐ **NO** ☐

2. **Do you currently have Cancer of any kind?**

If the above condition(s) is/are present, answer questions 2a-2b   If **NO** ☐ go to question 3

2a.   Does your cancer diagnosis include any of the following types: lung/bronchogenic, multiple myeloma (cancer of **YES** ☐ **NO** ☐
plasma cells), head, and/or neck?

2b.   Are you currently receiving cancer therapy (such as chemotheraphy or radiotherapy)? **YES** ☐ **NO** ☐

3. **Do you have a Heart or Cardiovascular Condition?** *This includes Coronary Artery Disease, Heart Failure,*
Diagnosed Abnormality of Heart Rhythm

If the above condition(s) is/are present, answer questions 3a-3d   If **NO** ☐ go to question 4

3a.   Do you have difficulty controlling your condition with medications or other physician-prescribed therapies? **YES** ☐ **NO** ☐
(Answer **NO** if you are not currently taking medications or other treatments)

3b.   Do you have an irregular heart beat that requires medical management? **YES** ☐ **NO** ☐
(e.g., atrial fibrillation, premature ventricular contraction)

3c.   Do you have chronic heart failure? **YES** ☐ **NO** ☐

3d.   Do you have diagnosed coronary artery (cardiovascular) disease and have not participated in regular physical **YES** ☐ **NO** ☐
activity in the last 2 months?

4. **Do you have High Blood Pressure?**

If the above condition(s) is/are present, answer questions 4a-4b   If **NO** ☐ go to question 5

4a.   Do you have difficulty controlling your condition with medications or other physician-prescribed therapies? **YES** ☐ **NO** ☐
(Answer **NO** if you are not currently taking medications or other treatments)

4b.   Do you have a resting blood pressure equal to or greater than 160/90 mmHg with or without medication? **YES** ☐ **NO** ☐
(Answer **YES** if you do not know your resting blood pressure)

5. **Do you have any Metabolic Conditions?** *This includes Type 1 Diabetes, Type 2 Diabetes, Pre-Diabetes*

If the above condition(s) is/are present, answer questions 5a-5e   If **NO** ☐ go to question 6

5a.   Do you often have difficulty controlling your blood sugar levels with foods, medications, or other physician- **YES** ☐ **NO** ☐
prescribed therapies?

5b.   Do you often suffer from signs and symptoms of low blood sugar (hypoglycemia) following exercise and/or **YES** ☐ **NO** ☐
during activities of daily living? Signs of hypoglycemia may include shakiness, nervousness, unusual irritability,
abnormal sweating, dizziness or light-headedness, mental confusion, difficulty speaking, weakness, or sleepiness.

5c.   Do you have any signs or symptoms of diabetes complications such as heart or vascular disease and/or **YES** ☐ **NO** ☐
complications affecting your eyes, kidneys, **OR** the sensation in your toes and feet?

5d.   Do you have other metabolic conditions (such as current pregnancy-related diabetes, chronic kidney disease, or **YES** ☐ **NO** ☐
liver problems)?

5e.   Are you planning to engage in what for you is unusually high (or vigorous) intensity exercise in the near future? **YES** ☐ **NO** ☐

Figure 3.7   *(continued)*

Reprinted with permission from the PAR-Q+ Collaboration and the authors of the PAR-Q+ (Dr. Darren Warburton, Dr. Norman Gledhill, Dr. Veronica Jamnik, and Dr. Shannon Bredin).

2018 PAR-Q+

6.   Do you have any Mental Health Problems or Learning Difficulties? *This includes Alzheimer's, Dementia, Depression, Anxiety Disorder, Eating Disorder, Psychotic Disorder, Intellectual Disability, Down Syndrome*

If the above condition(s) is/are present, answer questions 6a-6b   If **NO** ☐ go to question 7

6a.	Do you have difficulty controlling your condition with medications or other physician-prescribed therapies? (Answer **NO** if you are not currently taking medications or other treatments)	YES☐ NO☐
6b.	Do you have Down Syndrome **AND** back problems affecting nerves or muscles?	YES☐ NO☐

7.   Do you have a Respiratory Disease? *This includes Chronic Obstructive Pulmonary Disease, Asthma, Pulmonary High Blood Pressure*

If the above condition(s) is/are present, answer questions 7a-7d   If **NO** ☐ go to question 8

7a.	Do you have difficulty controlling your condition with medications or other physician-prescribed therapies? (Answer **NO** if you are not currently taking medications or other treatments)	YES☐ NO☐
7b.	Has your doctor ever said your blood oxygen level is low at rest or during exercise and/or that you require supplemental oxygen therapy?	YES☐ NO☐
7c.	If asthmatic, do you currently have symptoms of chest tightness, wheezing, laboured breathing, consistent cough (more than 2 days/week), or have you used your rescue medication more than twice in the last week?	YES☐ NO☐
7d.	Has your doctor ever said you have high blood pressure in the blood vessels of your lungs?	YES☐ NO☐

8.   Do you have a Spinal Cord Injury? *This includes Tetraplegia and Paraplegia*

If the above condition(s) is/are present, answer questions 8a-8c   If **NO** ☐ go to question 9

8a.	Do you have difficulty controlling your condition with medications or other physician-prescribed therapies? (Answer **NO** if you are not currently taking medications or other treatments)	YES☐ NO☐
8b.	Do you commonly exhibit low resting blood pressure significant enough to cause dizziness, light-headedness, and/or fainting?	YES☐ NO☐
8c.	Has your physician indicated that you exhibit sudden bouts of high blood pressure (known as Autonomic Dysreflexia)?	YES☐ NO☐

9.   Have you had a Stroke? *This includes Transient Ischemic Attack (TIA) or Cerebrovascular Event*

If the above condition(s) is/are present, answer questions 9a-9c   If **NO** ☐ go to question 10

9a.	Do you have difficulty controlling your condition with medications or other physician-prescribed therapies? (Answer **NO** if you are not currently taking medications or other treatments)	YES☐ NO☐
9b.	Do you have any impairment in walking or mobility?	YES☐ NO☐
9c.	Have you experienced a stroke or impairment in nerves or muscles in the past 6 months?	YES☐ NO☐

10.   Do you have any other medical condition not listed above or do you have two or more medical conditions?

If you have other medical conditions, answer questions 10a-10c   If **NO** ☐ read the Page 4 recommendations

10a.	Have you experienced a blackout, fainted, or lost consciousness as a result of a head injury within the last 12 months **OR** have you had a diagnosed concussion within the last 12 months?	YES☐ NO☐
10b.	Do you have a medical condition that is not listed (such as epilepsy, neurological conditions, kidney problems)?	YES☐ NO☐
10c.	Do you currently live with two or more medical conditions?	YES☐ NO☐

PLEASE LIST YOUR MEDICAL CONDITION(S) AND ANY RELATED MEDICATIONS HERE: _____

_____

> ## GO to Page 4 for recommendations about your current medical condition(s) and sign the PARTICIPANT DECLARATION.

Figure 3.7   *(continued)*

2018 PAR-Q+

☑ **If you answered NO to all of the FOLLOW-UP questions (pgs. 2-3) about your medical condition, you are ready to become more physically active - sign the PARTICIPANT DECLARATION below:**

▶ It is advised that you consult a qualified exercise professional to help you develop a safe and effective physical activity plan to meet your health needs.

▶ You are encouraged to start slowly and build up gradually - 20 to 60 minutes of low to moderate intensity exercise, 3-5 days per week including aerobic and muscle strengthening exercises.

▶ As you progress, you should aim to accumulate 150 minutes or more of moderate intensity physical activity per week.

▶ If you are over the age of 45 yr and **NOT** accustomed to regular vigorous to maximal effort exercise, consult a qualified exercise professional before engaging in this intensity of exercise.

⬤ **If you answered YES to one or more of the follow-up questions about your medical condition:**

You should seek further information before becoming more physically active or engaging in a fitness appraisal. You should complete the specially designed online screening and exercise recommendations program - the **ePARmed-X+ at www.eparmedx.com** and/or visit a qualified exercise professional to work through the ePARmed-X+ and for further information.

⚠ **Delay becoming more active if:**

✓ You have a temporary illness such as a cold or fever; it is best to wait until you feel better.

✓ You are pregnant - talk to your health care practitioner, your physician, a qualified exercise professional, and/or complete the ePARmed-X+ **at www.eparmedx.com** before becoming more physically active.

✓ Your health changes - talk to your doctor or qualified exercise professional before continuing with any physical activity program.

⬤ You are encouraged to photocopy the PAR-Q+. You must use the entire questionnaire and NO changes are permitted.
⬤ The authors, the PAR-Q+ Collaboration, partner organizations, and their agents assume no liability for persons who undertake physical activity and/or make use of the PAR-Q+ or ePARmed-X+. If in doubt after completing the questionnaire, consult your doctor prior to physical activity.

PARTICIPANT DECLARATION

⬤ All persons who have completed the PAR-Q+ please read and sign the declaration below.

⬤ If you are less than the legal age required for consent or require the assent of a care provider, your parent, guardian or care provider must also sign this form.

I, the undersigned, have read, understood to my full satisfaction and completed this questionnaire. I acknowledge that this physical activity clearance is valid for a maximum of 12 months from the date it is completed and becomes invalid if my condition changes. I also acknowledge that the community/fitness center may retain a copy of this form for records. In these instances, it will maintain the confidentiality of the same, complying with applicable law.

NAME _____   DATE _____

SIGNATURE _____   WITNESS _____

SIGNATURE OF PARENT/GUARDIAN/CARE PROVIDER _____

—————— **For more information, please contact** ——————
www.eparmedx.com
Email: eparmedx@gmail.com

Citation for PAR-Q+
Warburton DER, Jamnik VK, Bredin SSD, and Gledhill N on behalf of the PAR-Q+ Collaboration. The Physical Activity Readiness Questionnaire for Everyone (PAR-Q+) and Electronic Physical Activity Readiness Medical Examination (ePARmed-X+). Health & Fitness Journal of Canada 4(2):3-23, 2011.

Key References
1. Jamnik VK, Warburton DER, Makarski J, McKenzie DC, Shephard RJ, Stone J, and Gledhill N. Enhancing the effectiveness of clearance for physical activity participation; background and overall process. APNM 36(S1):S3-S13, 2011.
2. Warburton DER, Gledhill N, Jamnik VK, Bredin SSD, McKenzie DC, Stone J, Charlesworth S, and Shephard RJ. Evidence-based risk assessment and recommendations for physical activity clearance: Consensus Document. APNM 36(S1):S266-s298, 2011.
3. Chisholm DM, Collis ML, Kulak LL, Davenport W, and Gruber N. Physical activity readiness. British Columbia Medical Journal. 1975;17:375-378.
4. Thomas S, Reading J, and Shephard RJ. Revision of the Physical Activity Readiness Questionnaire (PAR-Q). Canadian Journal of Sport Science 1992;17:4 338-345.

The PAR-Q+ was created using the evidence-based AGREE process (1) by the PAR-Q+ Collaboration chaired by Dr. Darren E. R. Warburton with Dr. Norman Gledhill, Dr. Veronica Jamnik, and Dr. Donald C. McKenzie (2). Production of this document has been made possible through financial contributions from the Public Health Agency of Canada and the BC Ministry of Health Services. The views expressed herein do not necessarily represent the views of the Public Health Agency of Canada or the BC Ministry of Health Services.

Figure 3.7   *(continued)*

Reprinted with permission from the PAR-Q+ Collaboration and the authors of the PAR-Q+ (Dr. Darren Warburton, Dr. Norman Gledhill, Dr. Veronica Jamnik, and Dr. Shannon Bredin).

Table 3.2 General Warm-Up

Exercise		Time/reps
1. Low- to moderate-intensity exercise (jogging, cycling, or rowing at a pace during which the client or athlete can easily hold a conversation)		5 minutes
2. Bodyweight squats		10 times
3. Bodyweight walking lunges		10 times
4. Arm circles		10 times
5. Walking hamstring stretches (knee tucks)		10 times

Exercise		Time/reps
6. Arm swings		10 times
7. Walking quadricep stretches (heel kicks)		10 times
8. Push-ups		10 times
9. Bodyweight squat jumps		10 times

the assessment may need to be repeated.

SUMMARY

A wide variety of factors influence the selection of assessments. The needs of the client or athlete and coach or fitness professional must be considered while being aware that the availability of some resources, including time, may be limited. Assessment selection involves the determination of the basic physical fitness attributes necessary to contend with the movement patterns and metabolic requirements of the sport or activity of interest. This alignment can be supported by an understanding of the individual, task, and environmental constraints that exist as well as the basic principles of assessment, including validity and reliability. Following client or athlete screening, familiarization, pretesting guidelines, warm-up, and delivery procedures will support successful completion of the selected assessments. Finally, identification of assessments with normative data allows for the coach or fitness professional to engage in an informed evaluation of the client's or athlete's physical fitness profile as part of the continuous improvement process.

PART II

ASSESSMENT PROTOCOLS

The second section of this book provides assessment protocols for the basic fitness attributes covered in part I, including anthropometric and body composition, flexibility and balance, agility and sprinting, power, muscular strength and endurance, and cardiorespiratory fitness. The assessments are comprehensively presented with example scripts, research notes, and normative data. The final chapter has a slightly different format in order to highlight the concept of monitoring training, which is typically conducted on a more frequent basis than the assessment of basic fitness attributes.

CHAPTER 4

Anthropometrics and Body Composition

"Most of the world will make decisions by either guessing or using their gut. They will be either lucky or wrong."

Suhail Doshi, CEO, Mixpanel

Anthropometric measurements and body composition are commonly used to evaluate the general health of clients or athletes. The importance of these values varies greatly depending on the sporting context and goals of the individuals being evaluated. Extreme anthropometric values, such as a high body mass index or waist-to-hip ratio, are used as red flags for disease risk classification, while segmental circumferences and skinfold thicknesses may be used for comparative purposes and to estimate changes in body composition and aesthetics. Many people focus on body fat percentages; however, we often rely on estimation equations developed in small groups of people that have yet to be truly vetted with respect to their ability to track changes over time. Therefore, whenever possible, it is suggested that the actual measured values be recorded and evaluated. Because body composition and its relationship to performance is highly individualized, the terms *low* and *high* are used in this chapter rather than *suboptimal* and *outstanding*. The assessments covered in this chapter are as follows:

- Weight, height, and body mass index (11, 15)
- Segmental circumferences (8, 11)
- Skinfold assessment (body fat percentage, fat mass, and fat-free mass) (8, 11)
- Bioelectrical impedance analysis (8)

WEIGHT, HEIGHT, AND BODY MASS INDEX

Purpose

Body weight and standing height provide standard physical measures of the client or athlete. Body mass index is typically used for health risk classification but may also be used as a general indicator of body size relative to height.

Outcomes

Body weight in pounds (lb) or kilograms (kg); standing height in inches (in.) or centimeters (cm); body mass index in kilograms per meters squared (kg/m^2)

Equipment Needed

Balance beam (or digital scale) and wall-based or freestanding stadiometer (height measuring device); or combined scale and stadiometer; calculator or nomogram

Before You Begin

The time of day selected to conduct height and weight testing should be standardized because variations in both occur throughout typical 24-hour periods. The client or athlete should be instructed to refrain from eating and to maintain adequate hydration for four to six hours prior to the assessment session. Ensure that the scale or stadiometer is positioned on a stable, flat surface. During assessments, it is suggested to have another person present to record the values and repeat them back for clarification. Appropriate consideration should be given to the privacy of the client or athlete, including access to changing rooms and the comfort level or familiarity with those present during the assessment procedures.

Protocol

Body Weight

1. Begin the procedure by saying the following to the client or athlete: *"We are going to measure your body weight. Are you ready to begin? If so, please remove any unnecessary items of clothing, including shoes, socks, and jewelry."* Usually the weight of the necessary clothing (T-shirt and shorts), is minimal and it is recommended that similar clothing items be worn for each assessment. If a true nude weight is needed, the weight of the clothing can be taken separately and subtracted from the clothed weight.

2. Verify that the scale reads zero by consulting the digital readout for a digital scale or that the balance beam of a balance beam scale is centered when the sliding weight is placed at the zero mark.

3. Say to the client or athlete: *"Step onto the scale platform with feet shoulder-width apart and hands and arms at the side of the body. Please remain as still as possible until we have successfully recorded your body weight."*

4. Record the body weight value on the digital readout for a digital scale or the position of the sliding weight where the balance beam is centered using a balance beam scale to the closest 0.25 pound (0.11 kg).

5. Upon completing the assessment say, *"Thank you,"* and instruct the client or athlete: *"Step off of the scale."*

Standing Height

1. Begin the procedure by saying the following to the client or athlete: *"We are going to measure your body weight. Are you ready to begin? If so, please remove your shoes and socks as well as any headwear and accessories."*

2. Direct the client: *"Stand with your back to the measuring device [touching the wall for a wall-mounted stadiometer or the vertical column of a free-standing stadiometer/ medical scale] with your feet shoulder-width apart and hands and arms at the side of your body."*

3. Say to the client or athlete: *"Please look directly forward and try to keep your chin parallel with the ground."* If necessary, and after receiving confirmation to the question, *"May I help adjust your head into the appropriate position to determine your height?"* adjust the client's or athlete's jawline to horizontally align the lower portion of the eyes with the central opening of the ears.

4. Next, instruct the client or athlete: *"Stand as tall as possible and take a deep inward breath while I complete the measurement."* During this time, place the horizontal leveling arm at the highest point of the client's or athlete's head.

5. Record height to the closest 0.25 to 0.5 inch (0.64 to 1.27 cm).

6. Upon completing the assessment, direct the client or athlete: *"Step away from the stadiometer."*

Alternatives or Modifications

If sitting height or leg length is desired, repeat the standing height procedures but ask the client or athlete to be in the seated position with feet on the floor and the muscles of the lower body relaxed. Leg length can then be estimated by subtracting sitting height from standing height.

After You Finish

Body mass index can be manually calculated as body weight divided by standing height squared (as kg/m^2). You might need to first convert pounds to kilograms (pounds divided by 2.2) and inches to meters (inches multiplied by 0.254). An alternative to calculating body mass index is the use of the nomogram provided in figure 4.1.

Research Notes

While body mass index is typically used to classify health status by means of assessing if an individual is over- or underweight for a given height (see table 4.1), this approach may not be appropriate for those with excessive muscularity who would likely fall into the overweight or obese categories due to the inability to distinguish between body fat and muscle tissue. Body mass index certainly differs among athletes according to the sporting event. In track athletes, increases in body mass index can be seen when the competitive distances get shorter (or the average speeds become greater), with most 100-meter sprinters displaying values of approximately 24 kg/m^2, followed by 23 kg/m^2 in the 200-meter, 22-23 kg/m^2 in the 400-meter, 21 kg/m^2 in the 800-meter and 1500-meter, and 20 kg/m^2 in the 10,000-meter and marathon. Interestingly, there is much greater variation in body mass index in the shortest or fastest events than in the longer or slower events, indicating that certain biomechanical and physiological factors other than solely anthropometrics likely play a role in sprinting performance (17).

Figure 4.1 Nomogram for body mass index

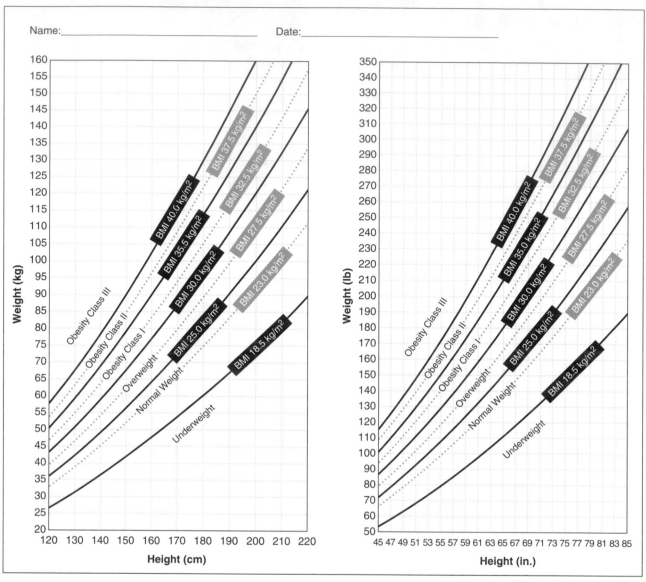

Name:_____   Date:_____

From D. Fukuda, *Assessments for Sport and Athletic Performance* (Champaign, IL: Human Kinetics, 2019). Data from World Health Organization, "Appropriate Body-Mass Index for Asian Populations and Its Implications for Policy and Intervention Strategies," *The Lancet* 363 (2004): 157-163.

Table 4.1 Body Mass Index (BMI) Classifications

Classification		BMI value
Underweight		<18.50
Normal weight		18.50-22.99 23.00-24.99
Overweight		25.00-27.49 27.50-29.99
Obesity	Class I	30.00-32.49 32.50-34.99
	Class II	35.00-37.49 37.50-39.99
	Class III	≥40.00

Data from World Health Organization, "Appropriate Body-Mass Index for Asian Populations and Its Implications for Policy and Intervention Strategies," *The Lancet* 363 (2004): 157-163.

Normative Data

Body weight classifications are provided for men in figure 4.2 and for women in figure 4.3. Table 4.1 provides the risk classifications for body mass index values, while figures 4.4 through 4.7 provide body mass index reference values across the lifespan and for select groups of male and female athletes.

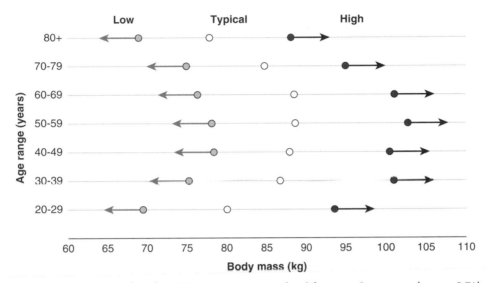

Figure 4.2 Body weight classifications across the lifespan for men: low—25th percentile; typical—50th percentile; high—75th percentile.

Data from (6).

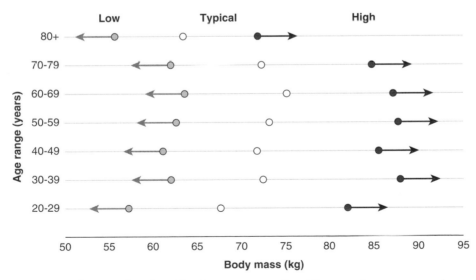

Figure 4.3 Body weight classifications across the lifespan for women: low—25th percentile; typical—50th percentile; high—75th percentile.

Data from (6).

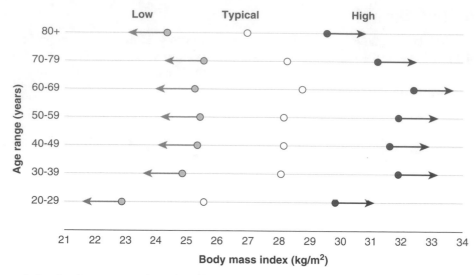

Figure 4.4 Body mass index classifications across the lifespan for men: low—25th percentile; typical—50th percentile; high—75th percentile.

Data from (6).

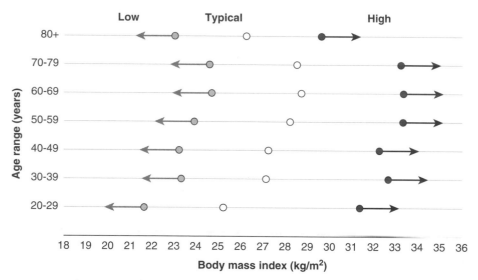

Figure 4.5 Body mass index classifications across the lifespan for women: low—25th percentile; typical—50th percentile; high—75th percentile.

Data from (6).

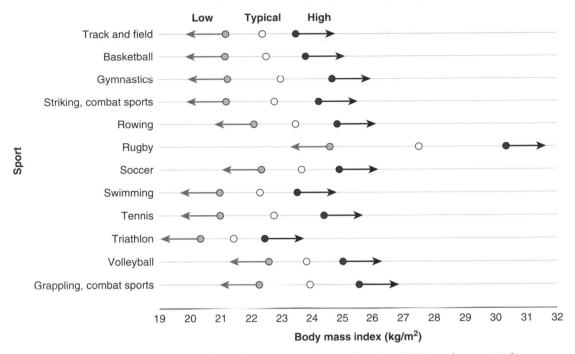

Figure 4.6 Body mass index values for select groups of male athletes: low—25th percentile; typical—50th percentile; high—75th percentile.

Data from (16).

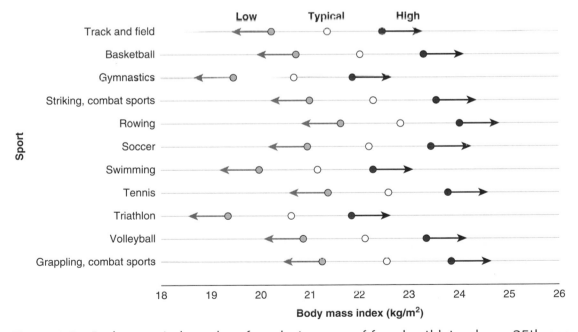

Figure 4.7 Body mass index values for select groups of female athletes: low—25th percentile; typical—50th percentile; high—75th percentile.

Data from (16).

SEGMENTAL CIRCUMFERENCES

Purpose

Assessment of segmental circumferences help evaluate health risks associated with regional mass (or fat) distribution through waist-to-hip ratio as well as anthropometric characteristics relative to segmental mass (arms, legs, and torso).

Outcomes

Circumference of specific segments of the body in inches (in.) or centimeters (cm); waist-to-hip ratio

Equipment Needed

Flexible measuring tape; calculator or nomogram

Before You Begin

The time of day selected to perform circumference assessments should be standardized. The client or athlete should be instructed to refrain from eating and to maintain adequate hydration for four to six hours prior to the assessment session. During assessments, it is suggested to have another person present to record the values and repeat them back for clarification. Appropriate consideration should be given to the privacy of the client or athlete, including access to changing rooms and the comfort level or familiarity with those present during the assessment procedures.

Protocol

1. Begin the procedure by saying the following to the client or athlete: *"We are going to measure the circumference of several parts of your body. Are you ready to begin? If so, please remove any unnecessary items of clothing, including shoes, socks, and jewelry."*

2. Once the client or athlete is prepared, continue by stating: *"After locating specific landmarks, we will use a measuring tape to determine the distance around certain segments of your body. Please remain relaxed and breathe normally while I'm completing the measurements."*

3. After identifying the appropriate landmarks on the right side of client's or athlete's body, as indicated in figure 4.8 and table 4.2, wrap the measuring tape around the segment of the body, ensuring that it is parallel to the ground while lying flat on the skin with no twists or bends and minimal compression of the underlying tissue (see figure 4.9). If a Gulick attachment is used, make sure that the spring-loaded mechanism is stretched to the same mark each time.

4. After attempting to place your eyes in line with the tape, record the measurement after the end of normal exhaled breath.

5. Work your way through each of the appropriate circumference locations and repeat each measurement until the recorded values are within 5 millimeters (~0.25 in.) of each other.

6. Upon completion of the assessment tell the client or athlete: *"Thank you for your cooperation."*

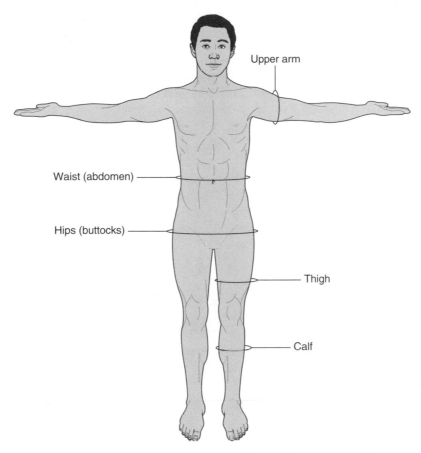

Figure 4.8 Visual representation of anatomical sites for segmental circumferences.

Table 4.2 Description of Anatomical Sites for Segmental Circumferences

Site	Description
Arm or upper arm (relaxed)	Located on the upper arm halfway between the shoulder and elbow joints; measured standing in a relaxed position and with arms at the side of body
Abdominal or waist	Located at the narrowest part of the torso between the ribs and the upper portion of the hip bone; measured in a relaxed standing position with arms at side of the body or folded across the chest and weight evenly distributed between the feet
Hip or gluteal	Located at the widest part of the hips and buttocks; measured in a relaxed standing position with arms at side of the body or folded across the chest and weight evenly distributed between the feet
Thigh or mid-thigh	Located halfway between the hip joint and the upper corner of the kneecap (patella) on the front of the upper leg; measured with arms at the side of body and standing in a relaxed position with weight evenly distributed between slightly separated feet
Calf	Located at the level of the maximal calf circumference taken while seated or with the foot placed on a raised box (with the knee and hip joints flexed to right angles); measured standing in a relaxed position with weight evenly distributed between slightly separated feet and arms at the side of body

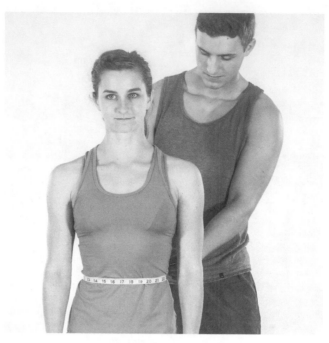

Figure 4.9 Circumference measurement example.

Alternatives or Modifications

The arm circumference measurement can also be completed at the largest portion of the upper arm in a flexed position.

After You Finish

The waist-to-hip ratio can be calculated by dividing the waist circumference (not to be confused with the abdominal circumference) by the hip circumference or by using the nomogram provided in figure 4.10. Waist-to-hip ratios are commonly used to differentiate between individuals who accumulate fat in the waist (apple or android body type) and individuals who accumulate fat in the hips (pear-shape or gynoid body type) as well as their relative risks for disease. The ratio is also an indicator of the relative distribution of mass, which likely affects an individual's center of gravity and a measure of balance termed postural stability. Segmental circumference values may be paired with skinfold thickness values from the same area of the body (covered in this chapter) to give a general estimate of the composition of the underlying tissues (fat and fat-free mass).

Research Notes

In the sport of rhythmic gymnastics, anthropometrics are highly related to performance outcomes. Interestingly, anthropometric values and aerobic capacity have been shown to equally contribute to the variability in competitive ranking scores while flexibility, power or explosiveness, and anaerobic capacity play lesser roles. Furthermore, while segmental circumferences may be similar between elite and non-elite gymnasts, the correlations with ranking scores earned during a national event appeared to be much greater for the elite competitors (5).

Normative Data

Figures 4.11 and 4.12 provide risk classifications for waist-to-hip ratio values in men and women, while figures 4.13 through 4.20 provide segmental circumference reference values for select groups of male and female athletes.

Figure 4.10   Nomogram for waist-to-hip ratio

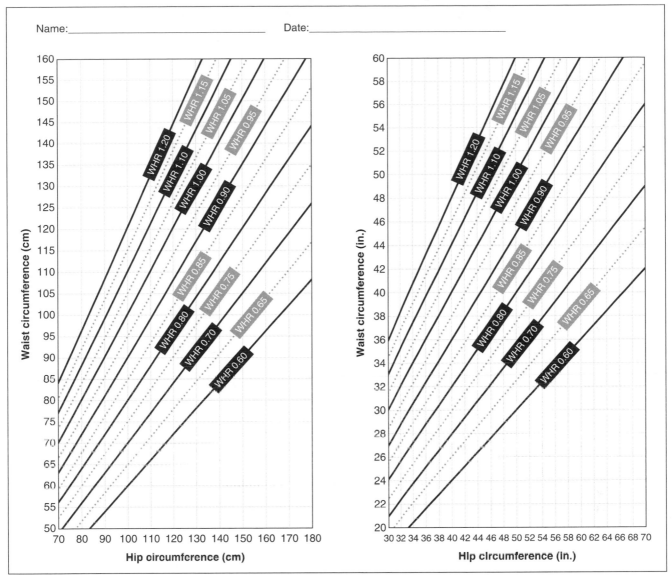

Name:_____   Date:_____

From D. Fukuda, *Assessments for Sport and Athletic Performance* (Champaign, IL: Human Kinetics, 2019).

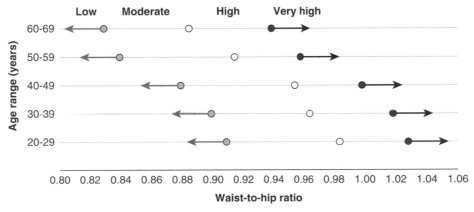

Figure 4.11   Waist-to-hip ratio health risk classifications across the lifespan for men.

Data from (8).

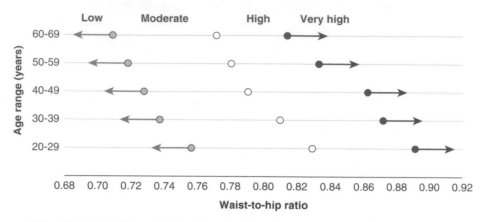

Figure 4.12 Waist-to-hip ratio health risk classifications across the lifespan for women.
Data from (8).

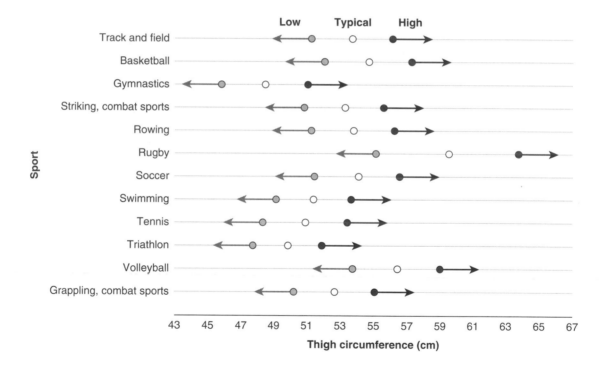

Figure 4.13 Thigh circumference values for select groups of male athletes: low—25th percentile; typical—50th percentile; high—75th percentile.
Data from (16).

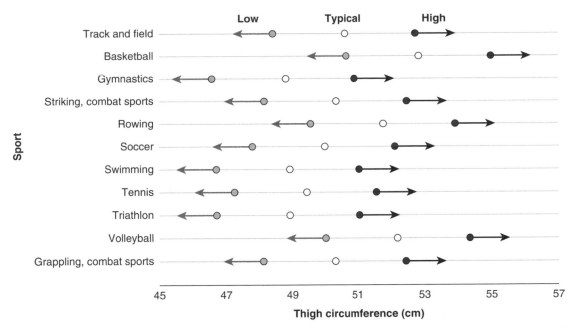

Figure 4.14 Thigh circumference values for select groups of female athletes: low—25th percentile; typical—50th percentile; high—75th percentile.

Data from (16).

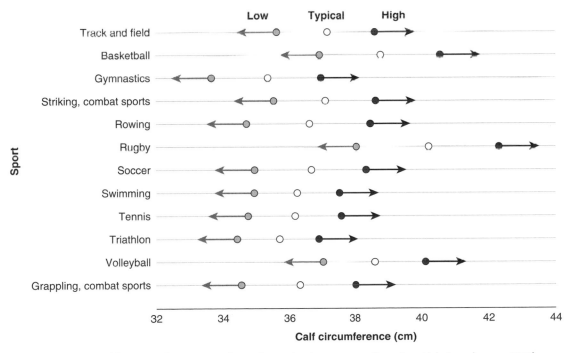

Figure 4.15 Calf circumference values for select groups of male athletes: low—25th percentile; typical—50th percentile; high—75th percentile.

Data from (16).

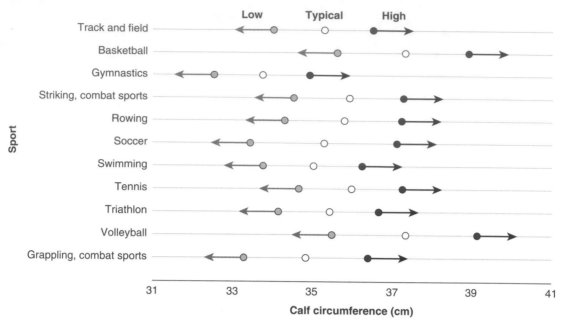

Figure 4.16 Calf circumference values for select groups of female athletes: low—25th percentile; typical—50th percentile; high—75th percentile.

Data from (16).

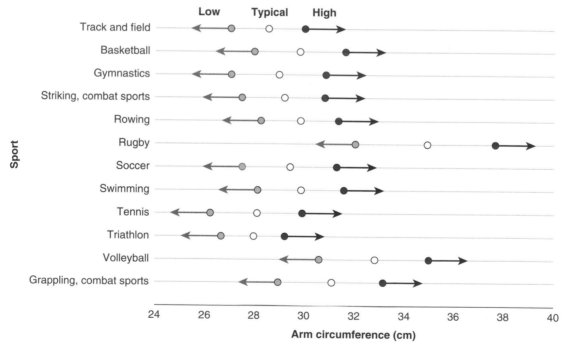

Figure 4.17 Arm circumference values for select groups of male athletes: low—25th percentile; typical—50th percentile; high—75th percentile.

Data from (16).

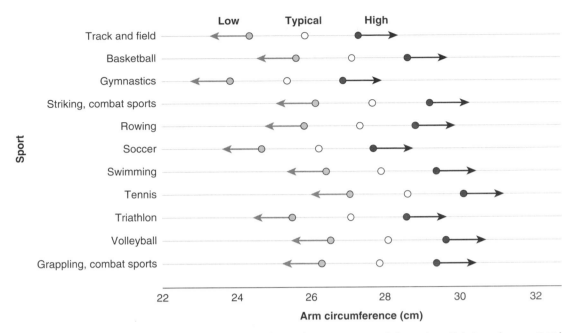

Figure 4.18 Arm circumference values for select groups of female athletes: low—25th percentile; typical—50th percentile; high—75th percentile.

Data from (16).

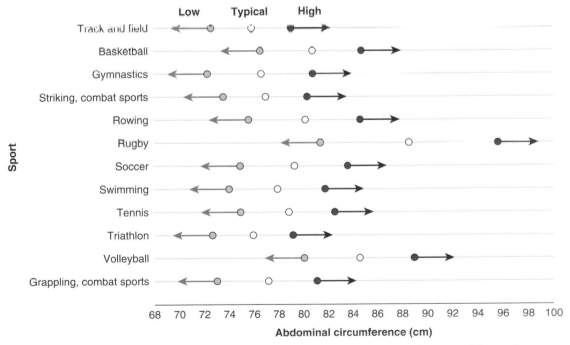

Figure 4.19 Abdominal circumference values for select groups of male athletes: low—25th percentile; typical—50th percentile; high—75th percentile.

Data from (16).

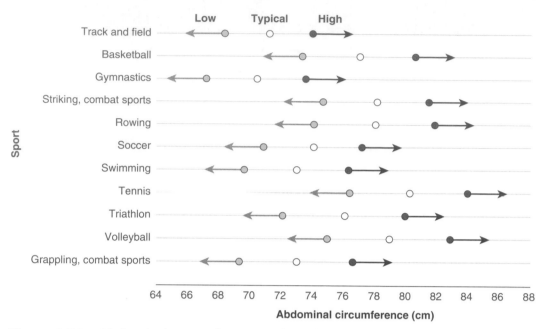

Figure 4.20 Abdominal circumference values for select groups of female athletes: low—25th percentile; typical—50th percentile; high—75th percentile.

Data from (16).

SKINFOLD ASSESSMENT

Purpose

Skinfold assessments provide an estimate of body composition.

Outcomes

Skinfold thicknesses in millimeters (mm), sum of measured skinfolds in millimeters (mm), estimated body fat percentage

Equipment Needed

Skinfold calipers, pen or marker, measuring tape

Before You Begin

The time of day selected for skinfold assessments should be standardized. The client or athlete should be instructed to refrain from eating and to maintain adequate hydration for four to six hours prior to the assessment session. The use of body lotion by the client or athlete will make skinfold assessments extremely difficult and should be avoided before testing. During assessments, it is suggested to have another person present to record the values and repeat them back for clarification. Appropriate consideration should be given to the privacy of the client or athlete, including access to changing rooms and the comfort level or familiarity with those present during the assessment procedures.

Protocol

1. Begin the procedure by saying to the client or athlete: *"We are going to measure your body fat percentage using skinfold calipers. Are you ready to begin? If so, please remove any unnecessary items of clothing or jewelry."*

2. Once the client or athlete is prepared, continue by stating: *"In order to get an accurate measurement, I will need to firmly pinch and hold your skin with my fingers, which may cause some discomfort. If at any point you are in pain and would like to take break from the procedure, please let me know. Please remain relaxed and breathe normally while I complete the measurements. Are you ready to begin?"*

3. After identifying the appropriate landmarks and marking the location of the specific skinfold on the right side of the body (see figure 4.21 and table 4.3), use your thumb and index finger to firmly pinch the skin and underlying fat in order pull it away from the underlying tissue.

4. While pulling the skin and fat away from the underlying tissue, place the jaws of the skinfold calipers approximately 1 centimeter (just less than 0.5 in.) below the fingers perpendicular to the fold.

5. Let the skinfold calipers settle into the skin for a few seconds and record the measurement while still pinching the fold (see figure 4.22 for an example of how skinfold calipers work).

6. Remove the jaws from the fold and release the skin.

7. Work your way through each of the appropriate skinfold locations and repeat each measurement until the recorded values are within 1 to 2 millimeters of each other.

8. The average of the two closest measurements can then be calculated.

9. Upon completion of the assessment tell the client or athlete: *"Thank you for your cooperation."*

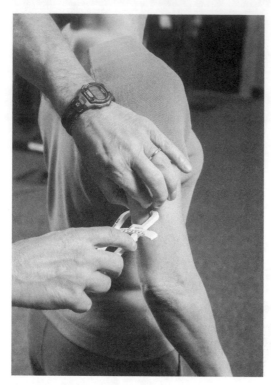

Figure 4.21 Example of skinfold thickness measurement.

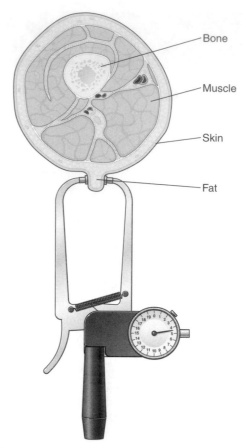

Figure 4.22 Measurement with skinfold calipers.

Table 4.3 Description of Anatomical Sites for Skinfold Thicknesses

Site	Description
Chest	Diagonal fold located halfway between the arm pit (axilla) and the nipple
Abdominal	Vertical fold located 2 cm (~0.75 in.) to the right of the belly button (umbilicus)
Triceps	Vertical fold located at the midline on the back of the upper arm halfway between the shoulder and elbow joints
Suprailiac	Diagonal fold located just above the upper front corner of the hip bone and 2-3 cm (~0.75-1.25 in.) toward the belly button (umbilicus)
Thigh	Vertical fold located halfway between the hip joint and the upper corner of the kneecap (patella) on the front of the upper leg taken while weight is shifted to the opposite (left) foot.

Alternatives or Modifications

While many different skinfold thickness sites exist, the coach or fitness professional may also be interested in the measurement of the calf in order to have a value corresponding to lower leg circumference. For the calf, measurement is taken at the vertical fold located on the inside of the lower leg at the level of the maximal calf circumference and is taken while seated or with the foot placed on a raised box while the knee and hip joints flex to right angles.

After You Finish

There are many conversion equations and formulas to estimate body fat percentage from skinfold thicknesses. Figure 4.23 provides a nomogram used to simplify this procedure by considering the client's or athlete's age and the sum of the skinfold thickness values for men (consisting of chest, abdominal, and thigh measurements) and women (consisting of tricep, suprailiac, and thigh measurements) as outlined in figure 4.21 and table 4.3. After body fat percentage values are calculated, they can be divided by 100 and multiplied by body weight to determine fat mass. Fat mass can then be subtracted from body weight to determine fat-free mass. With the depth and breadth, as well as questionable accuracy, in the large number of available equations to estimate body density (and then body fat percentage), the coach or fitness professional may wish to simply skip this conversion and just record the sum of skinfold values to gain a more accurate view of changes between assessments.

Research Notes

Competitive bodybuilders are judged by the appearance of their muscles, which usually requires drastic decreases in body fat while maintaining or increasing muscle size. Table 4.4 shows unpublished skinfold (SKF) data from a 12-month case study following the contest preparation and recovery of a natural bodybuilder (14). Contest preparation entails strict physical training and dietary regimens, while tracking of site-specific skinfold thicknesses may help identify progress, particularly when gold standard methods are unavailable.

Figure 4.23   Nomogram for body fat percentage using the sum of three skinfolds

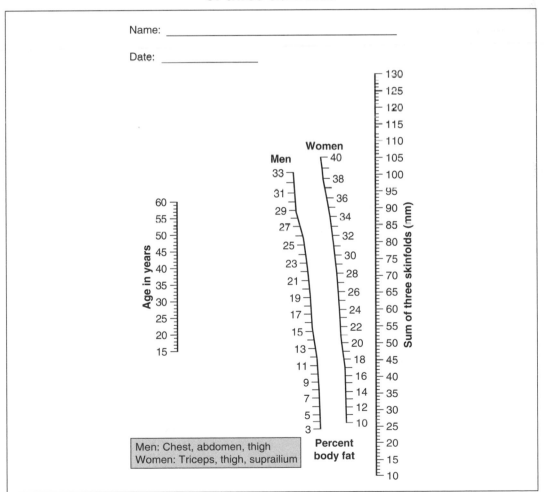

From W.B. Baun, M.R. Baun, and P.B. Raven, "A Nomogram for the Estimate of Percent Body Fat From Generalized Equations," *Research Quarterly for Exercise and Sport* 52, no. 3. (1981): 380-384. Reprinted by permission of Taylor & Francis Ltd.

Table 4.4 Skinfold Thicknesses and Body Mass Prior to and Following a Competitive Bodybuilding Event

	Months							Months					
	–6	–5	–4	–3	–2	–1	Event	+1	+2	+3	+4	+5	+6
Chest (mm)	3	3.5	3.5	3	3.5	3.5	2.25	3.5	6	3.5	4	5.5	6
Abdominal (mm)	15	13	8.5	5	6	5	4.5	9.5	11.5	11	12.5	12.25	9.5
Thigh (mm)	13	12	10	9.25	9	5.5	5.5	11.5	7.5	9	7	10.5	7
Sum of 3 SKF (mm)	31	28.5	22	17.25	18.5	14	12.25	24.5	25	23.5	23.5	28.25	22.5
Body weight (kg)	102.9	99.4	96.5	92.3	90.8	90.2	88.9	91.1	94.6	98.0	98.1	99.5	99.0

Normative Data

Due to the potential issues with selecting the appropriate body fat percentage estimation equations, it is recommended that coaches or fitness professionals use the measured skinfold thickness values in conjunction with either body weight or circumferences to evaluate generalized changes in body composition values of the client or athlete over time as outlined in figure 4.24. Body fat percentage classification values are provided in figure 4.25 for men and figure 4.26 for women.

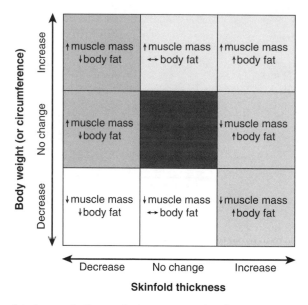

Figure 4.24 General interpretation of changes in body composition values relative to changes in body weight (or segmental circumferences) and skinfolds.

Adapted from S. Slater, S.M. Woolford, and M.J. Marfell-Jones, "Assessment of Physique." In *Physiological Tests for Elite Athletes,* 2nd ed., edited by R.K. Tanner and C.K. Gore for Australian Institute of Sport (Champaign, IL: Human Kinetics, 2013), 179.

BIOELECTRICAL IMPEDANCE ANALYSIS

Purpose

Bioelectrical impedance analysis is used to estimate body composition.

Outcomes

Estimated body fat percentage

Equipment Needed

Bioelectrical impedance analysis device

Before You Begin

The time of day selected should be standardized while exercise (approximately 12 hr) and alcohol consumption (roughly 48 hr) should be avoided before testing. The client or athlete should be instructed to refrain from eating and to maintain adequate hydration for four to six hours prior to the assessment session. It is also recommended that clients or athletes empty their bladder shortly in advance of the protocol. Appropriate consideration should be given to the privacy of the client or athlete, including access to changing rooms and the comfort level or familiarity with those present during the assessment procedures. The surface of the electrodes should be treated with the manufacturer-recommended wipes or cleaning solution between assessments.

Protocol

1. Begin the procedure by saying the following to the client or athlete: *"We are going to measure your body fat percentage using bioelectrical impedance analysis. Are you ready to begin? If so, please remove your shoes and socks as well as any metal objects."*

2. Using the standard prompts of the bioelectrical impedance analysis device, input the client's or athlete's relevant personal information, which typically includes some combination of age, height, weight (if not measured directly by the device), race, and level of physical activity.

3. Next, direct the client or athlete: *"Step onto the platform with your feet on the stainless-steel electrodes. Please remain as still as possible until we have successfully recorded your values."*

4. Record the relevant information, including the client's or athlete's personal information (age, height, weight, race, and level of physical activity) and estimated body fat percentage.

5. Upon completing the assessment, direct the client or athlete: *"Step off of the platform."*

Alternatives or Modifications

Some bioelectrical impedance analysis devices may use electrodes that require contact with the hands.

After You Finish

Because most bioelectrical impedance analysis devices rely on internal conversions, no additional calculations or use of equations are required. In extremely lean or obese individuals, estimated body fat percentage values from bioelectrical impedance analyses may be substantially different from those calculated using gold standard methods. Fat mass and fat-free mass can be determined using the same methods outlined in the skinfold assessment section.

Research Notes

Bioelectrical impedance analysis is one of the recommended body composition methods used to determine the minimum wrestling weight in high school athletes at the beginning of the competitive season. After verifying that the athlete is appropriately hydrated, body fat percentage is assessed using an approved bioelectrical impedance analysis device, which is then used to estimate body weight (and corresponding weight class) at 7 percent body fat for boys and 12 percent body fat for girls. For example, a male high school wrestler who weighs 175 pounds (79 kg) with 12 percent body fat would have a minimum wrestling weight of 166 pounds (75 kg), while a female high school wrestler who weighs 144 pounds (65 kg) with 15 percent body fat would have a minimum wrestling weight of 139 pounds (63 kg). In either case, the athletes would only be allowed to lose 1.5 percent of their body weight (this number varies depending on specific policies) from the initial assessment. Subsequently, this approach has been suggested as a means of minimizing the health risks associated with rapid weight loss in other combat sports (1).

It should be noted that body fat percentages provided by many bioelectrical impedance analysis devices rely on prediction equations that have substantial variability in athletes (12). Therefore, whenever possible, coaches or fitness professionals should look to use devices with more advanced technologies (bioelectrical impedance spectroscopy or multi-frequency bioelectrical impedance analysis rather than single-frequency bioelectrical impedance analysis) that are becoming less expensive and more readily available.

Normative Data

Body fat percentage classification values are provided in figure 4.25 for men and figure 4.26 for women.

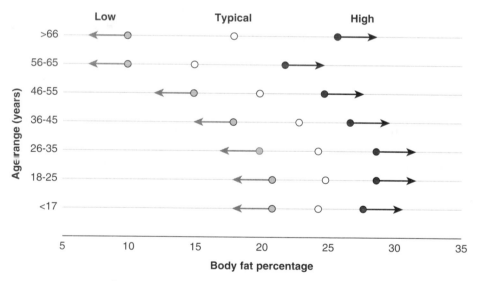

Figure 4.25 Percent body fat classifications across the lifespan for men.

Data from (1a).

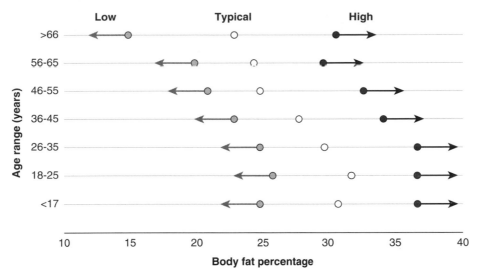

Figure 4.26 Percent body fat classifications across the lifespan for women.

Data from (13).

CHAPTER 5

Flexibility and Balance

"Not everything that can be counted counts, and not everything that counts can be counted."

Albert Einstein, Physicist

Flexibility and balance assessments may be used to evaluate general health and potentially mobility; however, their relationship with performance is not well understood. As such, results from evaluations of flexibility and balance are typically compared to minimum values that reflect acceptable levels of function. With respect to flexibility, extreme laxity (or looseness) at a given joint may increase the potential for injury. The process of aging is often coupled with declines in both flexibility and balance. While diminished balance may be of little concern for most healthy athletes and young people, assessments in those with limited functional mobility or those recovering from an injury play a crucial role in return-to-play or return-to-activity decisions. For this reason, it is important to collect baseline measures of balance for an athlete or client that can be used for comparison in the event of an injury. For example, the balance error

scoring system and tandem gait are commonly used to evaluate cognitive impairments related to concussions on the sideline following head injuries. Similar to body composition, flexibility and balance are highly individualized and must be interpreted in the context of the sport or activity of interest, so the terms *low* and *high* are used in this chapter rather than *suboptimal* and *outstanding*. The assessments covered in this chapter are as follows:

- Sit-and-reach test (12)
- Back-scratch test (12, 24)
- Shoulder elevation test (2, 12)
- Total body rotation test (24)
- Lumbar stability tests (14, 27)
- Functional reach test (26)
- Balance error scoring system (BESS) (22)
- Tandem gait test (1, 25)

SIT-AND-REACH TEST

Purpose

The sit-and-reach test measures a combination of hip and low back flexibility.

Outcome

Sit-and-reach length in centimeters or inches

Equipment Needed

Measuring stick and adhesive tape

Before You Begin

Secure a yardstick to the floor and place a strip of tape at the 23-centimeter (9.1 in.) mark. A standardized warm-up followed by moderate intensity stretching should be conducted prior to beginning the assessment.

Protocol

1. Begin the procedure by saying to the athlete or client: *"We are going to measure your hip and low back flexibility. Are you ready to begin? If so, please remove your shoes."*

2. Direct the client: *"Sit with the yardstick between your legs and place the bottom of your heels along the tape at the 23-centimeter (or 9.1-in.) mark. Keep your knees straight and your feet 30 centimeters or 10 to 12 inches apart"* (see figure 5.1).

3. Next, instruct the athlete or client: *"Now overlap your hands and fingers and slowly reach forward as far as possible along the yardstick. Once you've reached as far as you can, please hold that position for two seconds."*

4. Record the greatest length achieved to the nearest centimeter (or 0.25 in.) during the movement and ask the athlete or client to relax prior to making three more attempts.

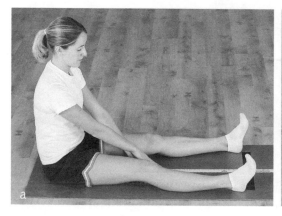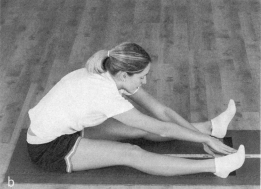

Figure 5.1 Sit-and-reach test.

Alternatives or Modifications

A sit-and-reach box with heels placed at the leading edge of the box may also be used (see figure 5.2a). For individuals who might experience discomfort during the standard protocols, the back-saver sit-and-reach test examines each leg separately with knee of the uninvolved leg bent and the heel placed on the floor. The back-saver sit-and-reach can be further modified by having the athlete or client sit on a bench with the foot of the uninvolved leg placed on the floor (see figure 5.2b).

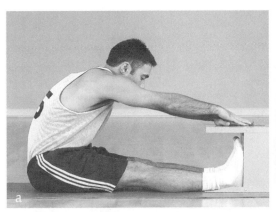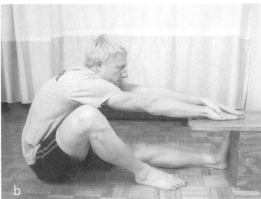

Figure 5.2 *(a)* Sit-and-reach and *(b)* modified back-saver approach.

After You Finish

The highest value of the trials (typically the fourth attempt) is the final result. If a sit-and-reach box is used and the heel placement is not at 23 centimeters (9.1 in.), a zero-point adjustment accounting for the difference may be needed to compare with normative data. For example, if the sit-and-reach box places the heel at 26 centimeters (10.2 in.), subtract 3 centimeters (1.2 in.) from the final result prior to making your comparison.

Research Notes

While much debate exists regarding the relationship between low-back pain and sit-and-reach values, considerations for sport- and activity-specific requirements may be particularly relevant. Within a given sport, positional characteristics may provide an indication of the potential for success. An analysis of the athletes participating in the National Hockey League Combine demonstrated that, while goalkeepers tended to possess greater body fat and lower strength and explosiveness than other positions, they had significantly greater sit-and-reach scores, which indicates the benefits that flexibility provide when attempting to block shots (35)

Normative Data

Sit-and-reach classification values are provided in figure 5.3 for boys, figure 5.4 for girls, figure 5.5 for men, and figure 5.6 for women.

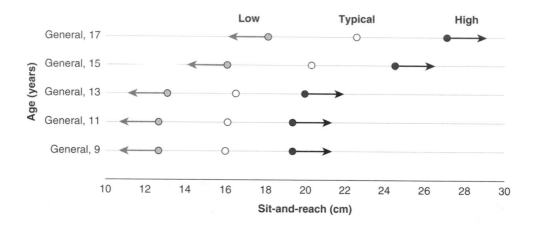

Figure 5.3 Sit-and-reach classifications for boys: low—30th percentile; typical—50th percentile; high—70th percentile.

Data from (34).

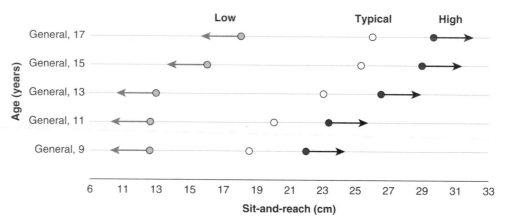

Figure 5.4 Sit-and-reach classifications for girls: low—30th percentile; typical—50th percentile; high—70th percentile.

Data from (34).

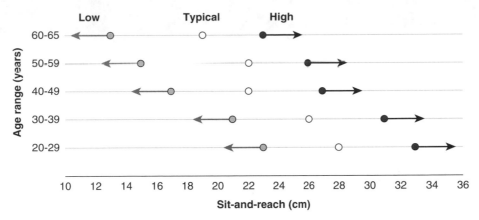

Figure 5.5 Sit-and-reach classifications across the lifespan for men: low—30th percentile; typical—50th percentile; high—70th percentile.

Data from (12).

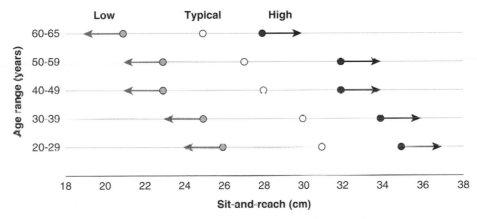

Figure 5.6 Sit-and-reach classifications across the lifespan for women: low—30th percentile; typical—50th percentile; high—70th percentile.

Data from (12).

BACK-SCRATCH TEST

Purpose

The back-scratch test is used to measure shoulder flexibility.

Outcome

The overlap or gap between the fingers in centimeters or inches

Equipment Needed

Ruler or yardstick; measuring tape

Before You Begin

A standardized warm-up, including arms swings, arm circles, and shoulder rotations, should be conducted prior to beginning the assessment.

Protocol

1. Begin the procedure by saying to the athlete or client: *"We are going to measure your shoulder flexibility by evaluating how far you can overlap your fingers behind your back. Are you ready to begin?"*

2. Direct the athlete or client: *"Raise your right elbow toward your right ear and reach down your back as far as possible. Now start with your left arm directly by your side and slowly move your elbow towards the middle of your back while reaching your left hand up as far as possible toward (or past) your right hand. Try to the hold this position for two seconds"* (see figure 5.7a).

3. While the athlete or client is completing the attempt, use a ruler or measuring tape to record the greatest finger overlap length achieved to the nearest centimeter or quarter inch (see figure 5.7b) and, prior to making three more attempts, instruct the client: *"Please bring both of your arms back to your side."* If the athlete or client is not able to overlap the fingers of the right and left hands, measure the gap between the fingers and record the result as a negative value.

4. Next, direct the client: *"Repeat the same procedure but with your left hand coming from above and your right hand coming from below."*

5. Once again, use a ruler to record the greatest finger overlap length achieved or gap between the fingertips to the nearest centimeter or quarter inch and, prior to making three more attempts, ask the client: *"Please bring both of your arms back to your side."*

After You Finish

The highest value of the trials (typically the fourth attempt) for each side are the final results. The individual values for the left and right sides can be evaluated or the average value from both sides can be calculated as follows:

$$\frac{\text{Right side score (in cm)} + \text{left side score (in cm)}}{2}$$

Research Notes

Many training programs attempt to incorporate both strength and aerobic components into a single concurrent exercise regimen. An 11-week intervention (with training 3 times per week) showed strength and aerobic improvements for women engaged in serial (consisting of a strength session followed by an aerobic session) and integrated (consisting of alternating sets

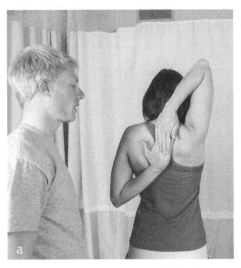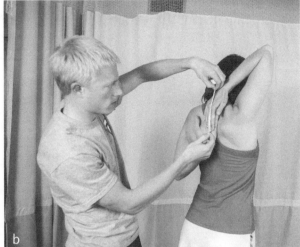

Figure 5.7 Back-scratch test.

of strength and aerobic training in a single session) concurrent exercise. However, the women in the serial exercise group exhibited no changes (or even potential decreases) in back-scratch scores while the women in the integrated exercise group showed significant increases (6). These results are interesting but should be interpreted with caution and within the context of the chosen activities of the athlete or client. For example, in the sport of judo, where a well-developed upper-body musculature may provide some competitive advantage, professional athletes have demonstrated lower back-scratch scores compared to recreational athletes (3).

Normative Data

Back-scratch classification values are provided in figure 5.8 for boys, figure 5.9 for girls, figure 5.10 for men, and figure 5.11 for women.

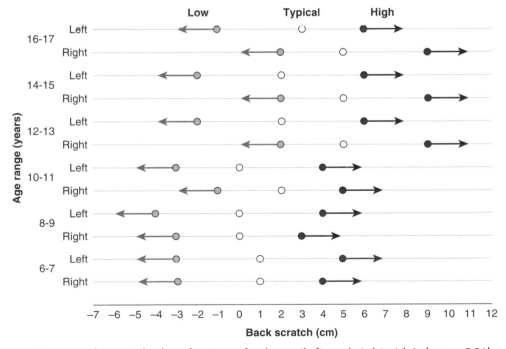

Figure 5.8 Back-scratch classifications for boys (left and right side): low—30th percentile; typical—50th percentile; high—70th percentile.

Data from (5)

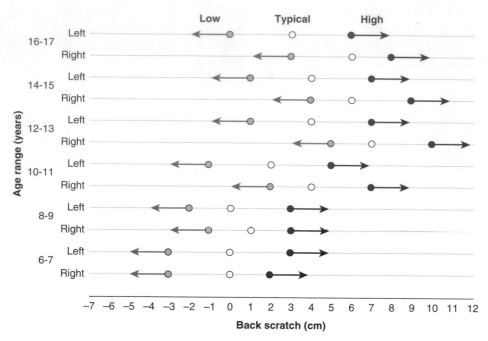

Figure 5.9 Back-scratch classifications for girls (left and right side): low—30th percentile; typical—50th percentile; high—70th percentile.

Data from (5)

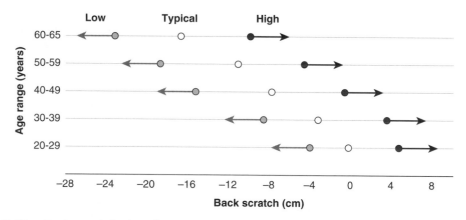

Figure 5.10 Back-scratch classifications across the lifespan for men: low—25th percentile; typical—50th percentile; high—75th percentile.

Data from (20)

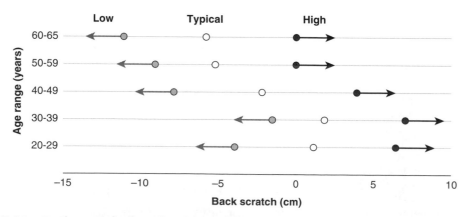

Figure 5.11 Back-scratch classifications across the lifespan for women: low—25th percentile; typical—50th percentile; high—75th percentile.

Data from (20)

SHOULDER ELEVATION TEST

Purpose

The shoulder elevation test measures wrist, chest, and shoulder flexibility during an overhead movement.

Outcome

Distance from the floor, in inches or centimeters, relative to arm length

Equipment Needed

Measuring stick; PVC pipe or wooden dowel

Before You Begin

A standardized warm-up, including arms swings, arm circles, and shoulder rotations, should be conducted prior to beginning the assessment.

Protocol

1. Begin the procedure by saying the following to the athlete or client: *"We are going to measure your chest and shoulder flexibility. Are you ready to begin?"*

2. Direct the athlete or client: *"Stand in a relaxed position while holding the PVC pipe with your thumbs toward its center and your hands approximately shoulder-width apart while I conduct the first measurement"* (see figure 5.12a).

3. Measure and record the athlete or client's arm length as distance between the top of the shoulder and the closest portion of the PVC pipe.

4. Next, instruct the athlete or client: *"Lie down with your stomach and chest on the floor. Raise your arms over your head while holding onto the PVC pipe with your thumbs toward its center and your hands approximately shoulder-width apart"* (see figure 5.12b).

5. Then say: *"Now keep your chin in contact with the floor and slowly attempt to raise the PVC pipe as far as possible off of the ground while I check the measurement."*

6. After you measure and record the distance between the floor and the bottom of the PVC pipe, direct the athlete or client: *"Return to the original position and relax."*

7. Repeat this measurement two additional times.

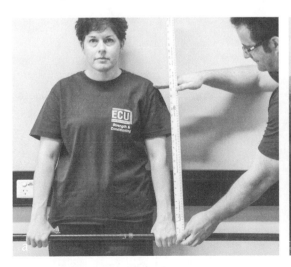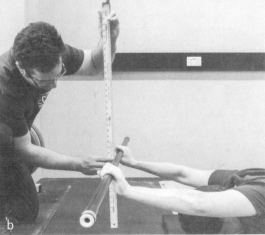

Figure 5.12 Shoulder elevation test.

After You Finish

Use the following formula with either centimeters or inches to calculate a score standardized with consideration of the arm length of the athlete or client.

$$\text{Shoulder elevation score} = \frac{\text{highest height achieved from the floor}}{\text{arm length}} \times 100$$

Research Notes

While the potential validity of the shoulder elevation test may be clear for overhead athletes, this assessment may also have health implications. For example, changes in shoulder elevation during military deployments have been reported to be significantly related to the number of medical visits for the upper extremities (36). Specifically, examinations of the hands, wrists, and shoulders by medical personnel tended to be most common in National Guard soldiers who exhibited the greatest decrease in shoulder elevation scores while deployed for 10 to 15 months.

Normative Data

Shoulder elevation classification values for men and women are provided in figure 5.13.

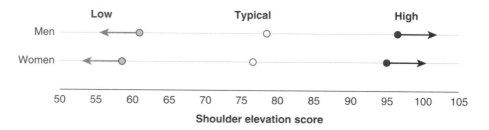

Figure 5.13 Normative data for the shoulder elevation test: low—30th percentile; typical—50th percentile; high—70th percentile.

Data from (19a)

TOTAL BODY ROTATION TEST

Purpose

The total body rotation test measures the flexibility of the trunk and several other joints that support this movement.

Outcome

Distance reached, in centimeters or inches, while conducting a total body rotation

Equipment Needed

Two measuring sticks; adhesive tape

Before You Begin

Using adhesive tape, secure two measuring sticks horizontally on a wall at a height approximately in line with the athlete's or client's shoulders. The measuring sticks should be parallel to each other and aligned at the 38-centimeter (15 in.) marks, but the top measuring stick should be positioned with its "0" end to the left and the bottom measuring stick should be upside-down and positioned with its "0" end to the right (see figure 5.14). Finally, place a strip of adhesive tape perpendicular to the wall at the 38-centimeter (15 in.) marks of the measuring sticks.

Request that the athlete or client remove any heavy or restrictive clothing. A standardized warm-up should be conducted prior to beginning the assessment.

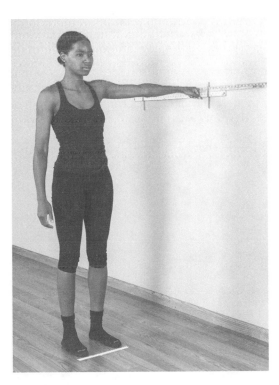

Figure 5.14   Alignment of measuring sticks for total body rotation test.

Protocol

1. Begin the procedure by saying the following to the athlete or client: *"We are going to measure your ability to rotate your body. Are you ready to begin? If so, please remove your shoes."*

2. Direct the athlete or client: *"Start standing with your left shoulder perpendicular to the wall and your toes along the tape on the floor. Make a fist with your left hand and adjust your body so that you are an arm's length away from the wall with your feet shoulder-width apart and knees slightly bent."*

3. After verifying the correct placement, instruct the athlete or client: *"Maintain this position and drop your left hand to your side. Make a fist with your right hand and raise your right arm parallel to the floor with your palm facing down. Now rotate to your right (away from the wall) while reaching your fist as far along the measuring stick as possible and hold that position for two seconds"* (see figure 5.15).

4. Record the greatest length achieved along the top yardstick by the knuckle of the right pinky or little finger to the nearest centimeter or quarter inch and, prior to making three more attempts, say to the client: *"Return to the starting position and relax."* As a reference, a score of 38 centimeters (15 in.) would reflect a 180-degree turn by the athlete or client.

5. Next, instruct the client: *"Repeat the same procedure but face the opposite direction with your right shoulder perpendicular to the wall and rotate to the left."*

6. Record the greatest length achieved along the bottom measuring stick by the knuckle of the left pinky or little finger to the nearest centimeter or quarter inch and, prior to making three more attempts, say to the client: *"Return to the starting position and relax."*

Alternatives or Modifications

For individuals who may become unstable during the assessments or have limited mobility, this test can also be modified to turn toward the wall rather than away (33).

After You Finish

The highest value of the trials (typically the fourth attempt) for each side are the final results. The individual values for the left and right sides can be evaluated, or the average value from both sides can be calculated as follows:

$$\frac{\text{Right side score (in cm)} + \text{left side score (in cm)}}{2}$$

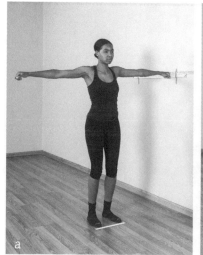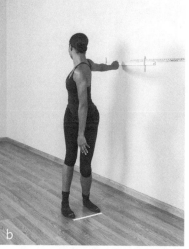

Figure 5.15 Total body rotation test.

Research Notes

Potentially due to their long-time adherence to movement-based exercise, experienced Tai Chi practitioners have exhibited greater total body rotation test scores compared to their sedentary older-adult counterparts (16). However, short-term exercise interventions may also have an influence on this measure. Middle-aged golfers demonstrated significant increases in total body rotation following an eight-week conditioning program consisting of strength, plyometric, and flexibility training (13).

Normative Data

Total body rotation classification values are provided in figure 5.16 for men and figure 5.17 for women.

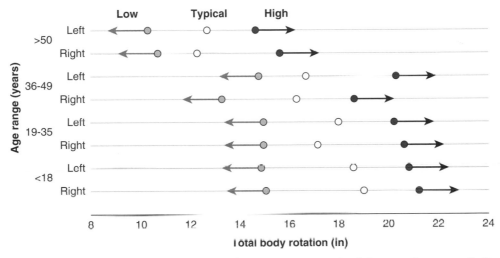

Figure 5.16 Total body rotation classifications across the lifespan for men (left and right side): low—30th percentile; typical—50th percentile; high—70th percentile.

Data from (15)

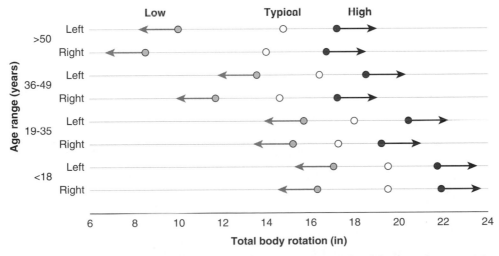

Figure 5.17 Total body rotation classifications across the lifespan for women (left and right side): low—30th percentile; typical—50th percentile; high—70th percentile.

Data from (15)

LUMBAR STABILITY TESTS

Purpose

Lumbar stability tests measure the endurance of the trunk muscles.

Outcome

Accumulated time, in seconds, until the athlete or client is unable to hold the desired position

Equipment Needed

Sturdy table; belts or an assistant to serve as a spotter; stool or chair; 60-degree wedge for adults (or 50 degrees for youth); stopwatch or timing device

Before You Begin

A standardized warm-up followed by moderate-intensity stretching should be conducted prior to beginning the assessment.

Protocol

Begin the procedure by saying the following to the athlete or client: "We are going to hold your trunk in several positions. Are you ready to begin?"

Trunk Extension

1. Direct the athlete or client: "Lie with your hips facing downward and your legs on top of the table. Adjust yourself so that your lower body (from the waist down) is supported by the table, and use your arms to support your upper body on the stool or chair" (see figure 5.18a).

2. Secure the athlete or client to the table with belts around the calves and thighs, or direct the spotter to hold the athlete's or client's ankles.

3. Next, explain to the athlete or client: "When I say 'Begin,' remove your arms from the stool or chair and cross them against your chest while keeping your body straight for as long as possible."

4. Verbally signal the athlete or client to begin and use the timing device to record how much time is accumulated until the horizontal position can no longer be maintained (see figure 5.18b).

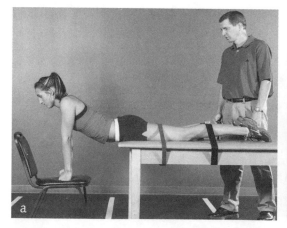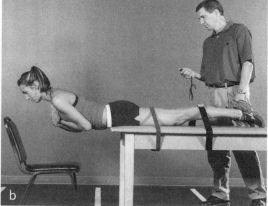

Figure 5.18 Trunk extension test.

Trunk Flexion

1. Direct the athlete or client: *"Sit on the table or floor with your arms crossed against your chest and your back against the wedge"* (see figure 5.19a).

2. Secure the athlete or client to the table with a belt across the feet, or direct another assessor to hold the athlete's or client's ankles.

3. Next, explain to the athlete or client: *"After I say 'Begin' and remove the wedge from your back, try not to move from this positon for as long as possible."*

4. Verbally signal the athlete or client to begin and use the timing device to record how much time is accumulated until the original position can no longer be maintained (see figure 5.19b).

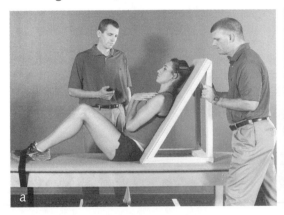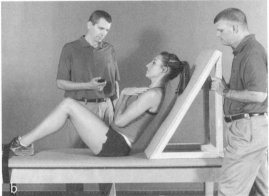

Figure 5.19 Trunk flexion test.

Side Bridge

1. Direct the athlete or client: *"Lie on your right side on top of the table or floor and prop yourself up on your right elbow. Keep both legs straight and place your top foot in front of your bottom foot for support."*

2. Next, explain to the athlete or client: *"When I say 'Begin,' lift your hips off the table or floor and keep your body, from your feet to your shoulders, straight for as long as possible. Continue to use your right elbow for support and place your left arm across your chest with your left hand on your right shoulder"* (see figure 5.20).

3. Verbally signal the athlete or client to begin and use the timing device to record how much time is accumulated until the hips touch the table or floor.

4. Next, direct the athlete or client: *"Repeat the same procedure but on your left side."*

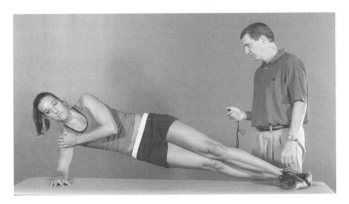

Figure 5.20 Side bridge test.

Alternatives or Modifications

Each of the lumbar stability assessments can be conducted on its own as deemed appropriate by the coach or fitness professional.

After You Finish

In order to evaluate potential deficits among the individual muscle groups, ratios can be calculated by dividing the endurance times from the trunk flexion and side bridge tests by the endurance time from the trunk extension test.

Research Notes

Due to the repetitive stresses on the body incurred by competitive gymnasts, low back pain is common, with as many as 86 percent of athletes reporting this issue (17). After completing a 10-week trunk muscle training intervention (twice weekly lasting approximately 15 minutes, including isometric holds with bodyweight as well as manual resistance and various abdominal exercises, female collegiate gymnasts improved endurance time during side bridge (+50%), trunk extension (+10%), and trunk flexion (+32%) assessments (10). Furthermore, no new issues related to low back pain were reported over the course of the competitive season.

Normative Data

Normative data for endurance ratios are provided in table 5.1, endurance times for trunk extension in figure 5.21, trunk flexion in figure 5.22, right side bridge in figure 5.23, and left side bridge in figure 5.24.

Table 5.1 Endurance Ratios for the Trunk Stability Tests

	Ratio	Flexion/extension	Side bridge right extension	Side bridge left extension
Adult	Male	0.99	0.64	0.66
	Female	0.79	0.38	0.40
18 years	Male	0.98	0.62	0.60
	Female	0.79	0.30	0.30
16 years	Male	0.93	0.50	0.48
	Female	0.92	0.37	0.38
14 years	Male	0.85	0.53	0.52
	Female	0.71	0.43	0.43
12 years	Male	0.73	0.47	0.42
	Female	0.59	0.30	0.32
10 years	Male	0.83	0.53	0.50
	Female	0.73	0.47	0.42
8 years	Male	1.11	0.47	0.47
	Female	0.73	0.39	0.32

Data from (7, 8, 21)

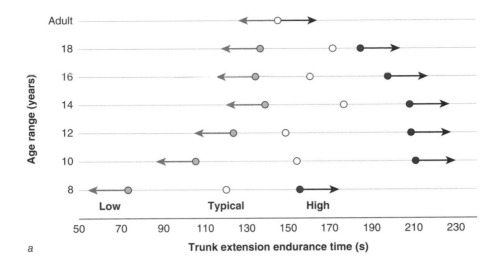

a

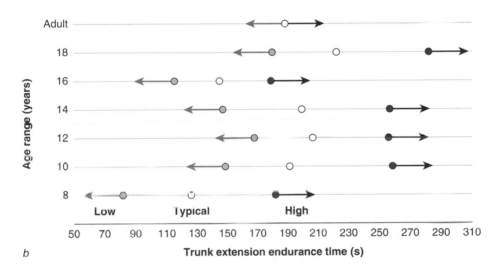

b

Figure 5.21 Normative data for trunk extension endurance in *(a)* males and *(b)* females: low—25th percentile; typical—50th percentile; high—75th percentile.

Data from (7, 8, 21)

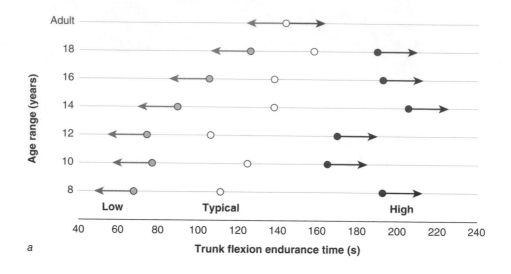

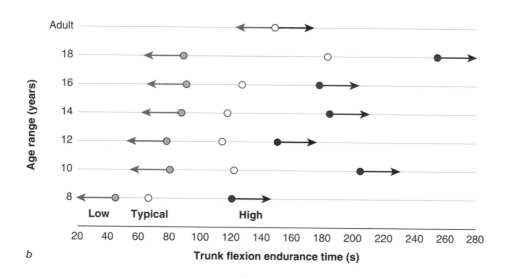

Figure 5.22 Normative data for trunk flexion endurance in *(a)* males and *(b)* females: low—25th percentile; typical—50th percentile; high—75th percentile.

Data from (7, 8, 21)

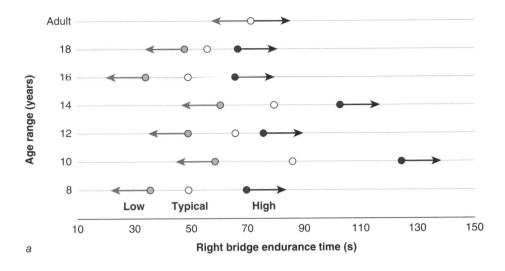

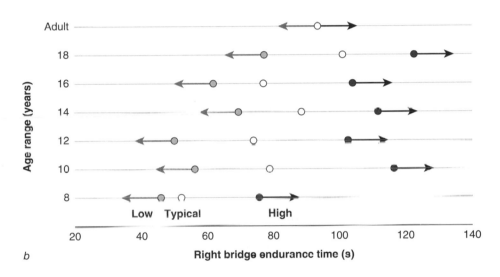

Figure 5.23 Normative data for right side bridge endurance in (a) females and (b) males: low—25th percentile; typical—50th percentile; high—75th percentile.

Data from (7, 8, 21).

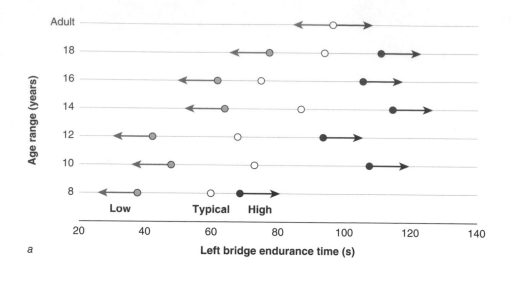

a

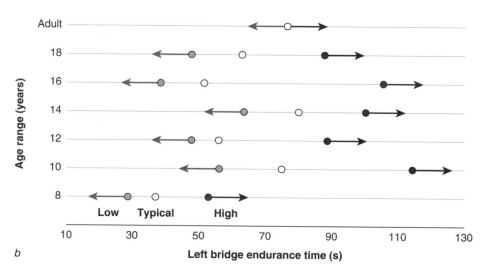

b

Figure 5.24 Normative data for left side bridge endurance in *(a)* males and *(b)* females: low—25th percentile; typical—50th percentile; high—75th percentile.

Data from (7, 8, 21).

FUNCTIONAL REACH TEST

Purpose

The functional reach test measures dynamic balance.

Outcome

Distance reached in centimeters or inches

Equipment Needed

Measuring stick; adhesive tape

Before You Begin

Using adhesive tape, secure a measuring stick horizontally on a wall at a height approximately in line with the athlete's or client's shoulders.

Protocol

1. Begin the procedure by saying to the athlete or client: *"We are going to measure your ability to reach with your arms. Are you ready to begin? If so, please remove your shoes."*

2. Direct the athlete or client: *"Start standing with your back straight and feet shoulder-width apart. With your shoulders perpendicular to the wall, adjust your body so that when your arms are straight ahead, your fingertips are located at the zero end of the measuring stick."*

3. Next, explain to the athlete or client: *"After I say 'Begin,' reach along the stick as far as possible without losing your balance while I record your score"* (see figure 5.25).

4. Record the greatest length achieved along the measuring stick to the nearest centimeter or quarter inch and, prior to making two more attempts, instruct the client or athlete: *"Return to the starting position and relax."*

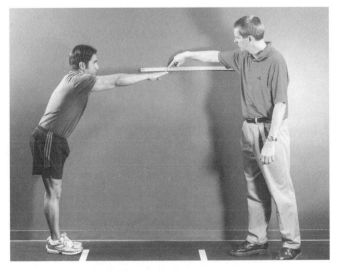

Figure 5.25 Positioning during the functional reach test.

Alternatives or Modifications

A lateral reach test can also be conducted wherein the athlete or client begins with his or her back to the wall and attempts to reach as far as possible along the measuring stick while keeping his or her feet in contact with the ground.

After You Finish

The highest value of the three trials is the final result.

Research Notes

While the functional reach test is commonly used to assess potential deficiencies of dynamic balance in older adults, this assessment may provide insight into improvements following interventions in younger people. For example, completing 12 weeks of Swiss ball training, 3 times per week, resulted in functional reach test improvements, along with increased flexibility, strength, and endurance, in previously sedentary women (with an average age of 36 years old) (32).

Normative Data

Functional reach test classification values are provided in figure 5.26 for men and figure 5.27 for women.

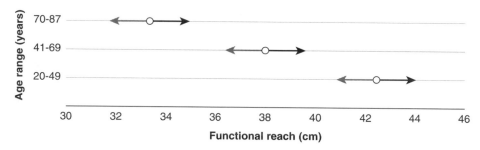

Figure 5.26   Descriptive (average) values for the functional reach test for men across the lifespan.

Data from (9)

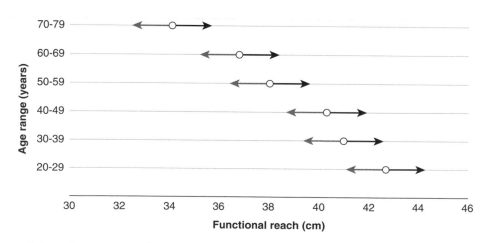

Figure 5.27   Descriptive (average) values for the functional reach test for women across the lifespan.

Adapted from (18).

BALANCE ERROR SCORING SYSTEM

Purpose

The balance error scoring system (BESS) measures static postural stability.

Outcome

Number of balance errors during different stances and surfaces

Equipment Needed

Medium density foam pad (approximately 50 cm x 40 cm x 6 cm); stopwatch or timing device; an assistant to serve as a spotter

Before You Begin

Identify the athlete's or client's dominant leg by asking which leg they would use to kick a ball. (The opposite leg would then be the nondominant leg.)

Protocol

Begin the procedure by saying to the athlete or client: *"We are going to measure your ability to balance under several conditions using different stances on firm and soft surfaces. Are you ready to begin? If so, please remove your shoes."*

Parallel Stance Test

1. Explain to the athlete or client: *"For the first test, you will simply need to stand still with your feet together, your hands on your hips, and your eyes closed for a period of 20 seconds. During this time, I will be evaluating how much you move. If your feet move out of position, open your eyes, return to the starting position, close your eyes, and continue the test"* (see figure 5.28a).

2. When the athlete or client appears to be comfortable with the initial instructions, say: *"When I say 'Begin,' close your eyes and we will start the test."*

3. Verbally signal the athlete or client to begin and record a point (up to a total of 10) whenever one of the following occurs.
   - the hands leave the hips
   - the eyes are opened
   - stepping, stumbling, or falling occurs
   - the client or athlete is out of position for longer than five seconds
   - major bending at the hip joint occurs (>30 degrees in any direction)
   - the forefoot or heel is lifted

4. Following completion of the test (after 20 seconds has passed) on the stable surface, instruct the client: *"Return to the starting position and relax. Next, you will complete the same test but will stand on the foam pad"* (see figure 5.28b).

Single-Leg Stance Test

1. Explain to the athlete or client: *"For the next test, you will stand still while balancing on your nondominant leg with your hands on your hips and your eyes closed for a period of 20 seconds. During this time, I will be evaluating how much you move. If your feet move out of position, open your eyes, return to the starting position, close your eyes, and continue the test"* (see figure 5.29a).

2. When the athlete or client appears comfortable with the initial instructions, continue: *"When I say 'Begin,' close your eyes and we will start the test."*

3. Verbally signal the athlete or client to begin and record a point (up to a total of 10) whenever one of the following occurs:
   - the hands leave the hips
   - the eyes are opened
   - stepping, stumbling, or falling occurs
   - the client or athlete is out of position for longer than five seconds
   - major bending at the hip joint occurs (>30 degrees in any direction)
   - the forefoot or heel is lifted

4. Following completion of the test (after 20 seconds has passed) on the stable surface, direct the client: *"Return to the starting position and relax. Next, you will complete the same test but will stand on the foam pad"* (see figure 5.29b)

Tandem Stance Test

1. Explain to the athlete or client: *"For the next test, you will stand still with the foot of your nondominant leg directly in front of the foot of your dominant leg while keeping your hands on your hips and your eyes closed for a period of 20 seconds. During this time, I will be evaluating how much you move. If your feet move out of position, open your eyes, return to the starting position, close your eyes, and continue the test"* (see figure 5.30a).

2. When the athlete or client appears comfortable with the initial instructions, continue: *"When I say 'Begin,' close your eyes and we will start the test."*

3. Verbally signal the athlete or client to begin and record a point (up to a total of 10) whenever one of the following occurs:
   - the hands leave the hips
   - the eyes are opened
   - stepping, stumbling, or falling occurs
   - the client or athlete is out of position for longer than five seconds
   - major bending at the hip joint occurs (>30 degrees in any direction)
   - the forefoot or heel is lifted

4. Following completion of the test (after 20 seconds has passed) on the stable surface, direct the client: *"Return to the starting position and relax. Next, you will complete the same test but will stand on the foam pad"* (see figure 5.30b).

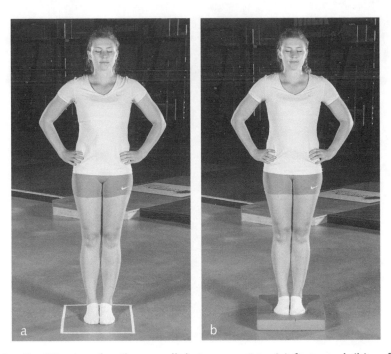

Figure 5.28 Positioning for the parallel stance using *(a)* firm and *(b)* soft conditions.

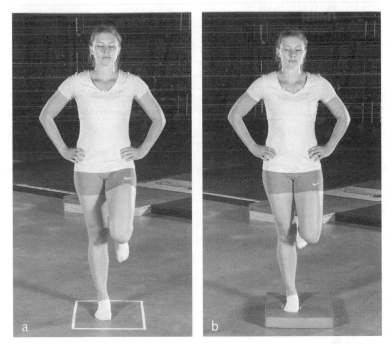

Figure 5.29 Positioning for the single-leg stance using *(a)* firm and *(b)* soft conditions.

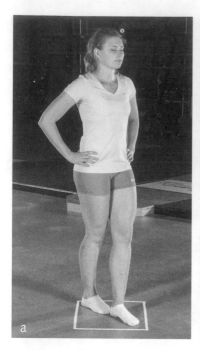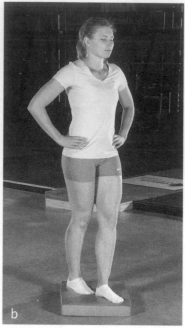

Figure 5.30 Positioning for the tandem stance using *(a)* firm and *(b)* soft conditions.

Alternatives or Modifications

The modified balance error scoring system (BESS) test, which includes only the stable and firm surface versions of the parallel, single-leg, and tandem stances, is part of the Sport Concussion Assessment Tool, 3rd Edition (SCAT3) protocol that can be conducted on the sideline immediately following a potential head injury (1).

The ability to maintain the single-leg stance for an extended period of time (maximum of 45 seconds) with the eyes either open or closed is also used as a measure of static balance.

After You Finish

Add up the total scores from each stance and surface condition with a maximum of 10 errors per 20-second test.

Research Notes

BESS scores are generally evaluated on an individual basis to identify potential deficits in postural stability; however, female collegiate gymnasts have been shown to perform better than basketball players (4). Subsequently, improved BESS scores were reported in female high school basketball players following six weeks of a "neuromuscular-training program that included plyometric, functional-strengthening, balance, and stability-ball exercises" (23).

Normative Data

BESS score classification values are provided in figure 5.31 for men and figure 5.32 for women.

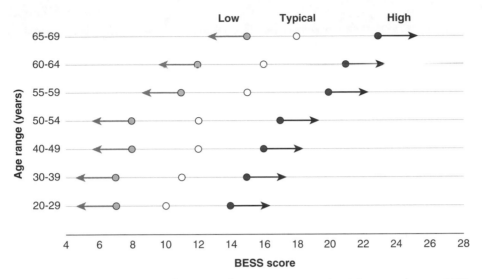

Figure 5.31 BESS score classifications for men across the lifespan: low—25th percentile; typical—50th percentile; high—75th percentile.

Data from (19).

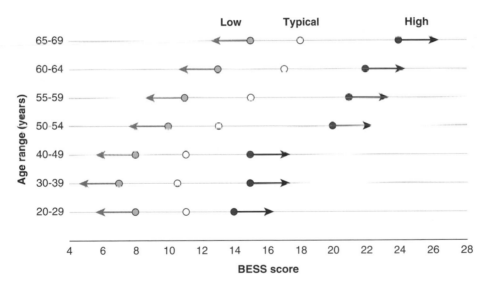

Figure 5.32 BESS score classifications for women across the lifespan: low—25th percentile; typical—50th percentile; high—75th percentile.

Data from (19).

TANDEM GAIT TEST

Purpose

The tandem gait test measures a combination of dynamic balance, speed, and coordination.

Outcome

Time, in seconds, needed to complete the required movement pattern

Equipment Needed

Measuring tape; adhesive tape

Before You Begin

Use adhesive tape and measuring tape to mark a 3-meter (9.8-ft) line on the floor as well as 0.25-meter (9.8-in.) perpendicular lines indicating the beginning and end of the 3 meters (9.8 ft).

Protocol

1. Begin the procedure by saying to the athlete or client: *"We are going to measure how quickly you walk heel to toe along this line. Are you ready to begin? If so, please remove your shoes and stand at one end of the line."*

2. Next, explain to the athlete or client: *"When I say 'Begin,' place the hands on the hips and move forward in an alternating heel-to-toe fashion from this starting point to the other end of the line. After you've cleared the perpendicular line at the end, turn around and resume the alternating heel-to-toe movement until you reach the starting point again. If you cannot maintain the heel-to-toe movement, lose your balance, fail to complete the turn, or step off the line, we will stop the test and try again"* (see figure 5.33).

3. Verbally signal the athlete or client to begin and use the timing device to record how much time passes while the assessment is completed.

4. After the athlete or client has completed the initial test, say, *"Return to the starting position and relax."*

5. After a brief rest, have the athlete or client make three more attempts with a brief rest between each attempt.

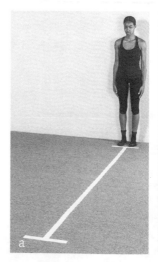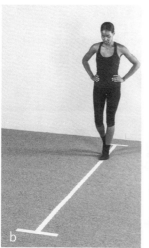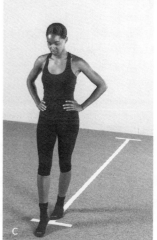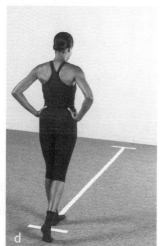

Figure 5.33   Positioning during the tandem gait test.

After You Finish

The fastest value of the four trials is the final result.

Research Notes

Tandem gait time has been shown to be less affected than single-leg stance time following moderate and high intensity exercise (31), which has implications for the selection of sideline protocols for concussion assessment during sport. Consequently, tandem gait is an optional assessment included in the Sport Concussion Assessment Tool, 3rd edition (SCAT3) (1). In support, youth soccer athletes who were evaluated for concussion symptoms following a potential head injury during a game exhibited significantly slower tandem gait times (and lower BESS scores) than uninjured athletes (11).

Normative Data

A tandem gait score of greater than 14 seconds has been recommended as the potential cutoff point for diminished functional movement capacities; however, support for this may be limited in high school athletes (29). Descriptive values for tandem gait scores are provided in figure 5.34.

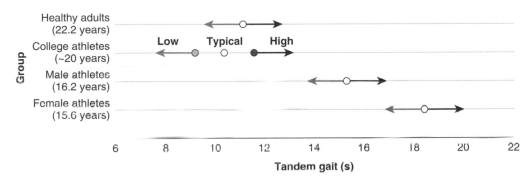

Figure 5.34 Descriptive values for tandem gait scores: low—25th percentile; typical—50th percentile; high—75th percentile.

Data from (25, 29, 30)

CHAPTER 6

Agility and Sprinting

"The goal is to turn data into information, and information into insight."

Carly Fiorina, former executive, president, and chair of Hewlett-Packard Co.

The results of agility and sprint assessments are commonly used as indicators of sport performance. Agility tests involve rapid change-of-direction skills executed over varying distances that can be either planned or unplanned/reactive, with the latter providing an additional measure of decision making and perceptual motor abilities. Straight-line sprint tests contain components of both acceleration and speed, which vary depending on the distance covered and the abilities of the athlete or client. Therefore, coaches or fitness professionals should consider the movement patterns of the sport or activity of interest when selecting the distance(s) to be examined. The agility and sprint assessments included in this chapter are presented exclusively with the use of handheld timing devices (i.e., stopwatches). However, the assessments may also be conducted with electronic timing systems, which typically require the athlete or client to begin slightly behind the starting line to initiate the timing sequence and often result in slower results. The assessments covered in this chapter are as follows:

- 5-10-5 test (pro agility or 20-yard shuttle run) (23, 32)
- T-test (23, 32)
- Three-cone drill (23)
- Y-shaped reactive agility test (15)
- Hexagon agility test (24, 32)
- Straight-line sprint (9, 32)
- Repeated sprint ability test (2, 33)
- Repeated change-of-direction test (2, 33)
- 300-yard shuttle run (7, 22)

5-10-5 TEST

Purpose

The 5-10-5 test (also called *pro agility* or *20-yard shuttle run*) measures multidirectional speed and planned change-of-direction abilities.

Outcome

Time, in seconds, needed to complete the required movement pattern

Equipment Needed

Cones or markers; adhesive tape or field paint; timing device; measuring tape

Before You Begin

Use the adhesive tape or field paint to make three parallel lines (long enough to allow the athlete or client to run and turn within them) each separated by 5 yards (15 ft; 4.6 m), and place cones or markers at each end of the parallel lines to serve as additional indicators (see figure 6.1). Also note that a standardized warm-up followed by three to five minutes of rest and recovery should be conducted prior to the assessment.

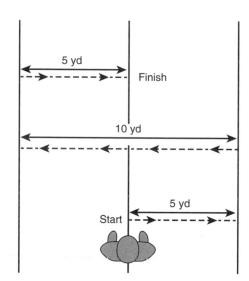

Figure 6.1   Setup for the 5-10-5 test.

Protocol

1. Begin the procedure by saying to the athlete or client: *"We are going to measure how quickly you can complete a series of planned movements. Are you ready to begin? If so, please stand straddling the middle cone or marker, which will be the start and finish position."*

2. Next, explain to the athlete or client: *"You will start this test with your feet shoulder-width apart and knees slightly bent. When I say 'Go,' turn and sprint to your right until you can touch the line with your right hand. After touching the far right line with your right hand, turn to your left and sprint past the middle line until you can touch the far left line with your left hand. After touching the far left line with your left hand, turn back to your right and sprint past the middle line to complete the test."*

3. Position yourself so that you can clearly view the start and finish line. Verbally signal the athlete or client, *"3, 2, 1, go,"* and use the timing device to record how much time is accumulated (to the nearest 0.01 second) while they complete the assessment. If the athlete or client does not touch the lines with the correct hand, stop the time and repeat the assessment.

4. After the athlete or client has completed the initial test, say, *"Return to the starting position and relax,"* prior to making two more attempts, each separated by three to five minutes of rest and recovery.

Alternatives or Modifications

The 5-10-5 test can also be started from a three- or four-point stance or completed while carrying an implement. Additional modifications include initially turning to the left, completing trials turning in both directions, or contacting lines with the foot rather than the hand.

After You Finish

The fastest value of the three trials is the final result.

Research Notes

Position-specific requirements exist in professional baseball, and fielding performance is a major indicator of success. Outfielders have to defend a much larger area of the playing field than infielders and are often required to make rapid change-of-direction movements during the initial response to a batted ball and after making a catch and turning to make a throw. Subsequently, the time needed to complete the 5-10-5 test has been shown to be significantly related to fielding performance in major league outfielders but not infielders (16).

Normative Data

Test classification values for the 5-10-5 test are provided in figure 6.2 for National Collegiate Athletic Association Division I athletes and figure 6.3 for the National Football League Scouting Combine.

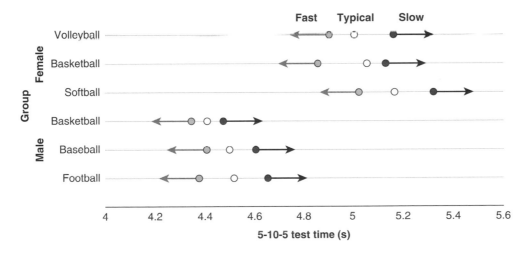

Figure 6.2 The 5-10-5 test time classifications for National Collegiate Athletic Association (NCAA) Division I college athletes: fast—70th percentile; typical—50th percentile; slow—30th percentile.

Data from (13).

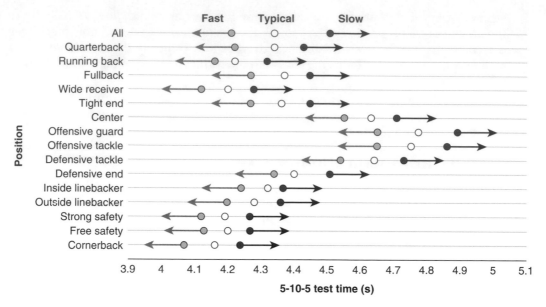

Figure 6.3 The 5-10-5 test time classifications from the National Football League (NFL) Scouting Combine: fast—70th percentile; typical—50th percentile; slow—30th percentile.

Data from (18).

Purpose

The T-test measures multidirectional speed and planned change-of-direction abilities.

Outcome

Time, in seconds, needed to complete the required movement pattern

Equipment Needed

Cones or markers; adhesive tape or field paint; timing device; measuring tape

Before You Begin

Use the adhesive tape or field paint and cone A to make a start/finish line. Place cone B 10 yards (30 ft; 9.1 m) directly in front of cone A, cone C 5 yards (15 ft; 4.6 m) to the left of cone B, and cone D 5 yards to the right of cone B, forming a "T" shape (see figure 6.4). Also note that a standardized warm-up followed by three to five minutes of rest and recovery should be conducted prior to the assessment.

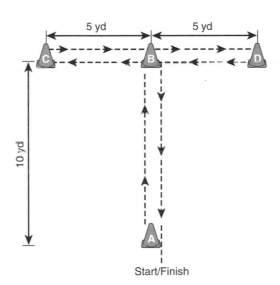

Figure 6.4 Setup for the T-test.

Protocol

1. Begin the procedure by saying to the athlete or client: *"We are going to measure how quickly you can complete a series of planned movements. Are you ready to begin? If so, please stand behind cone A, which will be the start and finish position."*

2. Next, explain to the athlete or client: *"You will start this test with your feet shoulder-width apart, knees slightly bent, and one foot on the start/finish line. When I say 'Go,' sprint forward and touch the bottom of cone B with your right hand. After touching cone B, side shuffle to your left and touch the bottom of cone C with your left hand. After touching cone C, side shuffle past cone B and touch the bottom of cone D with your right hand. Then side shuffle back and touch the bottom of cone B with your left hand, before backpedaling past cone A at the finish line to complete the test."*

3. Position yourself so that you can clearly view the start/finish line. Verbally signal the athlete or client "*3, 2, 1, go,*" and use the timing device to record how much time is accumulated (to the nearest 0.01 second) while they complete the assessment. If the athlete or client does not touch the base of the cones, crosses feet while shuffling, or cannot remain facing forward, stop the time and repeat the assessment.

4. After the athlete or client has completed the initial test, say, "*Return to the starting position and relax,*" prior to making two more attempts, each separated by three to five minutes of rest and recovery.

Alternatives or Modifications

The T-test can also be completed with an initial turn to the right, switching which hand touches the cones, or by having the athlete or client perform a sport-specific movement at the outer cones.

After You Finish

The fastest value of the three trials is the final result.

Research Notes

T-test performance is associated with various types of strength but has been shown to be primarily determined by the ability to produce braking (eccentric) force in female basketball players (31). Furthermore, indicative of the physical requirements in the sport of volleyball, T-test times have also been shown to be significantly related to playing level in junior male and female volleyball players while differentiating between male and female athletes (4).

Normative Data

T-test classification values are provided in figure 6.5 for college-aged individuals and figure 6.6 for National Collegiate Athletic Association Division III football and elite high school soccer athletes. Descriptive values for the T-test in various athletes are provided in figure 6.7.

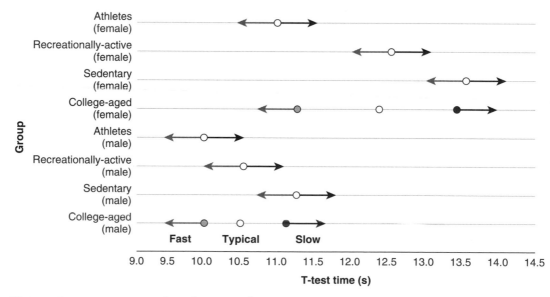

Figure 6.5   T-test time classifications for college-aged individuals: fast—75th percentile; typical—50th percentile; slow—25th percentile.

Data from (20).

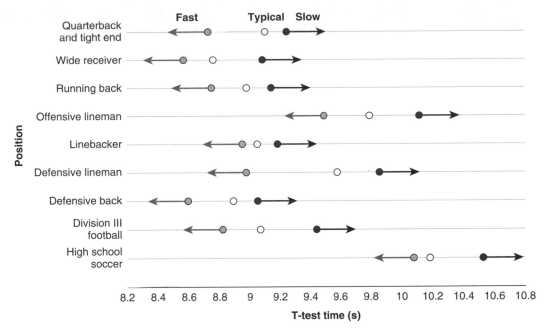

Figure 6.6 T-test time classifications for NCAA Division III football and elite high school soccer athletes: fast—70th percentile; typical—50th percentile; slow—30th percentile.

Data from (13).

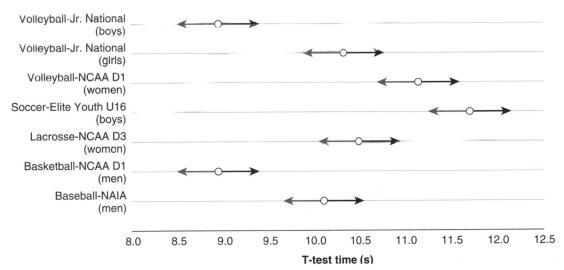

Figure 6.7 Descriptive (average) T-test times for various athletes.

Data from (32).

THREE-CONE DRILL

Purpose

The three-cone drill measures multidirectional speed and planned change-of-direction abilities.

Outcome

Time, in seconds, needed to complete the required movement pattern

Equipment Needed

Cones or markers; adhesive tape or field paint; timing device; measuring tape

Before You Begin

Use the adhesive tape or field paint and cone A to make a start/finish line. Place cone B 5 yards (15 ft; 4.6 m) directly in front of cone A, and cone C 5 yards (15 ft; 4.6 m) to the right of cone B, forming an upside down "L" shape (see figure 6.8). Also note that a standardized warm-up followed by three to five minutes of rest and recovery should be conducted prior to beginning the assessment.

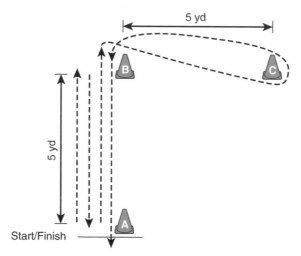

Figure 6.8 Setup for the three-cone drill.

Protocol

1. Begin the procedure by saying to the athlete or client: *"We are going to measure how quickly you can complete a series of movements. Are you ready to begin? If so, please stand behind the starting line at cone A, which will be the start and finish position."*

2. Next, explain to the athlete or client: *"You will start this test with your feet shoulder-width apart, knees slightly bent, and one foot on the start/finish line. When I say 'Go,' sprint forward and touch cone B. After touching cone B, turn around, sprint back to the start line, and touch cone A. After touching cone A, turn around again, and sprint past cone B before circling around cone C. Then sprint back around cone B and through cone A at the finish line to complete the test."*

3. Position yourself so that you can clearly view the start/finish line. Verbally signal the athlete or client "*3, 2, 1, go,*" and use the timing device to record how much time is accumulated (to the nearest 0.01 second). If the athlete or client knocks over any of the cones, stop the time and repeat the assessment.

4. After the athlete or client has completed the initial test, say, "*Return to the starting position and relax,*" prior to making two more attempts, each separated by three to five minutes of rest and recovery.

Alternatives or Modifications

While the three-cone drill is typically conducted using a planned right-hand turn, it can be completed with a planned left-hand turn or as an unplanned/reactive agility test with a left or right signal given midway between cones A and B (14). The three-cone drill can also be started from a three- or four-point stance, or completed while carrying an implement.

After You Finish

The fastest value of the three trials is the final result.

Research Notes

Performance in the three-cone drill has shown to be better in American football players who were drafted in the NFL Scouting Combine than those were not drafted, which appeared to be consistent across positions (28). Furthermore, three-cone drill data from the NFL Combine suggests that change-of-direction skills in professional football players have improved when comparing athletes who entered the NFL draft between 1999 and 2001 and between 2008 and 2010 (25).

Normative Data

Three-cone drill test classification values are provided in figure 6.9 for the NFL Scouting Combine.

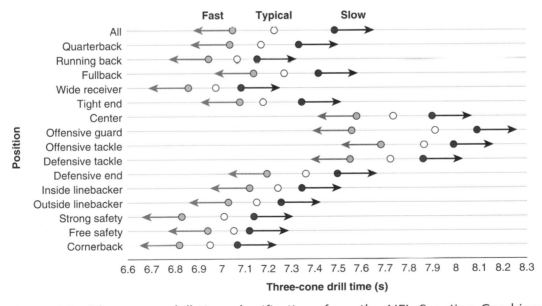

Figure 6.9 Three-cone drill time classifications from the NFL Scouting Combine: fast—70th percentile; typical—50th percentile; slow—30th percentile.

Data from (18).

Y-SHAPED REACTIVE AGILITY TEST

Purpose

The Y-shaped agility test measures multidirectional speed and unplanned change-of-direction abilities.

Outcome

Time, in seconds, needed to react to an external stimulus and complete the required movement pattern

Equipment Needed

Cones or markers; adhesive tape or field paint; timing device; measuring tape; goniometer or protractor; two evaluators

Before You Begin

Use the adhesive tape or field paint and cones or markers to make a starting line. Place a second set of cones or markers 5 meters (16.4 ft) directly in front of the starting line and two sets of cones 5 meters (16.4 ft) to the left and right at 45-degree angles from the second line to form a "Y" shape (see figure 6.10). Also note that a standardized warm-up followed by three to five minutes of rest and recovery should be conducted prior to beginning the assessment.

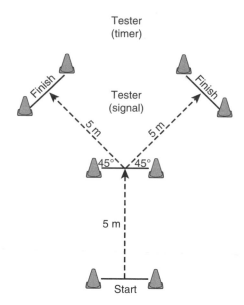

Figure 6.10 Setup for the Y-shaped reactive agility test.

Protocol

1. Begin the procedure by saying to the athlete or client: *"We are going to measure how quickly you can complete a series of unplanned movements. Are you ready to begin?"*

2. Next, explain to the athlete or client: *"You will start this test with your feet shoulder-width apart, knees slightly bent, and one foot on the start line. When I say 'Go,' sprint forward to the second set of cones or markers and look to the evaluator placed ahead of you for a signal. The evaluator will raise his or her right or left hand in the air and you will adjust your sprint to proceed through the cones or markers in this direction to complete the test."* Note: This protocol has been modified from the original version to accommodate the use of a handheld timing device and human signaling rather than timing gates and light indicators.

3. Position one evaluator approximately 8.5 meters (27.9 ft) from the start line (between the two finish lines), who will provide the direction signal. A second evaluator will be positioned roughly 13 meters (42.7 ft) from the start line (with both finish lines directly in view), who will then verbally signal the athlete or client "*3, 2, 1, Go*" and use the timing device to record how much time is accumulated (to the nearest 0.01 second). If the athlete or client appears to anticipate the direction of the turn or guess the wrong direction, stop the time and repeat the assessment.

4. After the athlete or client has completed the initial test, say, "*Return to the starting position and relax,*" prior to making five more attempts (three to the right and three to the left), each separated by three to five minutes of rest and recovery.

Alternatives or Modifications

A planned version can also be conducted with the athlete or client directed to the left or right prior to starting the test. A variety of sprinting distances and change-of-direction angles have been used. With the availability of more sophisticated technology, light or video stimuli may be used as directional indicators and high-speed cameras can specifically track decision-making time (6).

After You Finish

The fastest value of the three trials in each direction is the final result.

Research Notes

Several studies have shown that reactive agility tests more clearly differentiate between competitive levels of athletes than change-of-direction skill (unplanned agility) tests (15, 19, 27). For example, results from the Y-shaped reactive agility tests were found to be 6 percent faster in semiprofessional basketball players than amateur players, with no noticeable differences between these groups in a planned version of the test (15). These findings support the importance of perceptual motor skills and decision making in the sport of basketball.

Normative Data

Due to the widespread nature of the existing protocols and technology used during reactive agility testing, normative or descriptive data are limited. Figure 6.11 provides a general interpretation of the results from planned (change-of-direction) and unplanned/reactive agility tests.

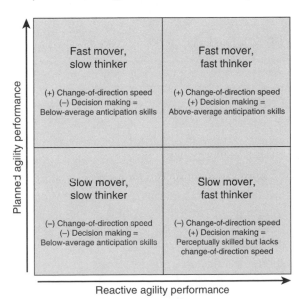

Figure 6.11 General interpretation of the results from planned (change-of-direction) and unplanned/reactive agility tests. A (–) sign indicates poor or slow performance; a (+) sign indicates superior or fast performance.

Data from (5).

HEXAGON AGILITY TEST

Purpose

The hexagon agility test measures multidirectional speed and planned change of direction during jumping.

Outcome

Time, in seconds, needed to complete the required movement pattern

Equipment Needed

Cones or markers; adhesive tape or field paint; timing device; measuring tape; goniometer or protractor

Before You Begin

Use the adhesive tape or field paint to make three parallel two-foot (0.6 m) lines each separated by 1.73 feet (0.53 m), with the middle line serving as the start/finish position. Connect the outer lines with four additional two-foot (0.6 m) lines with 120-degree angles between them to form a hexagon (see figure 6.12). Note that a standardized warm-up followed by three to five minutes of rest and recovery should be conducted prior to beginning the assessment.

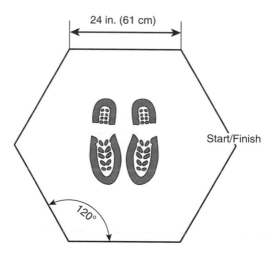

Figure 6.12   Setup for the hexagon agility test.

Protocol

1. Begin the procedure by saying to the athlete or client: *"We are going to measure how quickly you can complete a planned series of hopping movements. Are you ready to begin? If so, please stand on the line in the middle of the hexagon, which will serve as the start and finish position."*

2. Next, explain: *"When I say 'Go,' quickly perform a double-legged jump over and back on the line directly in front of you. Then continue to jump over each side of the hexagon in a clockwise order for a total of three full rotations as quickly as possible without stopping."*

3. Position yourself so that you can clearly view the start/finish line. Verbally signal the athlete or client *"3, 2, 1, go,"* and use the timing device to record how much time is accumulated (to the nearest 0.01 second). If the athlete or client does not fully cross the line while jumping, takes unnecessary steps or hops, cannot remain facing forward, or loses balance, stop the time and repeat the assessment.

4. After the athlete or client has completed the initial test, say, *"Return to the starting position and relax,"* prior to making two more attempts, each separated by three to five minutes of rest and recovery.

Alternatives or Modifications

A single-legged version of the hexagon agility test can be performed with the unengaged leg not touching the ground for the duration of the assessment. It may be useful to identify the athlete's or client's dominant leg by asking which leg they would use to kick a ball. (The opposite leg would then be the nondominant leg.)

After You Finish

The fastest value or the average of the three trials is the final result.

Research Notes

In the sport of figure skating, junior and senior skaters have been shown to perform better during the hexagon agility test than novice skaters, which may result from the increasing demand placed on advanced athletes with respect to jumping sequences and footwork (29). Singles skaters also appeared to be more agile than synchronized skaters, potentially identifying an opportunity for improvements in these athletes (29).

Normative Data

Hexagon agility test classification values are provided in figure 6.13 for college-aged individuals.

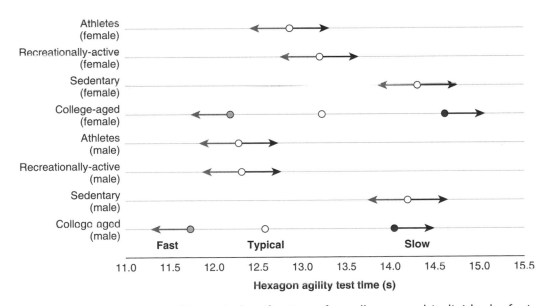

Figure 6.13 Hexagon agility test classifications for college-aged individuals: fast—75th percentile; typical—50th percentile; slow—25th percentile.

Data from (20).

STRAIGHT-LINE SPRINT

Purpose

Straight-line sprint tests are used to evaluate speed and acceleration over various distances.

Outcome

Time, in seconds, needed to cover the required distance

Equipment Needed

Cones or markers; adhesive tape or field paint; timing device; measuring tape

Before You Begin

Place two markers the selected distance apart (40 yards or meters will be used for this explanation). Place additional markers at 10 yards (or meters, or other intervals of interest) into the overall selected distance and 5 yards (or meters) past the finish line to remind the athlete or client to sprint through the entire test (see figure 6.14). Note that a standardized warm-up, including several practice runs with moderate effort, followed by three to five minutes of rest and recovery should be conducted prior to beginning the assessment.

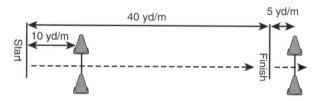

Figure 6.14   Setup for a 40-yard (or meter) straight-line sprint test.

Protocol

1. Begin the procedure by saying to the athlete or client: *"We are going to measure how quickly you can sprint 40 yards (or meters). Are you ready to begin? If so, please stand behind the starting line."*

2. Next, explain: *"You will start this test with your feet shoulder-width apart, knees slightly bent, and one foot on the start line. When I say 'Go,' sprint forward as fast as possible to the opposite line and slow down past the next cone to complete the test."*

3. Evaluators will be positioned at the 10-yard (or meter) marker (or the other intervals of interest) and the finish line. The evaluator located at the finish line opposite the athlete or client will verbally signal the athlete or client *"3, 2, 1, go,"* and all of the evaluators will use a timing device to record how much time is accumulated (to the nearest 0.01 second).

4. After the athlete or client has completed the initial test, say, *"Return to the starting position and relax,"* prior to making two more attempts, each separated by three to five minutes of rest and recovery.

Alternatives or Modifications

Coaches or fitness professionals should select sport- or activity-appropriate distances (5, 10, 20, 30, 40, 60 yards or meters). Sprint tests can also be started from a three- or four-point stance. If the ability to quickly attain maximal speed or velocity (acceleration) is important for the sport or activity of interest, it may be helpful to conduct several shorter and longer tests or to attain times from various points throughout a single assessment. Reminder: hand timing can result in faster times than timing gates.

After You Finish

The 10-yard split time recorded during a 40-yard test may be used as an indication of acceleration, while the difference between the overall 40-meter time and the 10-meter time, also known as a 30-meter *flying sprint*, can be used as an indication of maximal speed. The fastest times (overall, split, flying) of the three trials are the final results.

Research Notes

Improvements in lower-body strength are thought to be related to improvements in sprint speed (26). Interestingly, five weeks of either single-legged (unilateral) or standard (bilateral) squat training completed by rugby athletes resulted in decreased 40-meter sprint times but not in 10-meter sprint times (30). The authors suggested that this may indicate that adaptations related to strength improvements may take longer to translate into enhanced short distance sprinting than those related to the longer distance or that distance-specific sprint training may have been needed.

Normative Data

Sprint time classification values and descriptive data across several distances and in various populations are provided in figure 6.15 through figure 6.22.

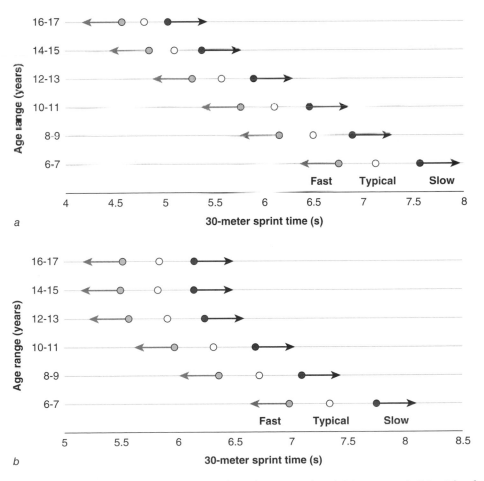

Figure 6.15 Thirty-meter sprint time classifications for (a) boys and (b) girls: fast—70th percentile; typical—50th percentile; slow—30th percentile.

Data from (0).

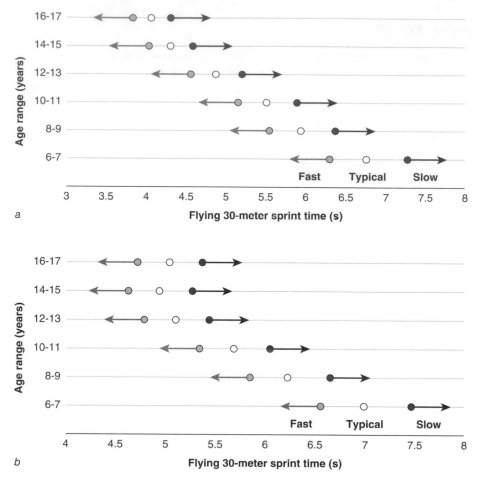

Figure 6.16 Flying 30-meter sprint time classifications for (a) boys and (b) girls: fast—70th percentile; typical—50th percentile; slow—30th percentile.

Data from (3).

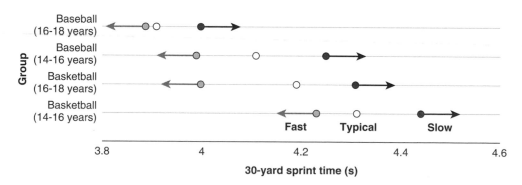

Figure 6.17 Thirty-yard sprint time classifications for male youth baseball and basketball athletes: fast—70th percentile; typical—50th percentile; slow—30th percentile.

Data from (13).

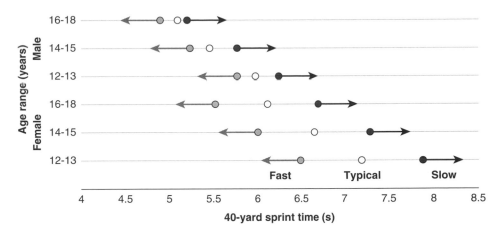

Figure 6.18 Forty-yard sprint time classifications for youths aged 12 to 18 years: fast—70th percentile; typical—50th percentile; slow—30th percentile.

Data from (9).

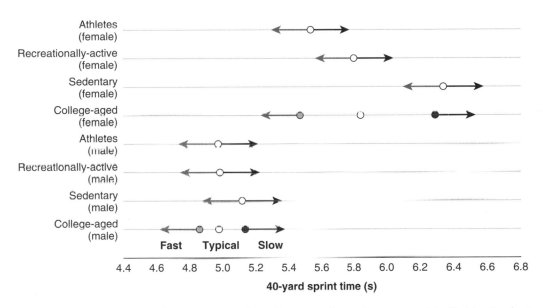

Figure 6.19 Forty-yard sprint time classifications for college-aged individuals: fast—75th percentile; typical—50th percentile; slow—25th percentile.

Data from (20).

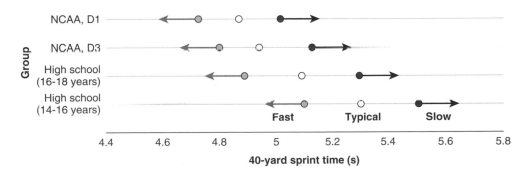

Figure 6.20 Forty-yard sprint time classifications for male American football athletes: fast—70th percentile; typical—50th percentile; slow—30th percentile.

Data from (13).

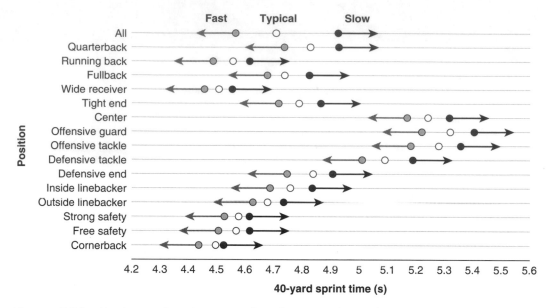

Figure 6.21 Forty-yard sprint time classifications from the NFL Scouting Combine (electronic timing system): fast—70th percentile; typical—50th percentile; slow—30th percentile.

Data from (18).

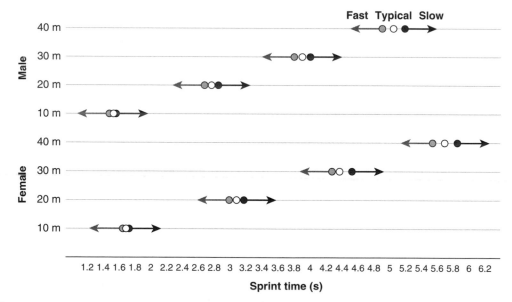

Figure 6.22 Forty-meter sprint times (and 10-meter splits) classifications from male professional and female elite soccer players (electronic timing system): fast—75th percentile; typical—50th percentile; slow—25th percentile.

Data from (10).

REPEATED SPRINT ABILITY TEST

Purpose

The repeated sprint ability (RSA) test measures the ability to perform several straight-line sprints separated by minimal recovery periods.

Outcome

Time, in seconds, needed to complete the required movement pattern

Equipment Needed

Cones or markers; adhesive tape or field paint; measuring tape; goniometer or protractor; at least two evaluators; at least two timing devices

Before You Begin

Place two parallel lines or sets of markers 20 meters (65.6 ft) apart, with both designated as start/finish lines, and two cones approximately 10 meters (32.8 ft) past the start/finish lines to allow the athlete or client to slow down (decelerate) after each sprint (see figure 6.23).

A standardized warm-up—including several familiarization trials completed at increasing submaximal intensities, followed by three to five minutes of rest and recovery—should be conducted prior to the assessments. Completion of a single 20-meter (65.6 ft) sprint has also been recommended prior to the repeated sprint ability test to verify that maximal effort is given in the first sprint (>95% of 20 m sprint time).

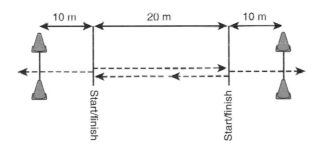

Figure 6.23 Setup for the repeated sprint ability test.

Protocol

1. Begin the procedure by saying to the athlete or client: *"We are going to measure how quickly you can complete a series of 20-meter sprints. Are you ready to begin? If so, please stand behind the closest start/finish line."*

2. Next, explain to the athlete or client: *"You will start this test with your feet shoulder-width apart, knees slightly bent, and one foot on the start/finish line. When I say 'Go,' sprint forward as fast as possible to the opposite start/finish line and slow down past the next cone. You will be given 25 seconds to turn, jog, and circle back before returning to the closest start/finish line to begin the next sprint in the opposite direction. You will complete a total of six sprints before finishing the test."*

3. Two evaluators will be positioned at each start/finish line. The evaluator located at the start/finish line opposite the athlete or client will verbally signal the athlete or client "3, 2, 1, go," and use a timing device to record how much time is accumulated (to the nearest 0.01 second) during each sprint, while another evaluator uses a separate timing device to monitor the 25-second rest and recovery periods.

Alternatives or Modifications

A version of this test using 10 sprints has also been proposed. Furthermore, the distances, number of sprints, and duration of rest and recovery periods used during repeated sprint ability tests have been altered to allow for sport-specific evaluations.

After You Finish

The best time of the six sprints, the average time of the six sprints, and the total time of the six sprints should be calculated and recorded.

Research Notes

Repeated sprint ability has been shown to be related to distances covered at high speeds during soccer matches (21) and provides a distinct measure separate from agility tests that focus on change of direction skills. Repeated sprint ability values have been shown to distinguish between recreationally active soccer players and competitive soccer athletes (33).

Normative Data

Descriptive values for the repeated sprint ability tests for recreationally active men and competitive male soccer athletes are provided in figure 6.24 and figure 6.25.

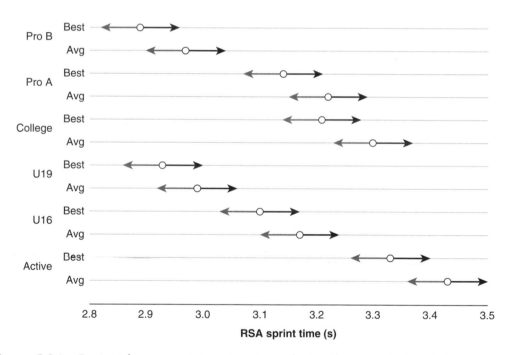

Figure 6.24 Best and average 20-meter times during the repeated sprint ability tests for recreationally active men and competitive male soccer players (electronic timing system).

Data from (33, 34).

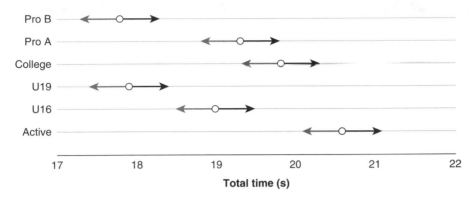

Figure 6.25 Total sprint times during the repeated sprint ability tests for recreationally active men and competitive male soccer players (electronic timing system).

Data from (33, 34).

Purpose

The repeated change-of-direction (RCOD) test measures the ability to perform several short sprints and turns separated by minimal recovery periods.

Outcome

Time, in seconds, needed to complete the required movement pattern

Equipment Needed

Cones or markers; adhesive tape or field paint; measuring tape; goniometer or protractor; at least two evaluators; at least two timing devices

Before You Begin

Place two parallel lines or sets of markers approximately 15.3 meters (50.2 ft) apart, with both being designated start/finish lines. Use cones or markers to configure five 4-meter (13.1 ft) lines with 100-degree angles between them and 50-degree angles from the start/finish lines. An additional set of cones should be placed approximately 4 to 5 meters (13.1 to 16.4 ft) past the start/finish lines to allow the athlete or client to decelerate after each change-of-direction drill (see figure 6.26).

A standardized warm-up—including several familiarization trials completed at increasing submaximal intensities, followed by three to five minutes of rest and recovery—should be conducted prior to beginning the assessment.

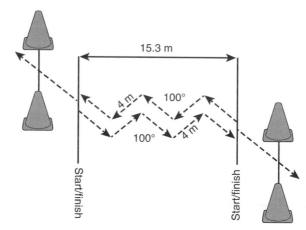

Figure 6.26 Setup for the repeated change-of-direction test.

Protocol

1. Approximately 15 minutes after completion of the repeated sprint ability test, begin the procedure by saying to the athlete or client: *"We are going to measure how quickly you can complete a series of change-of-direction drills. Are you ready to begin? If so, please stand behind the closest start/finish line."*

2. Next, explain: *"You will start this test with your feet shoulder-width apart, knees slightly bent, and one foot on the start/finish line. When I say 'Go,' sprint forward as fast as possible along the designated course during which you will make four sharp turns then sprint through the opposite start/finish line and slow down past the next cone. You will be given 25 seconds to turn, jog, and circle back before returning to the closest start/finish line to begin the next change-of-direction drill in the opposite direction. You will complete a total of six change-of-direction drills before finishing the test."* Note: this protocol has been

modified from the original version to accommodate the use of a handheld timing device and human signaling rather than timing gates and light indicators.

3. An evaluator will be positioned at each start/finish line. The evaluator located at the start/finish line opposite the athlete or client will verbally signal the athlete or client "*3, 2, 1, go,*" and use a timing device to record how much time is accumulated (to the nearest 0.01 second) during each change-of-direction drill, while another evaluator uses a separate timing device to monitor the 25-second rest and recovery periods.

Alternatives or Modifications

A version of this test using 10 change-of-direction drills has also been proposed.

After You Finish

The best time of the six change-of-direction drills, the average time of the six change-of-direction drills, and the total time of the change-of-direction drills should be calculated and recorded. The RCOD values can also be compared to RSA performance. For example, the RSA/RCOD index can then be calculated for the best time, average time, or total time as follows:

$$RSA/RCOD\ index = \frac{RSA\ time}{RCOD\ time}$$

Research Notes

RCOD and RSA/RCOD index values are shown to differ between recreationally active soccer players and competitive soccer athletes (33). The RSA/RCOD index may be similar among developing age-group soccer athletes, while specific test times improve from younger (U16) to older (U19/professional) groups (34). It has been proposed that deviations from the average RSA/RCOD index within a team or similar group of athletes may be used to identify training priorities. For example, for a group of soccer athletes with an average RSA/RCOD index of 0.59, those individuals with a value <0.59 should focus more on improving repeated change-of-direction skills, while those with a value of >0.59 should focus more on improving repeated sprint abilities (33).

Normative Data

Descriptive values for the repeated sprint ability and repeated change-of-direction tests for recreationally active men and competitive male soccer athletes are provided in figure 6.27 through figure 6.29. RSA/RCOD index values have been reported to be between 0.50 and 0.60; however, because these indices are likely related to playing and training styles and other factors, it is suggested that coaches or fitness professionals develop normative values for their own groups of athletes or clients.

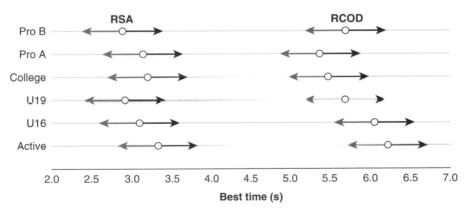

Figure 6.27 Best 20-meter times during the repeated sprint ability and repeated change-of-direction tests for recreationally active men and competitive male soccer players (electronic timing system).

Data from (33, 34).

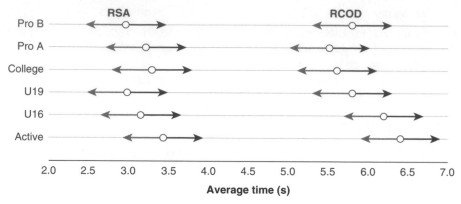

Figure 6.28 Average 20-meter times during the repeated sprint ability and repeated change-of-direction tests for recreationally active men and competitive male soccer players (electronic timing system).

Data from (33, 34).

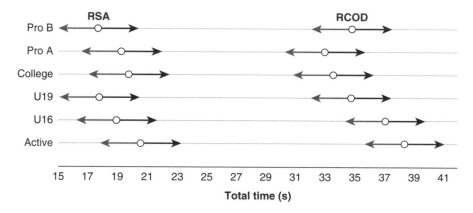

Figure 6.29 Total sprint times during the repeated sprint ability and repeated change-of-direction tests for recreationally active men and competitive male soccer players (electronic timing system).

Data from (33, 34).

300-YARD SHUTTLE RUN

Purpose

The 300-yard shuttle run tests the ability to complete consecutive straight-line sprints separated by a quick change of direction.

Outcome

Time, in seconds, needed to complete the required movement pattern

Equipment Needed

Cones or markers; adhesive tape or field paint; timing device; measuring tape

Before You Begin

Place two markers 25 yards (22.9 m) apart, with one being designated the start/finish line (see figure 6.30). Note that a standardized warm-up followed by three to five minutes of rest and recovery should be conducted prior to beginning the assessment.

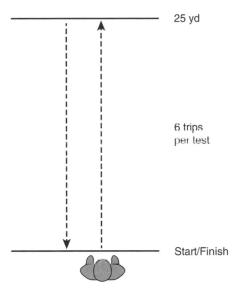

25 yd

6 trips
per test

Start/Finish

Figure 6.30   Setup for the 300-yard shuttle run.

Protocol

1. Begin the procedure by saying to the athlete or client: *"We are going to measure how quickly you can complete a series of 25-yard sprints. Are you ready to begin? If so, please stand behind the starting line."*

2. Next, explain: *"You will start this test with your feet shoulder-width apart, knees slightly bent, and one foot on the start/finish line. When I say 'Go,' sprint forward as fast as possible to the opposite marker. Once your foot has passed the marker, turn around and sprint back to the starting position. You will repeat this down-and-back pattern a total of 6 times (or 12 separate 25-yd sprints) to complete the test."*

3. Position yourself so that you can clearly view the start/finish line. Verbally signal the athlete or client *"3, 2, 1, go,"* and use the timing device to record how much time is accumulated (to the nearest 0.01 second) while they complete the assessment.

4. After the athlete or client has completed the initial test, say, *"Return to the starting position and relax,"* prior to making another attempt separated by three to five minutes of rest and recovery.

Alternatives or Modifications

The 300-yard shuttle run has also been conducted with the athlete or client wearing a weight vest (20 lb for those weighing ≤140 lb; 25 lb for those weighing 141 to 185 lb.; 30 lb for those weighing ≥186 lb). This version of the test has shown to be an indicator of injury risk in male soldiers (8).

After You Finish

The average of the two trials is the final result.

Research Notes

Dynamic warm-ups are often recommended prior to exercise due to the potential negative effects on subsequent performance following static stretching. In support, a four-week dynamic stretching routine (15 min of calisthenics and movement drills) conducted before practice by a group of NCAA Division I college wrestlers resulted in decreased 300-yard shuttle run times as compared to a static stretching group (15 min of various stretches held for 20 to 30 sec each) (11). These findings demonstrated that the benefits of engaging in regular dynamic warm-up routines extend past the subsequent exercise session and may provide long-term benefits.

Normative Data

Classification values for the 300-yard shuttle run are provided in figure 6.31 for NCAA Division I athletes. Descriptive values for the 300-yard shuttle run in various populations are provided in figure 6.32.

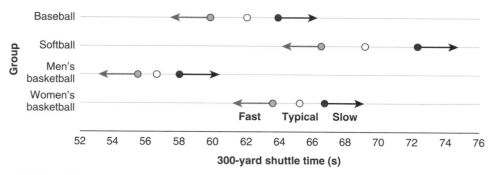

Figure 6.31 Classification values for the 300-yard shuttle run for NCAA Division I athletes.

Data from (12).

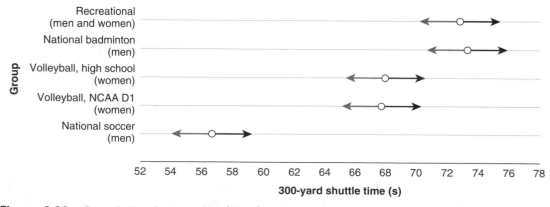

Figure 6.32 Descriptive (average) values for the 300-yard shuttle in various populations.

Data from (17).

CHAPTER 7

Power

> *"It is a capital mistake to theorize before one has data. Insensibly one begins to twist facts to suit theories, instead of theories to suit facts."*
>
> Sir Arthur Conan Doyle, author of Sherlock Holmes stories

While muscular strength and cardiovascular endurance are physical qualities commonly displayed by athletes, power or explosiveness tends to be a determining factor in successfully performing a variety of activities from nearly all sports to many daily functional tasks. Power is a function of body weight, the height achieved or distance covered, and the time it takes to complete a particular activity. The selection of appropriate power assessments will be dictated by the movement requirements of the targeted activity or sport, which may include distinctions between the upper and lower body, single-effort (or relatively stationary) and multiple-effort (cyclic motions, running, hopping, etc.) situations, and pushing and pulling actions.

Similar to the agility and sprint assessments covered in chapter 6, the power assessments included in this chapter are presented exclusively with the use of stopwatches, but they may be enhanced by using more advanced technol-ogy, such as mobile applications, contact mats, electronic timing systems, linear position transducers, or force plates. The assessments covered in this chapter are as follows:

- Vertical jump (or countermovement jump) test (19, 45)
- Standing long jump (or broad jump) test (19, 45)
- Single-leg triple hop test (37, 45, 54)
- Medicine ball chest pass test (5, 41)
- Forward overhead medicine ball throw test (58)
- Backward overhead medicine ball throw test (19, 46)
- Rotating medicine ball throw test (46)
- Stair sprint power (or Margaria-Kalamen) test (4, 32, 41)
- Rowing ergometer peak power test (21, 34)

VERTICAL JUMP TEST

Purpose

The vertical jump (also called the countermovement jump) test measures lower-body upward explosiveness or power.

Outcomes

Vertical jump height in centimeters or inches; estimated power output during jumping

Equipment Needed

Wall with enough vertical clearance to safely complete a maximal jump; measuring tape; chalk

Before You Begin

Follow the procedures outlined in chapter 4 to record the client's or athlete's body weight. Identify the client's or athlete's dominant hand, which is used for writing or throwing a ball. A standardized warm-up, including three to five practice jumps performed at moderate intensity (approximately 50% of estimated maximal effort), followed by three to five minutes of rest and recovery, should be conducted prior to beginning the assessment.

Protocol

1. Begin the procedure by saying to the client or athlete: *"We are going to measure how high you can jump. Are you ready to begin? If so, please cover the fingertips of your dominant hand with chalk"* (see figure 7.1a).

2. Next, direct the client or athlete: *"Stand with your dominant arm and torso next to the wall with equal weight on both feet."*

3. After the client or athlete has assumed the correct position, continue: *"Before you do the test, we need to determine your standing reach height. While keeping your feet firmly on the ground, reach up as high as possible above your head along the wall with the chalked hand and make a mark with your fingers. Then bring your arm back down to your side"* (see figure 7.1b).

4. Record the distance between the highest chalk mark and the floor as the standing reach height.

5. After determining the standing reach height, tell the client or athlete: *"When I say 'Go,' quickly perform a countermovement in which you squat down with your arms rapidly swinging back past your hips and then immediately reverse the movement to jump up as high as you can while reaching your chalked hand as high as possible along the wall. At your highest point, touch the wall with your fingertips to make a mark and then land safely back on the floor on both feet"* (see figure 7.2).

6. Position yourself so that you can clearly view the jump. Verbally signal the client or athlete *"3, 2, 1, go,"* and verify that the jump is begun with both feet flat on the ground, without taking a step, and that the client or athlete performs the countermovement, jumps as high as possible, and lands under control.

7. Record the distance to the closest centimeter or half inch between the highest chalk mark and the floor as the total jump height.

8. After the client or athlete has completed the initial vertical jump, say: *"Return to the starting position and relax,"* prior to making at least two more attempts, each separated by one minute of rest and recovery.

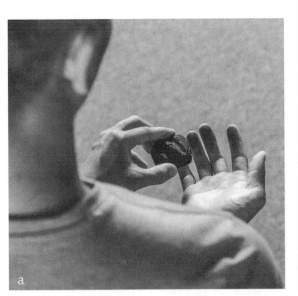
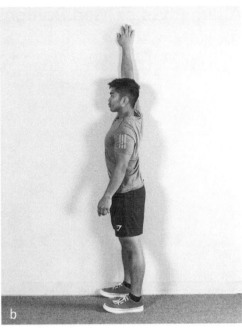

Figure 7.1 *(a)* Placement of chalk on fingers and *(b)* determining standing reach height with chalked hand.

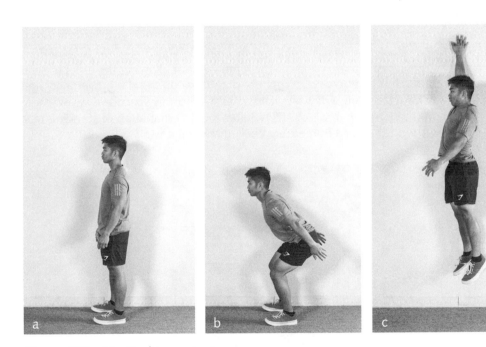

Figure 7.2 Vertical jump test.

Alternatives or Modifications

The squat jump test can also be used, during which the client or athlete is asked to achieve and hold a specified knee angle (approximately 90°) and arm position (in line with or behind the trunk) for a short period prior to executing the jump (see figure 7.3).

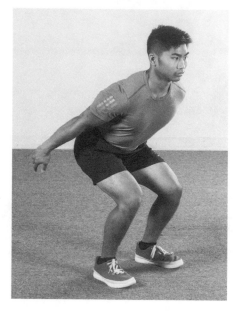

Figure 7.3   Squat jump test.

Modifications of the standard vertical jump test include allowing a step (or two, depending on the sport or activity of interest) prior to the jump and not allowing the arms to swing (hands on hips or with a bar or PVC pipe across the shoulders) during the movement. Jump testing can also be conducted using a device outfitted with uniformly spaced vanes extending from a vertical beam (see figure 7.4), which still requires the determination of standing reach height but does away with the need to measure chalk marks on a wall.

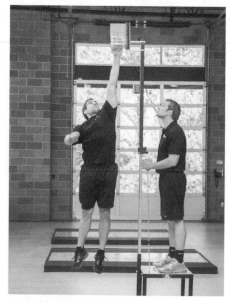

Figure 7.4   Use of a specifically outfitted vertical jump device for the vertical jump test.

After You Finish

The greatest recorded total jump height is the final result, and the vertical jump height can be calculated using the following formula:

Vertical jump height = total jump height − standing reach height

The coach or fitness professional may also choose to use the vertical jump height and the client's or athlete's body mass to estimate peak power output (48) using the following formula:

Peak power (watts) = 60.7 × jump height (cm) + 45.3 × body mass (kg) − 2,055

Evaluation of peak power during the vertical jump test allows the coach or fitness professional to gain a better understanding of the effects of a client's or athlete's body weight on jump performance. An alternative to calculating peak power output during the vertical jump test is the use of the nomogram provided in figure 7.5.

Figure 7.5 Nomogram for peak power output during a vertical jump test

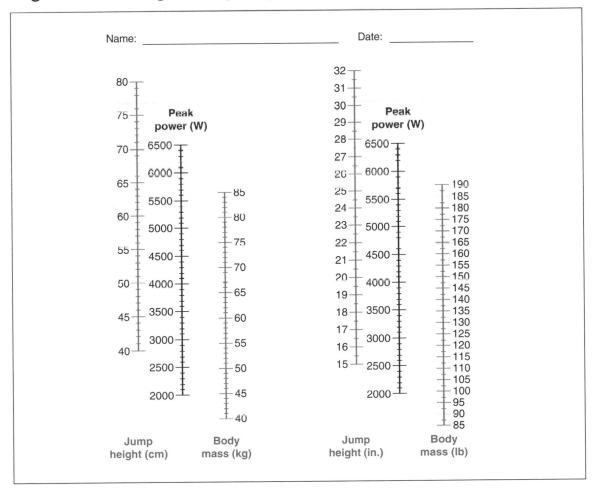

From D. Fukuda, *Assessments for Sport and Athletic Performance* (Champaign, IL: Human Kinetics, 2019). Using Sayers formula (48).

If both the vertical jump (with a countermovement executed before the jump) and squat jump tests are completed, the eccentric utilization ratio can be calculated with the following formula:

$$\text{Eccentric utilization ratio} = \frac{\text{vertical jump height}}{\text{squat jump height}}$$

The calculated eccentric utilization ratio provides an indication of how much the quick bend and rebound of the knees (termed the *stretch-shortening cycle*) executed before the jump contributes to the achieved height (12, 33). This value varies between individuals and likely depends on genetics, training status, and the activity or sport of interest.

Research Notes

Boys show somewhat steady improvements in vertical jump performance throughout the process of maturation, while girls demonstrate minimal improvements following puberty (22). In young male athletes, plyometric training has shown to be an effective approach to further increase vertical jump performance; however, it tends to be less beneficial between the ages of 13 and 16 years old for a variety of maturity-related reasons, potentially including adolescent awkwardness (35). Young female athletes have also demonstrated increased vertical jump with plyometric training, but the program may need to be continued for longer than 10 weeks (53).

Normative Data

Vertical jump classification values are provided in figure 7.6 for male high school athletes, figure 7.7 for the male general population and collegiate and professional athletes, figure 7.8 for the female general population and collegiate athletes, and figure 7.9 from the National Football League (NFL) Scouting Combine. Descriptive values for the eccentric utilization ratio in various sports are provided in figure 7.10.

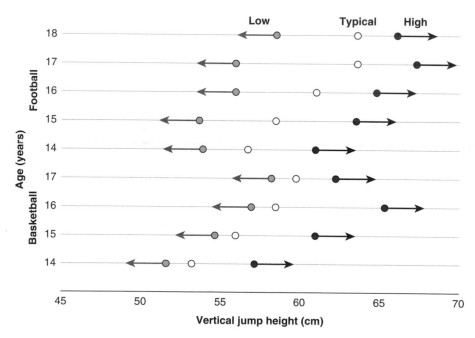

Figure 7.6 Vertical jump classifications for male high school American football and basketball players: high—70th percentile; typical—50th percentile; low—30th percentile.

Data from (16).

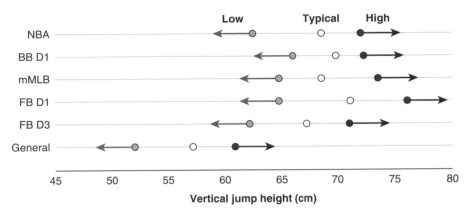

Figure 7.7 Vertical jump classifications for the male general adult population (General, 21-25 years old), National Collegiate Athletic Association (NCAA) Division I (FB D1) and III (FB D3) football players, minor and major league professional baseball players (mMLB), and NCAA Division (BB D1) and professional National Basketball Association (NBA) basketball players: high—70th percentile; typical—50th percentile; low—30th percentile.

Data from (16, 40).

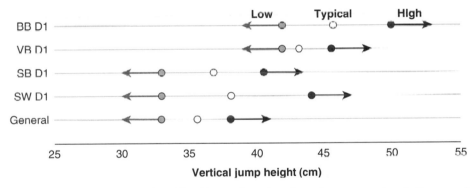

Figure 7.8 Vertical jump classifications for the female general adult population (General, 21-25 years old) and NCAA Division I swimming (SW D1), softball (SB D1), volleyball (VB D1), and basketball (BB D1) athletes: high—70th percentile; typical—50th percentile; low—30th percentile.

Data from (16, 40).

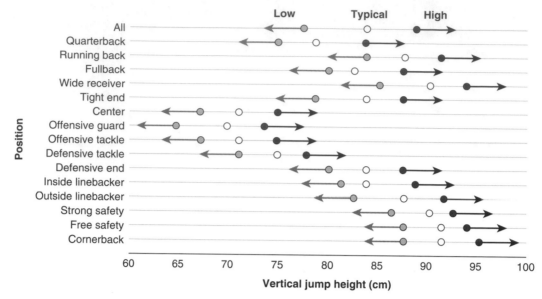

Figure 7.9 Vertical jump classifications from the NFL Scouting Combine: high—70th percentile; typical—50th percentile; low—30th percentile.

Data from (38).

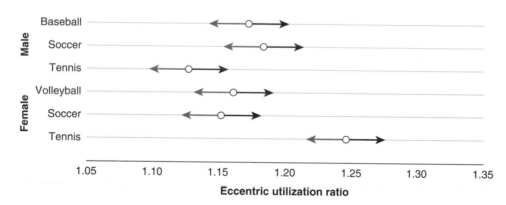

Figure 7.10 Descriptive (average) values for eccentric utilization ratio in various sports. Note: vertical jump and squat jumps were conducted with a PVC pipe placed across the shoulders.

Data from (55).

STANDING LONG JUMP TEST

Purpose

The standing long jump (also called the broad jump) test measures lower-body horizontal explosiveness or power.

Outcomes

Horizontal jump distance in centimeters or inches

Equipment Needed

Adhesive tape; measuring tape

Before You Begin

Place a 1-meter (3 ft) strip of adhesive tape on the ground to mark the starting line. A standardized warm-up, including three to five practice jumps performed at moderate intensity (approximately 50% of estimated maximal effort), followed by three to five minutes of rest and recovery, should be conducted prior to beginning the assessment.

Protocol

1. Begin the procedure by saying to the client or athlete: *"We are going to measure how far you can jump. Are you ready to begin? If so, please stand with your toes at the starting line."*

2. After the client or athlete has assumed the correct position, continue: *"When I say 'Go,' quickly perform a countermovement in which you bend your knees and rapidly swing your arms down past your hips prior to reversing the movement to maximally jump forward as far past the starting line as possible. Focus on landing safely back on both feet and hold this position so that your jump distance can be measured"* (see figure 7.11).

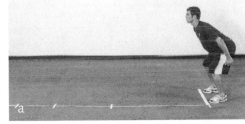
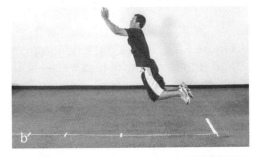
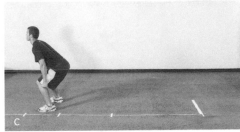

3. Position yourself so that you can clearly view the jump. Verbally signal the client or athlete *"3, 2, 1, go,"* and verify that the jump is begun with both feet flat on the ground and that the client or athlete performs a countermovement, jumps as far as possible, and lands under control without taking a step.

4. Record the distance to the closest centimeter or half inch between the starting line and the back of the client's or athlete's closest foot.

5. After the client or athlete has completed the initial standing long jump, say, *"Return to the starting position and relax,"* prior to making at least two more attempts, each separated by one minute of rest and recovery.

Figure 7.11 Standing long jump test.

Alternatives or Modifications

The standing long jump can also be performed without an arm swing by asking the client or athlete to keep hands on hips through the entire jump.

After You Finish

The longest recorded distance is the final result.

Research Notes

The force produced during a standing long jump has shown to be more closely related to sprint speed than the force produced during a vertical jump (7). Furthermore, standing long jump performance reportedly demonstrated a stronger relationship to 100-meter times recorded during competitive events than shorter distance (10-, 30-, and 50-meter) times recorded during speed testing sessions (26).

Normative Data

Standing long jump classification values are provided in figure 7.12 for the male general youth population and adult elite athletes, figure 7.13 for the female general youth population and adult elite athletes, and figure 7.14 from the NFL Scouting Combine.

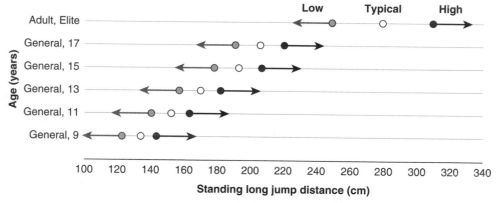

Figure 7.12 Standing long jump classifications for the male general youth population and adult elite athletes: high—70th percentile; typical—50th percentile; low—30th percentile.

Data from (2, 57).

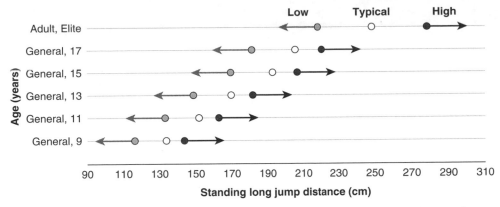

Figure 7.13 Standing long jump classifications for the female general youth population and adult elite athletes: high—70th percentile; typical—50th percentile; low—30th percentile.

Data from (2, 57).

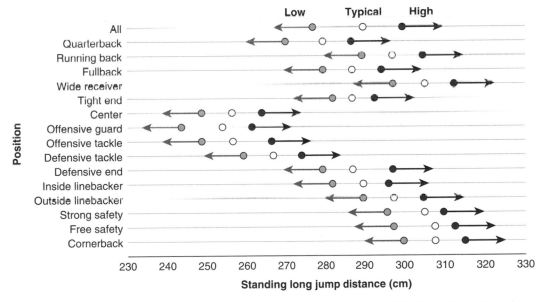

Figure 7.14 Standing long jump classifications from the NFL Scouting Combine: high—70th percentile; typical—50th percentile; low—30th percentile.

Data from (38).

SINGLE-LEG TRIPLE HOP TEST

Purpose

The single-leg triple hop test measures lower-body horizontal explosiveness or power on a single leg while providing leg-to-leg comparisons of balance, motor control, and strength.

Outcomes

Horizontal jump distance in centimeters or inches for each leg; side-to-side differences

Equipment Needed

Adhesive tape; measuring tape

Before You Begin

Place a one-meter (3 ft) strip of adhesive tape on the ground to mark the starting line. Identify the client's or athlete's dominant leg by asking which leg they would use for hopping or kicking a ball. A standardized warm-up, including practice hops performed at moderate intensity (approximately 50% of estimated maximal effort), followed by three to five minutes of rest and recovery, should be conducted prior to beginning the assessment.

Protocol

1. Begin the procedure by saying to the client or athlete: *"We are going to measure how far you can jump during several hops on one leg. Are you ready to begin? If so, please stand on your dominant leg with your toes at the starting line."*

2. After the client or athlete has assumed the correct position, continue by saying: *"When I say 'Go,' perform three single-legged hops as far forward past the starting line as possible. Use your arms for balance and focus on landing safely on two feet after the third hop. Afterward, hold the final position so that your jump distance can be measured"* (see figure 7.15 and figure 7.16).

3. Position yourself so that you can clearly view the jump. Verbally signal the client or athlete *"3, 2, 1, go,"* and verify that the hop begins with the foot flat on the ground and that the client or athlete lands under control on both feet without taking a step.

4. Record the distance to the closest centimeter or half inch between the starting line and the back of the client's or athlete's closest foot or heel.

5. After the client or athlete has completed the initial single-leg triple hop test, say, *"Return to the starting position and relax,"* prior to repeating the procedure with the opposite (nondominant) leg. The client or athlete will complete a total of three attempts per leg, with each attempt separated by 30 seconds to 1 minute of rest and recovery. The coach or fitness professional should also be keenly aware of the potential for a client or athlete to become fatigued during these tests and should be prepared to decrease the number of attempts if safety is compromised.

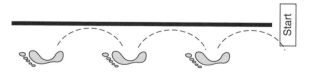

Figure 7.15 Foot placement for the single-leg triple hop test.

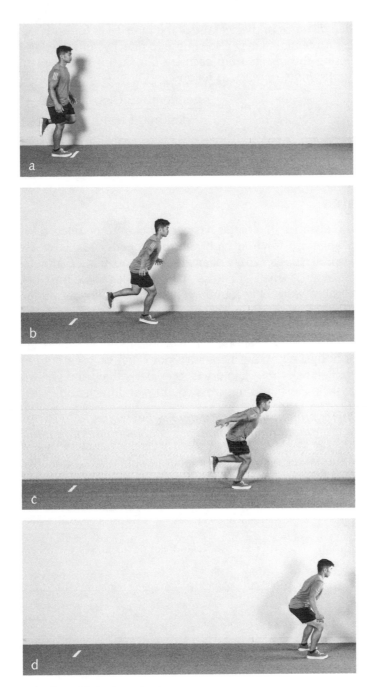

Figure 7.16 Single-leg triple hop test.

Alternatives or Modifications

The single-leg triple hop test can also be performed without an arm swing by asking the client or athlete to keep hands on hips through the series of hops, or with the client or athlete landing on one foot (rather than both feet) following the third and final hop. Additional versions of this test include adding a lateral (side-to-side) component to the standard distance test, which requires the client or athlete to perform three crossover hops (back and forth across a straight line) on a single leg.

After You Finish

The longest recorded distance or the average of the three trials for each leg is the final result. The coach or fitness professional may also choose to directly compare leg-to-leg differences or imbalances by using the results from each leg during the single-leg triple hop test and calculating the lateral symmetry index as follows:

$$\text{Lateral symmetry index} = \frac{\text{nondominant leg distance}}{\text{dominant leg distance}} \times 100$$

Lateral symmetry index values below 100 percent indicate that during the nondominant leg triple hop test, less distance was covered and some underlying between-leg performance differences exist.

Research Notes

Single-leg triple hop distance in athletes has been shown to be related to the vertical jump and the ability to generate force at high and low speeds (13) as well as short-distance (≤10 m [32.8 ft]) sprint speed (25). Collegiate male and female athletes perform better than high school male and female athletes in the single-leg triple hop; however, significant between-leg differences were only found in the female collegiate athletes (36). From an injury or sport readiness perspective, the symmetry index comparing triple hop distance between legs has shown to be reduced in female athletes who had been cleared to return to their sport after undergoing anterior cruciate ligament (ACL) reconstruction surgery (60). When adjusted for body weight, the symmetry index may be greater in athletes participating in sports with a high risk for ACL injury (soccer, basketball, and volleyball) than athletes participating in low-risk sports (diving, cross country, and track and field) (18).

Normative Data

Descriptive values for the single-leg triple hop test in various populations are provided in figure 7.17. While specific cutoffs are recommended (approximately 90%), healthy, active individuals may display lateral symmetry index values between 85 and 90 percent. Therefore, baseline measures and client or athlete tracking over time is advisable.

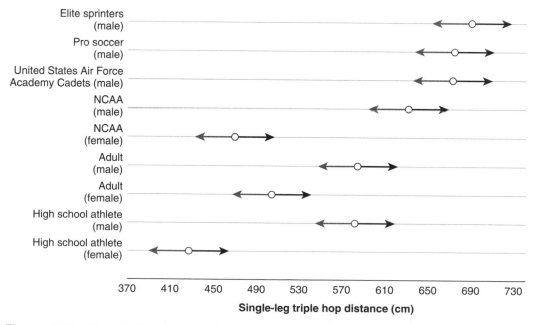

Figure 7.17 Descriptive (average) values for the single-leg triple hop test in various populations. Note: data taken from research studies employing a variety of different protocols (with and without arm swing, one- and two-foot landing, best performance or average of three trials, etc.) and only the greater distance of the two legs is reported.

Data from (36, 54).

MEDICINE BALL CHEST PASS TEST

Purpose

The medicine ball chest pass test measures upper-body explosiveness or power during a pushing movement.

Outcomes

Horizontal throwing distance in centimeters or inches

Equipment Needed

Adhesive tape; measuring tape; bench with 45-degree incline; adequate vertical and horizontal clearance to safely complete the assessment; medicine ball (6 kg [13.2 lb] for females, 9 kg [19.8 lb] for males); spotter

Before You Begin

Extend a measuring tape at least 25 feet (7.6 m) out from the starting point where the medicine ball would contact the client's or athlete's chest prior to a throwing attempt. Secure the measuring tape on the floor under the front support beam of the bench and lay it out in the direction of the throw. A standardized warm-up, including upper-body specific movements and practice throws performed at moderate intensity (approximately 50% of estimated maximal effort), followed by three to five minutes of rest and recovery, should be conducted prior to beginning the assessment.

Protocol

1. Begin the procedure by saying to the client or athlete: "We are going to measure how far you can throw a medicine ball. Are you ready to begin? If so, please pick up the medicine ball, take a seat on the bench, and then lean back so your torso and head are in contact with the bench. Check that your feet are flat on the floor a comfortable distance apart."

2. After the client or athlete has assumed the correct position, continue: "When I say 'Go,' bring the medicine ball to your chest with both hands and maximally push it away from your body as far as possible. Focus on releasing the medicine ball at a 45-degree angle relative to the floor so you can get the greatest distance" (see figure 7.18).

3. Position yourself so that you can clearly view the throw. Verbally signal the client or athlete "3, 2, 1, go," and verify that he or she remains in contact with the bench during the throw. A spotter placed near the end of the measuring tape should attempt to mark the landing point. (Alternatively, the ball can be covered with chalk to aid in identifying the proper location.) In order for an attempt to be counted, the medicine ball should land within 2 feet (0.6 m) of the measuring tape.

4. Record the distance to the closest centimeter or half inch between the starting point and the landing point.

5. After the client or athlete has completed the initial medicine ball pass, say, "Relax," prior to making at least two more attempts, each separated by two to three minutes of rest and recovery.

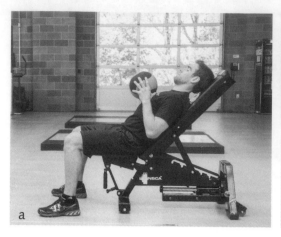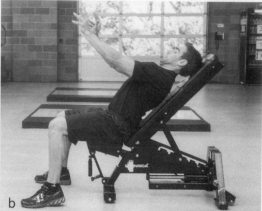

Figure 7.18   Medicine ball chest pass.

Alternatives or Modifications

The medicine ball chest pass may be conducted with the client or athlete seated on a chair (for example, in older adults, with a 3-kilogram [6.6 lb] medicine ball (14)) or a bench with a 90-degree incline, on the floor with knees either bent or extended and with the back against the wall (for example, in five- to six-year-old children with a 2-pound [0.9 kg], 8-inch [20 cm] diameter medicine ball (6)), and from a kneeling position. A seated one-armed version of this test that allows for side-to-side comparisons can also be completed.

After You Finish

The longest recorded distance is the final result.

Research Notes

Medicine ball chest pass performance has been shown to be highly related to power output during a bench press throw test (5) and a significant predictor variable for club head speed in golfers with single-figure handicaps (43). In collegiate American football players, medicine ball chest pass performance, using a bench with a 90-degree incline, was reported to increase following a 15-week (4 days per week) offseason resistance training program (17).

Normative Data

Due to the wide variety of assessment protocols employed and the size of medicine balls used, limited widespread normative data is available. Medicine ball chest pass classification values for college-aged men and women are provided in figure 7.19.

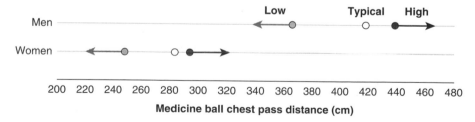

Figure 7.19   Medicine ball chest pass classifications for college-aged men and women: high—70th percentile; typical—50th percentile; low—30th percentile. A 6-kilogram (13.2 lb) medicine ball was used for females, and a 9-kilogram (19.8 lb) medicine ball was used for males.

Data from (5).

FORWARD OVERHEAD MEDICINE BALL THROW TEST

Purpose

The forward overhead medicine ball throw test measures total body explosiveness or power during a pushing or throwing and forward bending motion.

Outcomes

Horizontal throwing distance in centimeters or inches

Equipment Needed

Adhesive tape; measuring tape; adequate vertical and horizontal clearance to safely complete the assessment; medicine ball (various sizes; 2 kg is recommended for tennis athletes); spotter

Before You Begin

Place a 1-meter (3 ft) strip of adhesive tape on the ground to mark the starting line, and similar parallel strips every 0.5 meters (20 in.) up to a total distance appropriate for the client or athlete being evaluated to determine the landing point. A standardized warm-up, including upper-body-specific movements and practice throws performed at moderate intensities (approximately 50% of estimated maximal effort), followed by three to five minutes of rest and recovery, should be conducted prior to beginning the assessment.

Protocol

1. Begin the procedure by saying to the client or athlete: *"We are going to assess how far you can throw a medicine ball. Are you ready to begin? If so, please pick up the medicine ball and stand back behind the starting line with your feet parallel."*

2. After the client or athlete has assumed the correct position, continue: *"When I say 'Go,' bring the medicine ball up and back over your head with both hands and, without taking a step, throw the ball as far forward as possible. During the throwing motion, your back will slightly hyperextend; however, do not move your feet, focus on maintaining your balance, and throw the medicine ball straight ahead"* (see figure 7.20).

3. Position yourself so that you can clearly view the throw. Verbally signal the client or athlete *"3, 2, 1, go,"* and verify that he or she does not cross the starting line. A spotter placed a safe distance behind the client or athlete should attempt to mark the landing point. (Alternatively, the ball can be covered with chalk to aid in identifying the landing location.)

4. Record the distance to the closest centimeter or half inch between the starting line and the landing point.

5. After the client or athlete has completed the initial throw, say, *"Return to the start position and relax,"* prior to continuing attempts separated by one minute of rest and recovery until two consecutive throws are within 0.5 meters (20 in.) of each other.

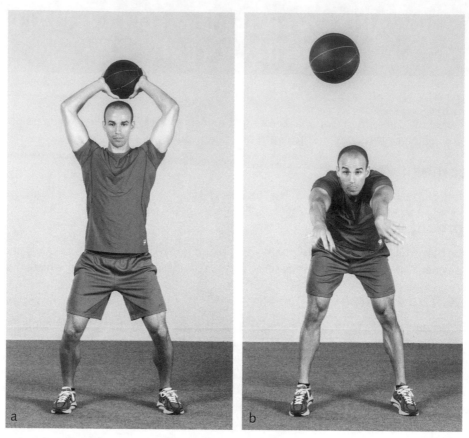

Figure 7.20 Forward overhead medicine ball throw.

Alternatives or Modifications

A standing version with a step or a kneeling version of the forward overhead medicine ball throw, which removes the influence of the lower body, may also be conducted.

After You Finish

The longest recorded distance is considered the final result.

Research Notes

Forward overhead medicine ball throw performance may be of particular relevance to athletes who are required to produce powerful movements with their arms overhead (termed *over-head athletes*). For example, youth tennis players demonstrated improved forward overhead medicine ball throw performance following eight weeks of twice-weekly plyometric training consisting of both upper- and lower-body exercise (10).

Backward overhead medicine ball throw performance likely differs by playing position in volleyball (29) and in soccer with forwards exhibiting greater throwing distances than defenders (27). Professional female volleyball players have shown improvements in this measure during a competitive season (28).

Normative Data

Forward overhead medicine ball throw classification values for elite tennis players are provided in figure 7.21. Descriptive values for the forward overhead medicine ball throw in volleyball players are provided in figure 7.22 and in male youth soccer players in figure 7.23 and figure 7.24.

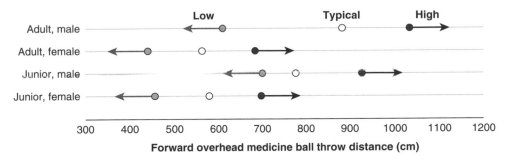

Figure 7.21 Forward overhead medicine ball throw classifications for elite tennis players. A 6-pound (2.7 kg) medicine ball was used.

Data from (9, 46).

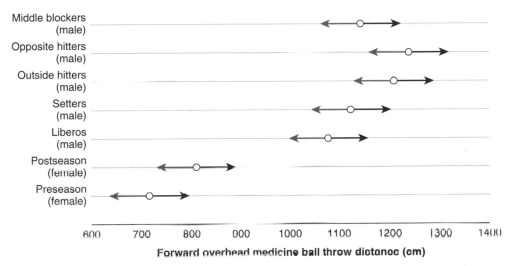

Figure 7.22 Descriptive (average) values for the forward overhead medicine ball throw in professional volleyball players. A 3-kilogram (6.6 lb) medicine ball was used.

Data from (28, 29).

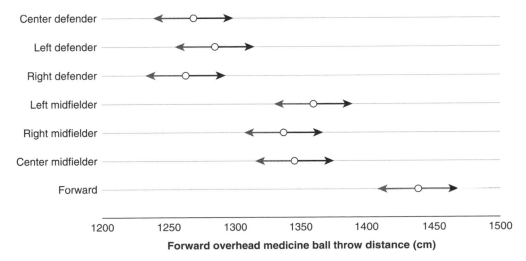

Figure 7.23 Descriptive (average) values for the forward overhead medicine ball throw in male youth soccer players separated by position. A 5-kilogram (11 lb) medicine ball was used.

Data from (27).

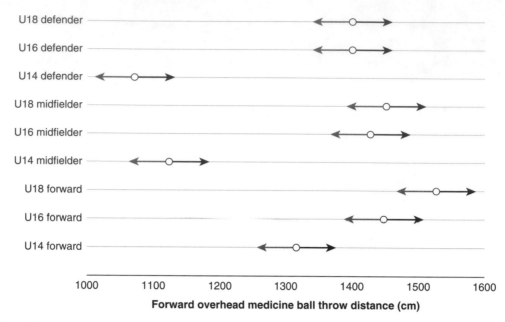

Figure 7.24 Descriptive (average) values for the forward overhead medicine ball throw in male youth soccer players separated by age group. A 5-kilogram (11 lb) medicine ball was used.

Data from (27).

BACKWARD OVERHEAD MEDICINE BALL THROW TEST

Purpose

The backward overhead medicine ball throw test measures total body explosiveness or power during a pushing or throwing and backward extending motion.

Outcomes

Horizontal throwing distance in centimeters or inches

Equipment Needed

Adhesive tape; measuring tape; adequate vertical and horizontal clearance to safely complete the assessment; medicine ball (various sizes); spotter

Before You Begin

Place a 1-meter (3 ft) strip of adhesive tape on the ground to mark the starting line, and similar parallel strips every 0.5 meters (20 in.) up to a total distance appropriate for the client or athlete being evaluated to determine the landing point. A standardized warm-up, including upper-body-specific movements and practice throws performed at moderate intensity (approximately 50% of estimated maximal effort), followed by three to five minutes of rest and recovery, should be conducted prior to beginning the assessment.

Protocol

1. Begin the procedure by saying to the client or athlete: "*We are going to measure how far you can throw a medicine ball. Are you ready to begin? If so, please pick up the medicine ball and stand behind the starting line.*"

2. After the client or athlete has assumed the correct position, continue: "*When I say 'Go,' extend your arms forward and bring the medicine ball to chest height directly in front of you with both hands, then quickly bend your knees and swing your arms and the medicine ball down between them. Without pausing or stopping, immediately reverse the movement to jump up and swing the medicine ball up, over, and backward over your head as forcefully as possible. Focus on keeping your arms straight throughout the movement and on landing safely after releasing the medicine ball*" (see figure 7.25).

3. Position yourself so that you can clearly view the throw. Verbally signal the client or athlete "*3, 2, 1, go,*" and verify that the knees do not bend past 90 degrees and shoulders do not lean too far forward. A spotter placed a safe distance behind the client or athlete should attempt to mark the landing point. (Alternatively, the ball can be covered with chalk to aid in identifying the landing location.)

4. Record the distance to the closest centimeter or half inch between the starting line and the landing point.

5. After the client or athlete has completed the initial throw, say, "*Return to the start position and relax,*" prior to continuing attempts separated by one minute of rest and recovery until two consecutive throws are within 0.5 meters (20 in.) of each other.

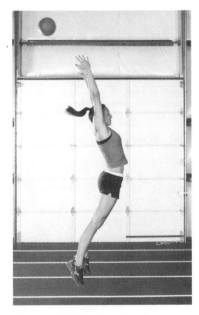

Figure 7.25 Backward overhead medicine ball throw.

Alternatives or Modifications

Some backward overhead medicine ball throw protocols require the client or athlete to maintain foot contact with the ground throughout the entire throwing motion. This approach potentially allows for greater control (and safety) but decreases the explosiveness of the maneuver resulting in shorter throwing distances. A seated version of the backward overhead medicine ball throw, which removes the influence of the lower body, may also be conducted.

After You Finish

The longest recorded distance is the final result.

Research Notes

Backward overhead medicine ball throw performance has been shown to be related to power output generated during a vertical jump in a variety of athletes, including volleyball players (50), football players (31), and wrestlers (51), as well as maximal strength during Olympic lifting (snatch and clean and jerk) (39).

Interestingly, backward overhead medicine ball throw distance is reportedly a significant predictor variable of cross-country skiing performance in boys (13-14 years old) but not in girls with whom 3,000-meter running time was the best predictor variable (52).

Normative Data

Backward overhead medicine ball throw classification values for elite tennis players are provided in figure 7.26. Descriptive values for the backward overhead medicine ball throw in various populations are provided in figure 7.27 and figure 7.28.

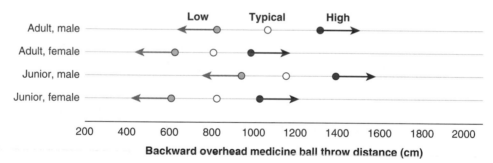

Figure 7.26 Backward overhead medicine ball throw classifications for elite tennis players. A 6-pound (2.7 kg) medicine ball was used.

Data from (9, 46).

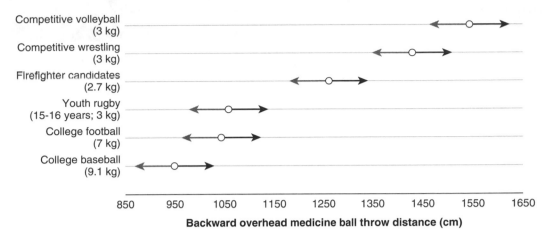

Figure 7.27 Descriptive (average) values for the backward overhead medicine ball throw in various male populations. Medicine ball size indicated as kilograms (kg).

Data from (3, 5a, 8, 31, 51).

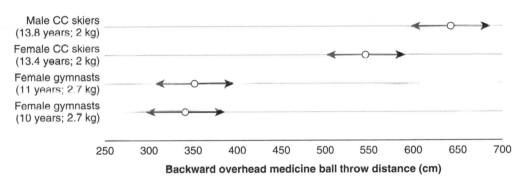

Figure 7.28 Descriptive (average) values for the backward overhead medicine ball throw in various female youth gymnasts and male and female cross-country skiers. Medicine ball size indicated as kilograms (kg).

Data from (47, 52).

ROTATING MEDICINE BALL THROW TEST

Purpose

The rotating medicine ball throw test measures upper-body explosiveness or power during a twisting motion.

Outcomes

Sideways throwing distance in centimeters or inches

Equipment Needed

Adhesive tape; measuring tape; adequate vertical and horizontal clearance to safely complete the assessment; medicine ball (various sizes); spotter

Before You Begin

Place a 1-meter (3 ft) strip of adhesive tape on the ground to mark the starting line, and similar parallel strips every 0.5 meters (20 in.) up to a total distance appropriate for the client or athlete being evaluated to determine the landing point. A standardized warm-up, including upper-body-specific movements and practice throws performed at moderate intensities (approximately 50% of estimated maximal effort), followed by three to five minutes of rest and recovery, should be conducted prior to beginning the assessment.

Protocol

1. Begin the procedure by saying the following to the client or athlete: *"We are going to measure how far you can throw a medicine ball. Are you ready to begin? If so, please pick up the medicine ball and stand sideways behind the starting line."*

2. After the client or athlete has assumed the correct position, continue by saying: *"When I say 'Go,' extend your arms forward and bring the medicine ball to chest height directly in front of you with both hands. Quickly rotate away from the starting line, then swing your arms and the medicine ball back toward the starting line before throwing it as far sideways as possible. Focus on keeping your arms straight and feet on the ground, maintaining your balance, and throwing the medicine ball in a straight line"* (see figure 7.29).

3. Position yourself so that you can clearly view the throw. Verbally signal the client or athlete "3, 2, 1, go," and verify that his or her feet do not cross the starting line. A spotter placed a safe distance behind the client or athlete should attempt to mark the landing point. (Alternatively, the ball can be covered with chalk to aid in identifying the landing location.)

4. Record the distance to the closest centimeter or half inch between the starting line and the landing point.

5. After the client or athlete has completed the initial throw, say, *"Return to the start position and relax,"* prior to testing the throw in the opposite direction and continuing attempts separated by one minute of rest and recovery until two consecutive throws on a given side are within 0.5 meters (20 in.) of each other.

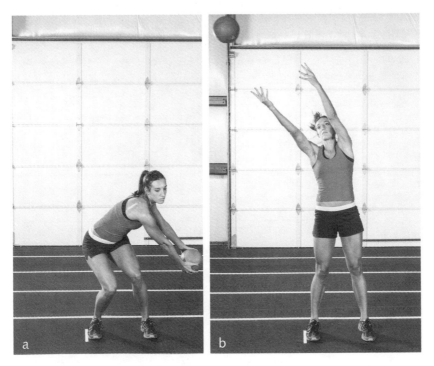

Figure 7.29 Rotating medicine ball throw.

Alternatives or Modifications

Kneeling or seated versions of the rotating medicine ball throw, which remove the influence of the lower body, have also been conducted. A sport-specific modification of this test, termed the *medicine ball hitter's throw*, requires that the athlete assume a typical batting stance and hold a 1-kilogram (2.2 lb) medicine ball with two hands at shoulder level prior to completing the throwing motion in a manner similar to swinging a baseball bat (56).

After You Finish

The longest recorded distance for each side is the final result.

Research Notes

Rotating medicine ball throw performance provides an indication of the ability to produce force during trunk rotation and both upper- and lower-body power output, which typically requires expensive, instrumented equipment and additional safety considerations (9). Rotating medicine ball throw performance has shown to correlate to the ability to produce rotational force in tennis players (9), club head speed in golfers (43), and cricket ball-throwing velocity in cricket players (11).

Normative Data

Rotating medicine ball throw classification values for elite tennis players are provided in figure 7.30. Descriptive values for the rotating medicine ball throw in young men and women with different-sized medicine balls are provided in figure 7.31.

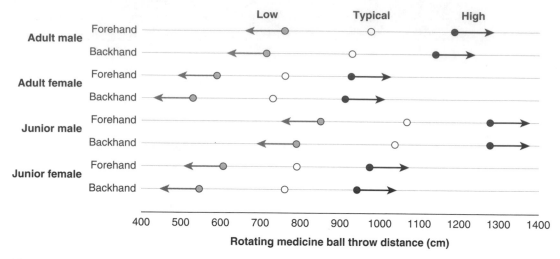

Figure 7.30 Rotating medicine ball throw classifications for elite tennis players. A 6-pound (2.7 kg) medicine ball was used.

Data from (9, 46).

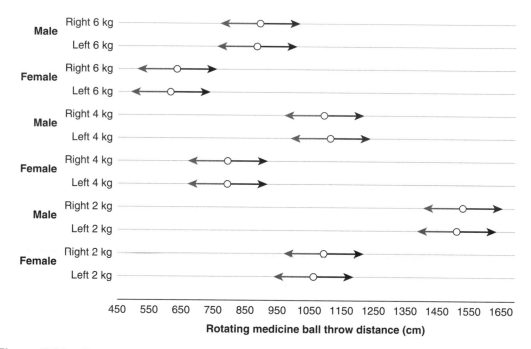

Figure 7.31 Descriptive (average) values for the rotating medicine ball throw in young men and women. Side indicated as right or left and medicine ball size indicated as kilograms (kg).

Data from (20, 46).

STAIR SPRINT POWER TEST

Purpose

The stair sprint power test (also called the Margaria-Kalamen test) measures lower-body power and explosiveness while running up an incline.

Outcomes

Time, in seconds, needed to complete the intended movement pattern; estimated average power output

Equipment Needed

Stairs with at least nine stair steps that are approximately 17 to 18.5 centimeters (0.170 to 0.185 m or 6.7 to 7.28 in.) high and 29 to 32 centimeters (0.29 to 0.32 m or 11.4 to 12.6 in.) deep with a lead-up length of approximately 6 meters (20 ft); adhesive tape; measuring stick or tape; timing device

Before You Begin

Follow the procedures outlined in chapter 4 to record the client's or athlete's body weight in kilograms. Verify the height of the steps and determine the vertical distance between the third and the ninth stair step in meters (typically 0.17 m × 6 stair steps = 1.02 m). Place a strip of adhesive tape on the ground six meters from the base of the staircase to serve as the starting line. A schematic for this version of the stair sprint power test is provided in figure 7.32. Also note that a standardized warm-up, including several practice stair sprints performed at moderate intensities (approximately 50 to 80% of estimated maximal effort), followed by three to five minutes of rest and recovery, should be conducted prior to beginning the assessment.

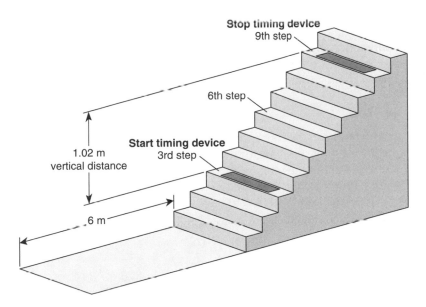

Figure 7.32 Setup for the stair sprint power test (Margaria-Kalamen test).

Adapted by permission from G.G. Haff and C. Dumke, *Laboratory Manual for Exercise Physiology,* 2nd ed. (Champaign, IL: Human Kinetics, 2019), 300.

Protocol

1. Begin the procedure by saying to the client or athlete: *"We are going to measure how quickly you can sprint up this staircase. Are you ready to begin? If so, please stand behind the starting line."*

2. Next, explain: *"When I say 'Go,' sprint forward and go up the staircase three steps at a time as fast as possible to complete the test."*

3. Position yourself so that you can clearly view the third and ninth stair steps. Verbally signal the client or athlete *"3, 2, 1, go,"* and start the timing device when the third stair step is reached and stop it when the ninth stair step is reached. Record this to the nearest 0.01 second.

4. After the client or athlete has completed the initial test, say, *"Return to the starting position and relax,"* prior to making two more attempts, each separated by two to three minutes of rest and recovery.

Alternatives or Modifications

An alternative version of the test can be performed when 6 meters of lead-up length is not available. In this test, the timing device begins when the client's or athlete's foot makes contact with the first step and stops when five strides at two stair steps per stride have been climbed. This version of the stair sprint test was established with 18.5-centimeter (0.185 m or 7.28 in.) stair steps, which equals a total vertical distance of 2.04 meters (0.185 meters × 11 stair steps).

After You Finish

The fastest recorded time is the final result. Coaches or fitness professionals can then calculate average power output using the following formula:

$$\text{Power (watts)} = \frac{\text{body weight (kg)} \times 9.807 \times \text{height (m)}}{\text{time (sec)}}$$

The height in this equation will be determined by the vertical distance between the first and final steps outlined in the assessment protocol (i.e., 1.02 m or 2.04 m). Coaches or fitness professionals can then divide the average power output by body weight to account for size differences between clients or athletes.

Research Notes

Power output calculated from the stair sprint power test was found to be more influential than the vertical jump or 50-meter sprint performance when evaluating explosiveness (or anaerobic power) in athletes and nonathletes engaged in plyometric training (59). Furthermore, the stair sprint power test performance has been shown to differentiate between playing positions in American football (15) and demonstrated to have a positive relationship with an on-ice sprint skate test in youth hockey players (42).

Normative Data

Stair sprint test power classification values are provided in figure 7.33. Descriptive values for stair sprint test power values relative to body mass in various groups are provided in figure 7.34.

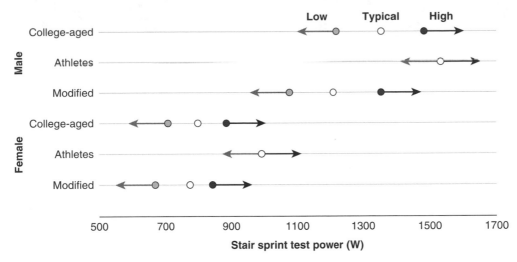

Figure 7.33 Stair sprint test classifications for various groups (electronic timing system): high—70th percentile; typical—50th percentile; low—30th percentile. Modified: see "Alternatives or Modifications" section for details.

Data from (1, 4, 30, 32).

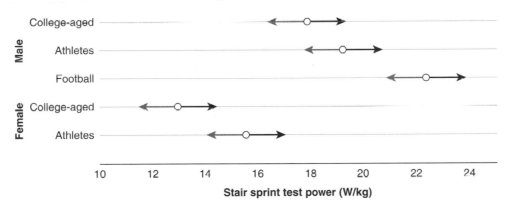

Figure 7.34 Descriptive values for the stair sprint test for various groups (electronic timing system). Reported in watts per kilogram of body weight (W/kg).

Data from (1, 30, 32, 49).

ROWING ERGOMETER PEAK POWER TEST

Purpose

The rowing ergometer peak power test measures whole-body power or explosiveness during a lower-body pushing motion and an upper-body/trunk-pulling motion.

Outcomes

Peak power output, in watts or watts per kilogram of body weight, during a rowing stroke

Equipment Needed

Rowing ergometer

Before You Begin

Follow the procedures outlined in chapter 4 to record the client's or athlete's body weight in kilograms. Set the adjustable resistance level to the highest setting: 10 for nonrowers (or 5 for trained rowers) and the on-board computer to display watts and strokes per minute. Review the basic elements of a rowing stroke with the client or athlete (preferably during a familiarization session prior to testing) as outlined in table 7.1. Also note that a standardized warm-up, including five minutes of rowing performed at moderate intensity (approximately 50 to 80% of estimated maximal effort), followed by three to five minutes of rest and recovery, should be conducted prior to beginning the assessment.

Table 7.1   Basic Elements of a Rowing Stroke

1. Start	2. Drive
• Arms are out in front of the torso with the elbows fully extended • Head is in a neutral position • Shoulders are level with the ground and in front of the hips • Shins are vertical and the knees are bent without going past 90° • Feet are fully in contact with the foot plate	• Extend the hips and knees to push with the legs to drive through the foot plate • Maintain upper-body position • As the hips and knees extend, lean the upper body back and pull the hands to the lower ribs
3. Finish	**4. Recovery**
• Hips and knees are fully extended with the handle near the lower ribs • Upper body is slightly reclined with support from the core muscles • Head is in a neutral position • Neck and shoulders are relaxed	• Reverse the movement of the drive • Elbows are extended with the arms out in front of the torso • Lean the upper body forward and bend the knees as the seat slides forward

Protocol

1. Begin the procedure by saying to the client or athlete: *"We are going to measure how hard you can pull during a rowing stroke. Are you ready to begin? If so, please have a seat on the rowing ergometer, tighten the foot plate straps around your feet, and grasp the handle with both hands."*

2. Next, explain: *"When I say 'Go,' pull on the handle while going completely through the start, drive, finish, and recovery phases for a total of six initial warm-up strokes followed by six all-out strokes, pulling as hard and fast as possible to complete the test"* (see figure 7.35).

3. Position yourself so that you can clearly view the performance monitor. Verbally signal the client or athlete *"3, 2, 1, go,"* and verify that the client or athlete maintains a stroke rate of 35 to 45 strokes per minute while recording the power outputs displayed by the on-board computer for each stroke.

4. After the client or athlete has completed the initial test, say, *"Return to the starting position and relax,"* prior to making at least one more attempt separated by three to five minutes of rest and recovery.

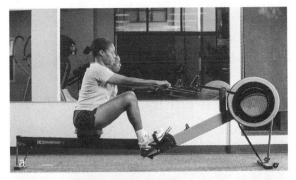
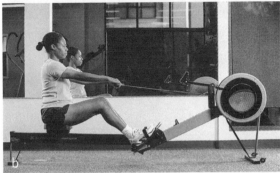
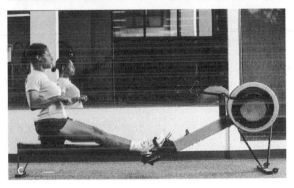

Figure 7.35 The (a) start, (b) drive, and (c) finish elements of a rowing stroke.

Alternatives or Modifications

Protocols containing up to 15 rowing strokes have been used to evaluate peak power, and the coach or fitness professional should verify that a relative plateau in power output has been achieved during the assessment.

After You Finish

The highest recorded peak power during a single stroke is the final result. Coaches or fitness professionals can then divide the peak power output by body weight to account for size differences between clients or athletes.

Research Notes

Peak power determined on a rowing ergometer has been shown to be related to bench pull and power clean performance in trained rowers (24). In a more varied group consisting of inactive and physically active men and women as well as rowing athletes, rowing ergometer peak power correlated significantly to countermovement jump peak power determined using a force plate (34).

Normative Data

Descriptive values for the rowing ergometer peak power test in various populations are provided in figure 7.36.

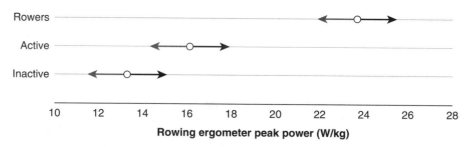

Figure 7.36 Descriptive (average) values for the rowing ergometer peak power test in male and female rowing athletes, physically active individuals, and physically inactive individuals. Reported in watts per kilogram of body weight (W/kg).

Data from (34).

CHAPTER 8

Muscular Strength and Endurance

> *"If the statistics are boring, then you've got the wrong numbers."*
>
> Edward R. Tufte, Statistician

Musculoskeletal fitness is commonly evaluated through the static (without movement) or dynamic (with movement) assessment of muscular strength and muscular endurance. Because muscular strength is an indicator of force production and contributes to power output (along with speed or velocity), it plays a large direct or indirect role in many activities of daily living, recreational endeavors, and sports performance. Furthermore, higher levels of muscular strength may provide a protective effect with respect to injury. While maximal dynamic strength can be safely measured using a one-repetition maximum (1RM) test in resistance-trained individuals, coaches or fitness professionals working with athletes or clients who have minimal training may elect to use a multiple-repetition maximum test or a static test (e.g., using a handgrip dynamometer) that can be generalized to more functional movements. Muscular endurance can also be measured via a static or dynamic test to evaluate general health and injury risk or as a measure of force production over an extended period of time (or during repeated movements). In particular, muscular endurance tests are included in many testing batteries focused on children, older adults, and occupational settings due to their relevance to day-to-day tasks and work-related duties. The movement pattern and muscle groups engaged will likely dictate which assessments are most appropriate for a given situation. The assessments covered in this chapter are as follows:

- One-repetition maximum strength test: back squat, leg press, bench press, and bench pull (21, 34)
- Multiple-repetition maximum strength test (21, 34)
- Maximal handgrip strength test (8)
- Static muscular endurance tests: prone bridge (or plank) (28); half-squat (or wall-sit) (22); and flexed-arm hang (or bent-arm hang) (29)
- Dynamic muscular endurance tests: partial curl-ups (or bent-knee sit-ups) (21); push-ups (21); squats (4); and pull-ups (29)
- YMCA bench press test (21)

ONE-REPETITION MAXIMUM STRENGTH TEST

Purpose

The one-repetition maximum (1RM) strength test measures the maximal strength of the muscle groups engaged during a single specified movement.

Outcomes

Maximum amount of weight lifted for a single repetition (termed *absolute strength*); maximum strength relative to body weight (termed *relative strength*)

Equipment Needed

Rack or stands; flat bench or leg press; barbell; safety locks; weight plates; spotters

Before You Begin

Follow the procedures outlined in chapter 4 to record the client's or athlete's body weight. Review the basic elements of the movement to be assessed (preferably during a familiarization session prior to testing) with the client or athlete and spotters as outlined in tables 8.1 through 8.4 and figures 8.1 through 8.4. These selections should be made with consideration for the muscle groups used, with the leg press and back squat used to evaluate the lower body and the bench press and bench pull used to evaluate the upper body, and the relevant movements (i.e., the bench press for pushing and the bench pull for pulling).

Clear the lifting area, place the supports at the appropriate height in order to hold the barbell at an easily accessible location for the client or athlete, lower the safety bars enough to allow for the full range of motion, and make sure that the collars are in working order. Verify that the selected spotters are of adequate size and strength to support the loads lifted by the client or athlete being evaluated. Prior to attempting the 1RM test, determine a phrase ("Take it") or action that will signal that the client or athlete cannot complete a repetition. Upon hearing or seeing this signal, the spotters should grasp the barbell and assist with reracking it on the supports.

A standardized general warm-up followed by three to five minutes of rest and recovery should be conducted prior to beginning the assessment. A specific lifting warm-up is built into the 1RM protocol.

Table 8.1 Back Squat Technique

1. Starting position (barbell on the rack)	2. Downward movement
Client or athlete • With the feet parallel, position the barbell across the shoulders or back and grip with the hands (with the palms forward and the thumbs wrapped underneath) a comfortable distance outside of the shoulders • Bring the elbows under the barbell with the chest up and the eyes forward before lifting it from the rack supports and taking a step or two backward • Reposition the feet to shoulder-width apart or wider and point the toes slightly outward *Two spotters* • Stand at each end of the barbell and grip with both hands (with the thumbs crossed below) • Coordinate with the client or athlete to assist with the liftoff of the barbell and release the hands but keep them in close proximity	*Client or athlete* • Keep the back straight, chest up, eyes forward, and elbows down; maintain the grip on the barbell • Slowly bend the knees and hips (similar to sitting in a chair) and lower the barbell in a smooth, controlled motion; maintain the heels on the floor and the knees over the feet • Continue the descent until the thighs are parallel with the ground, the back begins to bend excessively, or the heels begin to rise from the floor *Two spotters* • Without touching the barbell, mirror its downward movement using both hands (with the thumbs crossed below) • Keep the back straight while bending the knees and hips through the descent of the barbell
3. Upward movement	**4. Completion**
Client or athlete • Keep the back straight, chest up, eyes forward, and elbows down; maintain the grip on the barbell • Simultaneously extend the knees and hips and raise the barbell in a smooth, controlled motion until reaching the starting position *Two spotters* • Without touching the barbell, mirror its upward movement using both hands (with the thumbs crossed below) • Keep the back straight while extending the knees and hips through the ascent of the barbell	*Client or athlete* • Following completion of the intended number of repetitions and returning to the starting position, step forward and position the barbell back on the supports • Slightly bend the knees and lower the shoulders from under the racked barbell *Two spotters* • Grip the barbell with both hands to assist with placing the barbell back on the supports

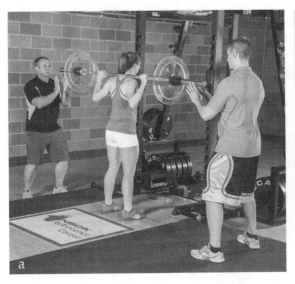 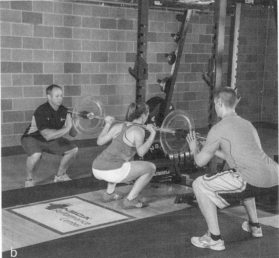

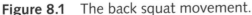

Figure 8.1 The back squat movement.

Table 8.2 Leg Press Technique

1. Starting position	2. Downward movement
Client or athlete • Take a seat in the machine with the back and buttocks flat on the support pads • Place the feet parallel hip-width apart with full contact on the platform and the toes pointing slightly outward • Grip the stationary handles located at the sides of the seat and straighten the knees (but do not lock them) • Let go of the stationary handles, release the support mechanism, and regrip the stationary handles *Two spotters* • Coordinate with the client or athlete to assist with the liftoff of the sled and release the hands but stay in close proximity	*Client or athlete* • Keep the back and buttocks flat on the support pads; maintain the grip on the stationary handles and the feet on platform • Slowly bend the knees and hips and lower the sled in a smooth, controlled motion • Continue the descent until the thighs are parallel with the platform *Two spotters* • Stand alert at the side of the sled during its downward movement and, if needed, be prepared to step in front of the sled to assist the client or athlete by supporting the platform
3. Upward movement	**4. Completion**
Client or athlete • Keep the back and buttocks flat on the support pads; maintain the grip on the stationary handles and the feet on platform • Slowly extend the knees (without locking them) and the hips, and raise the sled in a smooth, controlled motion • Continue the ascent until reaching the starting position *Two spotters* • Stand alert at the side of the sled during its upward movement and, if needed, be prepared to step in front of the sled to assist the client or athlete by supporting the platform	*Client or athlete* • Following completion of the intended number of repetitions and returning to the starting position, let go of the stationary handles and engage the support mechanism • Remove the feet and exit the seat *Two spotters* • Assist by supporting the platform until the support mechanism is engaged and the client has safely exited the seat

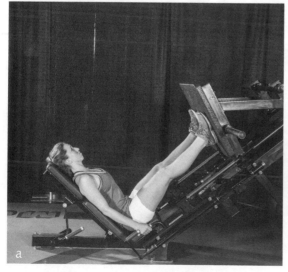 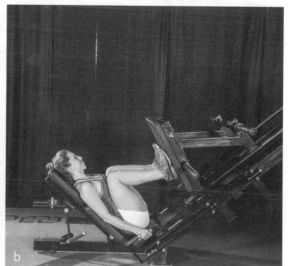

Figure 8.2 Leg press movement.

Table 8.3 Bench Press Technique

1. Starting position (barbell on the rack)	2. Downward movement
Client or athlete • Lie down on the bench facing up while making contact with the head and shoulders or back, with feet flat on the ground • Adjust the body so that the eyes are in line with the barbell; grip with the hands (palms forward and thumbs wrapped underneath) a comfortable distance outside of the shoulders • Extend the elbows and lift the barbell from the rack supports and position it over the chest *Spotter* • Stand at the client's or athlete's head and grip the barbell with both hands (with the palm of one hand facing forward and the other facing backward, and the thumbs wrapped underneath) • Coordinate with the client or athlete to assist with the liftoff of the barbell and release the hands but keep them in close proximity to the barbell	*Client or athlete* • Keep the head and shoulders or back in contact with the bench, and keep the feet on the ground • Ensure that the forearms are parallel with each other and perpendicular to the ground; maintain the position of the wrists • Slowly bend the elbows and lower the barbell in a smooth, controlled motion until contacting the lower portion of the chest *Spotter* • Without touching the barbell, mirror its downward movement with both hands (with the palm of one hand facing forward and the other facing backward, and the thumbs wrapped underneath) • Keep the back straight while bending the knees and hips along with the descent of the barbell
3. Upward movement	**4. Completion**
Client or athlete • Keep the head and shoulders/back in contact with the bench and the feet on the ground • Ensure that the forearms are parallel with each other and perpendicular to the ground; maintain the position of the wrists • Slowly extend the elbows and raise the barbell up and slightly backward in a smooth, controlled motion until reaching the starting position *Spotter* • Without touching the barbell, mirror its upward movement with both hands (with the palm of one hand facing forward and the other facing backward and the thumbs wrapped underneath) • Keep the back straight while extending the knees and hips through the ascent of the barbell	*Client or athlete* • Following completion of the intended number of repetitions and returning to the starting position, place the barbell back on the supports and release the hands *Spotter* • Grip the barbell with both hands (with the palm of one hand facing forward and the other facing backward, and the thumbs wrapped underneath) to assist with placing the barbell back on the supports • Note: For additional safety, particularly during heavier RM attempts, additional spotters can be placed on the ends of the barbell in a manner similar to the back squat.

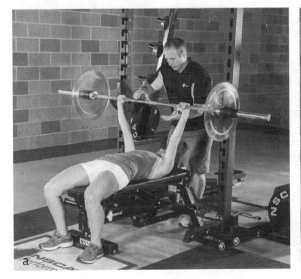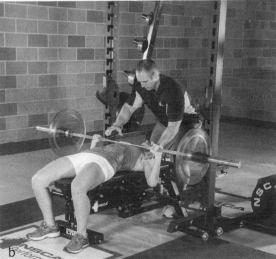

Figure 8.3 The bench press movement.

Table 8.4 Bench Pull Technique

1. Starting position	2. Upward movement
Client or athlete • Lie down on the bench facing down while making contact with the chest and head (or side of the head); keep the feet off of the ground • Adjust so that the barbell placed on the ground is at chest level, and grip with the hands (with the palms down and the thumbs wrapped underneath) a comfortable distance outside of the shoulders • Lift the barbell so that a small amount of ground clearance is available (the bench height must be set accordingly) *Spotter* • Assist with the positioning and initial liftoff	*Client or athlete* • Maintain bench contact with the chest and head (or side of the head) with the feet off of the ground with limited movement • From the hang position, bend the elbows until the barbell makes contact with the bottom of the bench in line with the lower chest *Spotter* • Verify contact between the barbell and bench
3. Downward movement	**4. Completion**
Client or athlete • Maintain bench contact with the chest and head (or side of the head), and keep the feet off of the ground with limited movement • Extend the elbows and lower the barbell to the hang position in a controlled manner without touching the ground	*Client or athlete* • Following completion of the intended number of repetitions and returning to the hang position, place the barbell back on the ground *Spotter* • Assist the client or athlete with returning the barbell to the ground

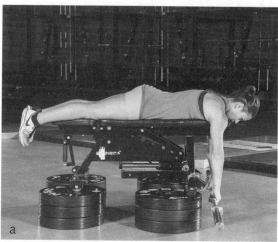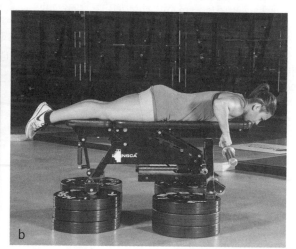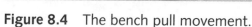

Figure 8.4 The bench pull movement.

Protocol

1. Begin the procedure by saying to the client or athlete: *"We are going to measure your strength during a single specific lifting movement. Are you ready to begin? If so, please get into the starting positon."*

2. Make sure to account for the weight of the unloaded barbell or sled and add a minimal amount of weight for the initial warm-up set.

3. Next, direct the client or athlete: *"Start with a warm-up set of 5 to 10 repetitions and focus on using proper technique. After the first warm-up set, you will rest for one minute."*

4. After one minute of rest:
   - Add an additional 10 to 20 pounds (5 to 9 kg) for bench press or bench pull.
   - Add an additional 30 to 40 pounds (14 to 18 kg) for back squat or leg press.

5. Continue by saying: *"Now complete another warm-up set of two to three repetitions with proper technique and then rest for a few minutes."*

6. After two to four minutes of rest:
   - Add an additional 10 to 20 pounds (5 to 9 kg) for bench press or bench pull.
   - Add an additional 30 to 40 pounds (14 to 18 kg) for back squat or leg press.

7. Tell the client or athlete: *"Now attempt to complete one repetition with proper technique. After your attempt, you will rest for a few minutes. Depending on your performance, we will add or remove some weight and try again."*

8. After two to four minutes of rest:
   - If the previous bench press or bench pull attempt was successful, add an additional 10 to 20 pounds (5 to 9 kg).
   - If the previous back squat or leg press attempt was successful, add an additional 30 to 40 pounds (14 to 18 kg)
   - If the previous bench press or bench pull attempt was unsuccessful, remove 5 to 10 pounds (2 to 5 kg).
   - If the previous back squat or leg press attempt was unsuccessful, remove 15 to 20 pounds (7 to 9 kg).

9. Continue attempts (repeat from step 7) until a 1RM value can be identified, preferably within three to five sets. Note: The load increases during 1RM testing can be larger for more experienced or stronger clients or athletes and potentially lower for those with less experience or baseline strength.

Alternatives or Modifications

If the client or athlete or the coach or fitness professional is relatively new to weight training or a particular movement pattern, the multiple-repetition maximum strength test protocol outlined in the next section may be more appropriate.

The estimated percentage of 1RM for a given number of repetitions is provided in table 8.5. For example, the client or athlete would be able to complete approximately three repetitions at roughly 93 percent of the 1RM, or 5 to 10 repetitions between 75 percent and 87 percent of the 1RM. Note that these estimated values do not consider specific muscle groups and will likely vary depending on the use of the upper versus lower body.

Table 8.5 Estimated Percentage of the One-Repetition Maximum (%1RM) for a Given Number of Repetitions

Repetitions	%1RM
1	100
2	95
3	93
4	90
5	87
6	85
7	83
8	80
9	77
10	75

Reprinted by permission from J.M. Sheppard and N.T. Triplett, "Program Design for Resistance Training." In *Essentials of Strength Training and Conditioning,* 4th ed., edited for the National Strength and Conditioning Association by G.G. Haff and N.T. Triplett (Champaign, IL: Human Kinetics, 2016), 452.

After You Finish

The greatest amount of weight lifted with good technique for a single repetition is the final result. In an effort to account for the size differences between clients or athletes, relative strength can be calculated by dividing the RM test result by body weight.

Research Notes

Considerations for body weight are relevant to the evaluation of maximal strength. For example, heavyweight powerlifters clearly dominate when examining absolute strength, whereas lightweight powerlifters possess greater relative strength. Which begs the question: Who is the strongest? Absolute strength is highly related to body weight, with larger individuals demonstrating greater strength values; however, a similar relationship exists between relative strength and body weight but in the opposite direction, with smaller individuals potentially demonstrating greater strength values. Ultimately, the actual application of strength and potentially the influence of power during a particular sport or activity will play a role in which approach is most valuable to the coach or fitness professional. Relative strength may be of particular importance in situations where a client or athlete is losing or gaining body weight to determine the influence of these changes on performance.

From a sports medicine perspective, weaker youth female athletes have approximately 9.5 times greater odds of traumatic knee injury than stronger female athletes as determined by 1RM back squat, while a similar increase in risk was not found for youth male athletes (31). The researchers who conducted this investigation reported a 1RM back squat cutoff of less than 105 percent of body weight for high versus low risk of injury in youth female athletes.

Normative Data

1RM strength classification values for male high school and collegiate athletes are provided in figure 8.5 (back squat) and figure 8.6 (bench press), and for female collegiate athletes in figure 8.7 (back squat) and figure 8.8 (bench press). Descriptive values for 1-RM bench pull in various populations are provided in figure 8.9. Relative maximum strength classifications for men are provided in figure 8.10 (leg press) and figure 8.11 (bench press), and women in figure 8.12 (leg press) and 8.13 (bench press).

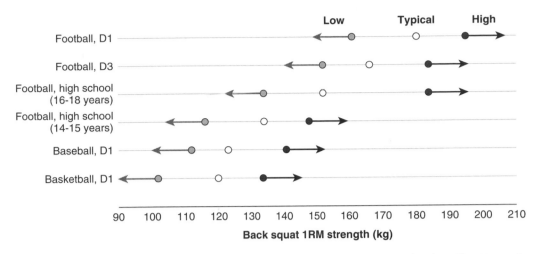

Figure 8.5 Back squat one-repetition maximum (1RM) strength classifications for male high school and National Collegiate Athletics Association athletes: high—70th percentile; typical—50th percentile; low—30th percentile.

Data from (14).

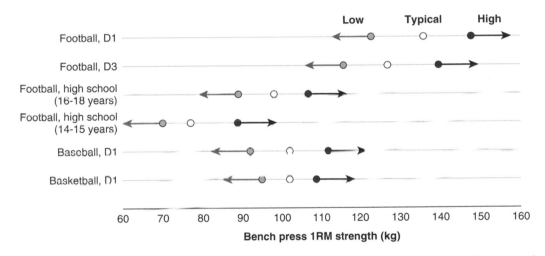

Figure 8.6 Bench press one-repetition maximum (1RM) strength classifications for male high school and National Collegiate Athletics Association athletes: high—70th percentile; typical—50th percentile; low—30th percentile.

Data from (14).

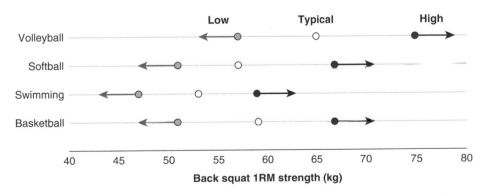

Figure 8.7 Back squat one-repetition maximum (1RM) strength classifications for female National Collegiate Athletics Association Division I athletes: high—70th percentile; typical—50th percentile; low—30th percentile.

Data from (14).

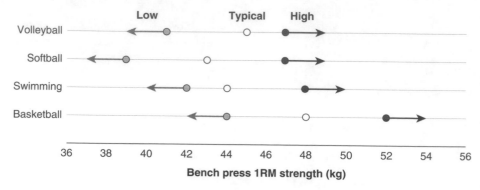

Figure 8.8 Bench press one-repetition maximum (1RM) strength classifications for female National Collegiate Athletics Association Division I athletes: high—70th percentile; typical—50th percentile; low—30th percentile.

Data from (14).

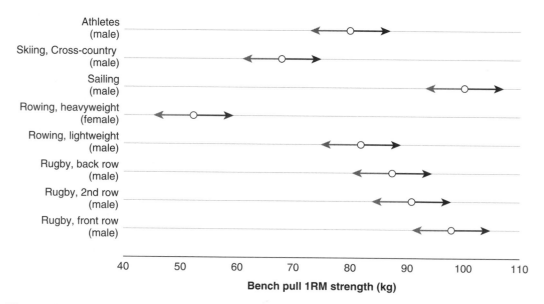

Figure 8.9 Descriptive (average) values for one-repetition maximum (1RM) bench pull strength in various populations.

Data from (15, 18, 25, 32, 37, 40).

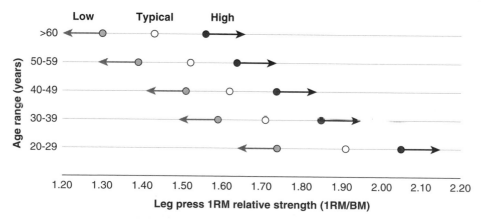

Figure 8.10 Leg press one-repetition maximum (1RM) strength relative to body mass (BM) classifications across the lifespan for men: high—70th percentile; typical—50th percentile; low—30th percentile.

Data from (11).

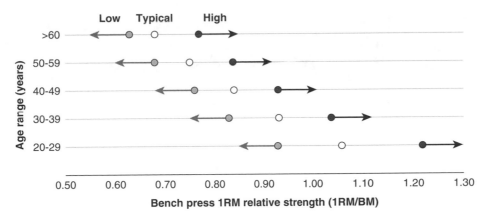

Figure 8.11 Bench press one-repetition maximum (1RM) strength relative to body mass (BM) classifications across the lifespan for men: high—70th percentile; typical—50th percentile; low—30th percentile.

Data from (11).

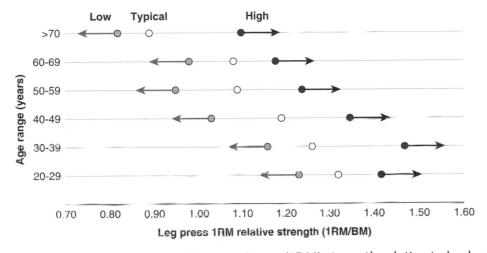

Figure 8.12 Leg press one-repetition maximum (1RM) strength relative to body mass (BM) classifications across the lifespan for women: high—70th percentile; typical—50th percentile; low—30th percentile.

Data from (11).

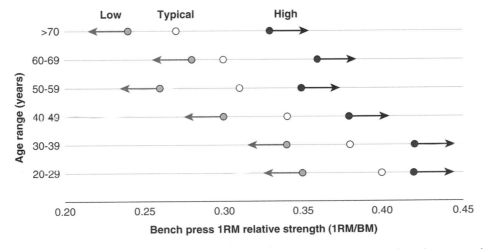

Figure 8.13 Bench press one-repetition maximum (1RM) strength relative to body mass (BM) classifications across the lifespan for women: high—70th percentile; typical—50th percentile; low—30th percentile.

Data from (11).

MULTIPLE-REPETITION MAXIMUM STRENGTH TEST

Purpose

The multiple-repetition maximum (RM) strength test measures the maximal strength of the muscle groups engaged during several specific movements.

Outcomes

Maximum amount of weight lifted for the intended number of repetitions (absolute strength); estimated one-repetition maximum (1RM); maximum strength relative to body weight (relative strength)

Equipment Needed

Rack or stands; flat bench or leg press; barbell; safety locks; weight plates; spotters

Before You Begin

Follow the procedures outlined in chapter 4 to record the client's or athlete's body weight. Review the basic elements of the movement to be assessed (preferably during a familiarization session prior to testing) with the client or athlete and spotters as outlined in tables 8.1 through 8.4 and figures 8.1 through 8.4. These selections should be made with consideration for the muscle groups used, with the leg press and back squat used to evaluate the lower body and the bench press and bench pull used to evaluate the upper body, and the relevant movements (i.e., the bench press for pushing and the bench pull for pulling). Next, determine the number of repetitions to be completed (preferably fewer than 10 repetitions due to a better estimation of "true" maximal strength; a 5-repetition maximum [5RM] will be used for this explanation).

Clear the lifting area, place the supports at the appropriate height in order to hold the barbell at an easily accessible location for the client or athlete, lower the safety bars enough to allow for the full range of motion, and make sure that the collars are in working order. Verify that the selected spotters are of adequate size and strength to support the loads lifted by the client or athlete being evaluated. Prior to attempting the multiple-RM test, determine a phrase ("Take it") or action that will signal that the client or athlete cannot complete a repetition. Upon hearing or seeing this signal, the spotters should grasp the barbell and assist with reracking it on the supports. A standardized general warm-up followed by three to five minutes of rest and recovery should be conducted prior to beginning the assessment. A specific lifting warm-up is built into the RM protocol.

Protocol

1. Begin the procedure by saying to the client or athlete: "We are going to measure your strength to perform five repetitions of an exercise. Are you ready to begin? If so, please get into the starting positon."

2. Make sure to account for the weight of the unloaded barbell or sled and add a minimal amount of weight for the initial warm-up set.

3. Next, direct the client or athlete: "Start with a warm-up set of 8 to 10 repetitions and focus on using proper technique. After the first warm-up set, you will rest for one minute."

4. After one minute of rest:
   - Add an additional 5 to 10 pounds (2.3 to 5 kg) for bench press or bench pull.
   - Add an additional 15 to 20 pounds (7 to 9 kg) for back squat or leg press.

5. Continue: *"Now complete another warm-up set of six to eight repetitions with proper technique and then rest for a few minutes."*

6. After two to four minutes of rest:
   - Add an additional 5 to 10 pounds (2.3 to 5 kg) for bench press or bench pull.
   - Add an additional 15 to 20 pounds (7 to 9 kg) for back squat or leg press.

7. Tell the client or athlete: *"Now attempt to complete five repetitions with proper technique. After your set, you will rest for a few minutes. Depending on your performance, we will add or remove some weight and try again."*

8. After two to four minutes of rest:
   - If the previous bench press or bench pull attempt was successful, add an additional 5 to 10 pounds (2.3 to 5 kg).
   - If the previous back squat or leg press attempt was successful, add an additional 15 to 20 pounds (7 to 9 kg).
   - If the previous bench press or bench pull attempt was unsuccessful, remove 2.5 to 5 pounds (1 to 2.3 kg).
   - If the previous back squat or leg press attempt was unsuccessful, remove 5 to 10 pounds (2.3 to 5 kg).

9. Continue attempts (repeat from step 7) until a 5RM value can be identified, preferably within three to five sets. Note: The load increases during multiple RM testing can be larger for more experienced or stronger clients or athletes and potentially lower for those with less experience or baseline strength.

Alternatives or Modifications

Multiple RM tests evaluating between five-repetition maximum (5RM) and 10-repetition maximum (10RM) strength are recommended due to being more closely related to one-repetition maximum (1RM) strength and less influenced by muscular endurance. For those individuals with a higher level of experience, a three-repetition maximum (3RM) may also be appropriate.

After You Finish

The greatest amount of weight lifted with good technique for the intended number of repetitions is the final result. In an effort to account for the size differences between clients or athletes, relative strength can be calculated by dividing the RM test result by body weight.

While the results of the RM test can be simply recorded and used to track change or make comparisons, coaches or fitness professionals can use the number of repetitions completed and the load lifted to estimate the client's or athlete's 1RM with one of the following formulas.

General 10RM or less; in pounds (6)

$$\text{Predicted 1RM (lb)} = \frac{\text{xRM}}{[1.0278 - (\text{reps to fatigue} \times 0.0278)]}$$

Here is an example for a client or athlete with a 5RM of 145 pounds.

$$\text{Predicted 1RM (lb)} = \frac{145 \text{ lb}}{[1.0278 - (5 \text{ reps} \times 0.0278)]} = \frac{145 \text{ lb}}{[1.0278 - (0.139)]} = \frac{145 \text{ lb}}{[0.8888)]} = 163.1 \text{ lb}$$

Bench press or back squat 10RM or less; in kilograms (42)

$$\text{Predicted 1RM (kg)} = \frac{100 \times \text{xRM}}{48.8 + (53.8 \times (e^{-0.075 \times \text{number of repetitions}}))}$$

Note that e is a mathematical term that is roughly equal to 2.71828

Here is an example for a client or athlete with a 10RM of 75 kilograms.

$$\text{Predicted 1RM (kg)} = \frac{100 \times 75 \text{ kg}}{48.8 + (53.8 \times e^{-0.075 \times 10 \text{ reps}})} = \frac{7{,}500 \text{ kg}}{48.8 + (53.8 \times e^{-0.75})]}$$

$$= \frac{7{,}500 \text{ kg}}{48.8 + (53.8 \times 0.472)} = \frac{7{,}500 \text{ kg}}{48.8 + (25.4)} = \frac{7{,}500 \text{ kg}}{74.2} = 101.1 \text{ kg}$$

Leg press 5RM; in kilograms (30)

$$\text{Predicted 1RM (kg)} = (1.09703 \times 5\text{RM}) + 14.2546$$

Here is an example for a client or athlete with a 5RM of 100 kilograms.

$$\text{Predicted 1RM (kg)} = (1.09703 \times 100 \text{ kg}) + 14.2546$$

$$= (109.703) + 14.2546 = 124.0 \text{ kg}$$

The calculation of the predicted 1RM can also be facilitated by using the conversion nomograms provided in figure 8.14. There are inherent limitations to predicting 1RM values, including considerations for the equipment used, number of repetitions performed, age, sex, and training status; however, this conversion may provide the ability to compare the results to published normative data and to set training loads as percentages of estimated maximum strength. Coaches or fitness professionals may also simply elect to use results from a 3RM strength test for training prescription and other comparisons.

Research Notes

Maximal strength may have a direct or indirect relationship with sports performance. Interestingly, bench press and back squat 3RM strength has been shown to be more highly correlated with tackling ability in rugby athletes than measures of upper- and lower-body power output (35). The same researchers demonstrated that rugby athletes with the greatest 3RM strength improvements following eight weeks of resistance training also had the greatest improvements in tackling performance (36).

Normative Data

Descriptive values for 3RM back squat, 3RM bench press, and 3RM bench pull strength in various populations are provided in figure 8.15 through figure 8.17.

Figure 8.14 Conversion nomograms for estimating one-repetition maximum (1RM) strength from five-repetition (5RM) and 10-repetition maximum (10RM) bench press or back squat and 5RM leg press assessments

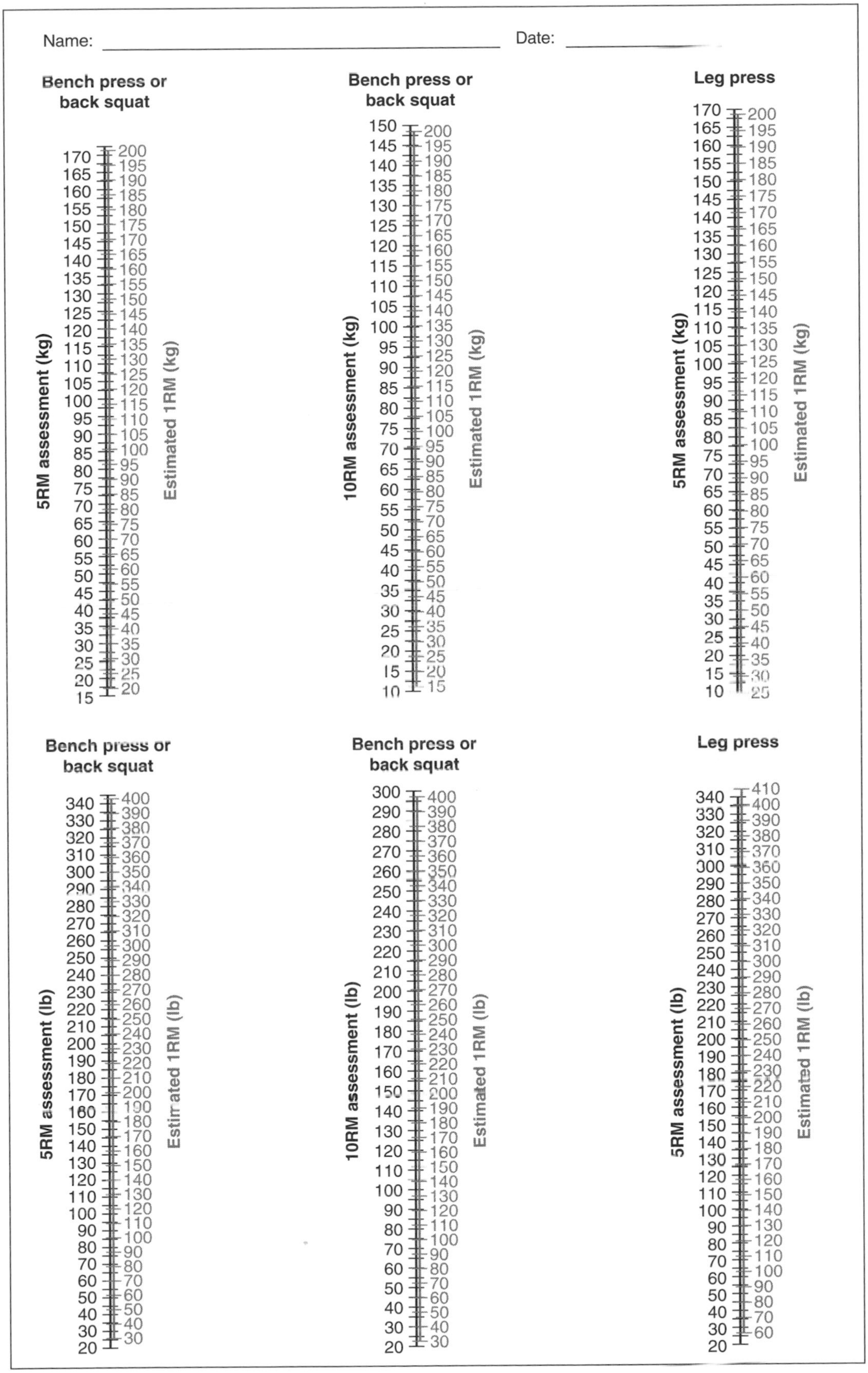

From D. Fukuda, *Assessments for Sport and Athletic Performance* (Champaign, IL: Human Kinetics, 2019). Using Wathen (42) and Reynolds (30) formulas.

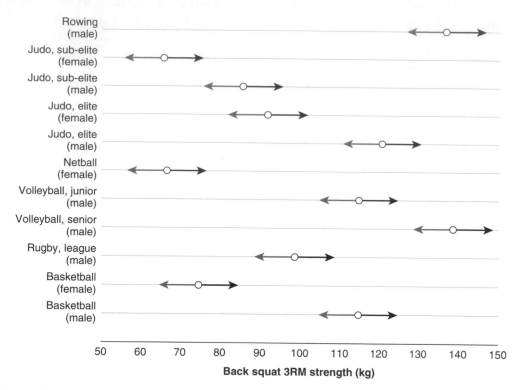

Figure 8.15 Descriptive (average) values for three-repetition maximum (3RM) back squat strength in various populations.

Data from (38).

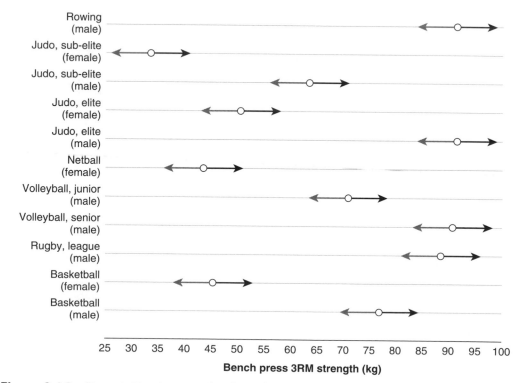

Figure 8.16 Descriptive (average) values for three-repetition maximum (3RM) bench press strength in various populations.

Data from (38).

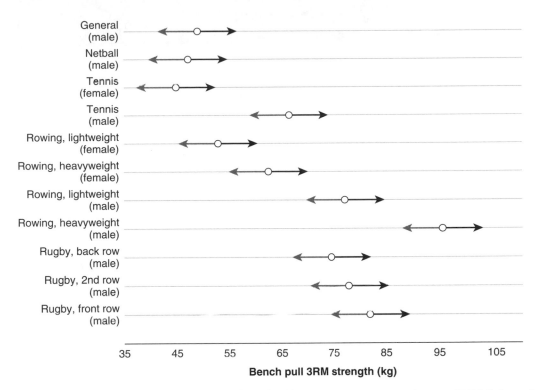

Figure 8.17 Descriptive (average) values for three-repetition maximum (3RM) bench pull strength in various populations.

Data from (38, 40).

MAXIMAL HANDGRIP STRENGTH TEST

Purpose

The maximal handgrip strength test measures static strength of the forearm muscles.

Outcomes

Maximum static strength, in kilograms or pounds, generated during gripping

Equipment Needed

Handgrip strength measuring device (or handgrip dynamometer)

Before You Begin

Follow the procedures outlined in chapter 4 to record the client's or athlete's body weight in kilograms or pounds. Adjust the handle of the measuring device so that the middle portion of the athlete or client's middle finger is at a right angle (90°) and record the appropriate settings for both hands. A standardized warm-up followed by three to five minutes of rest and recovery should be conducted prior to beginning the assessment.

Protocol

1. Begin the procedure by saying to the client or athlete: *"We are going to measure your grip strength. Are you ready to begin? If so, please stand with your feet parallel and shoulder-width apart with your arms at your sides, and grip the measuring device with one hand."*

2. Verify that the measuring device reads zero and say: *"Keep your arm at your side with your palm facing toward your thigh"* (see figure 8.18).

3. Next, explain: *"When I say 'Squeeze,' breathe out while gripping the measuring device as hard as possible until I say 'Relax' to complete the test."*

4. Verbally signal to the client or athlete, *"Squeeze, squeeze, squeeze, and relax,"* while verifying that he or she remains stationary.

5. Record the greatest strength value achieved from the measuring device and say: *"Repeat the same procedure with your opposite hand,"* prior to making two or three more attempts with each hand separated by approximately one minute of rest and recovery.

Alternatives or Modifications

The maximal handgrip strength test can also be performed with the elbow bent at a right angle (90°) in a standing or seated position; however, lower strength values should be expected compared to when the measuring device is held with the arm straight and next to the thigh.

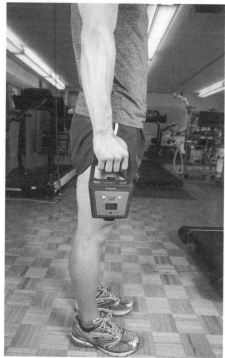

Figure 8.18 Setup for the maximal handgrip strength test with arm straight and measuring device held next to the thigh.

After You Finish

The greatest strength value achieved with either hand is the final result. In an effort to account for size differences between clients or athletes, relative strength can be calculated by dividing the maximal handgrip strength test result by body weight.

The sum (right + left) or average [(right + left)/2] of values from both hands can also be calculated, and coaches or fitness professionals may choose to make side-to-side comparisons of maximal handgrip strength.

Research Notes

Maximal handgrip strength has been shown to be a general measure of overall strength (44) and has wide relevance to the evaluation of children and older adults as well as certain sporting environments. For example, handgrip strength is related to freestyle swimming performance and implement velocity in a number of sports, including tennis, hockey, golf, baseball, and softball (9).

Normative Data

Maximal handgrip strength classification values are provided for boys in figure 8.19, girls in figure 8.20, adult men in figure 8.21, and adult women in figure 8.22. Maximal handgrip strength values relative to body mass for the same group are provided in figure 8.23 through figure 8.26.

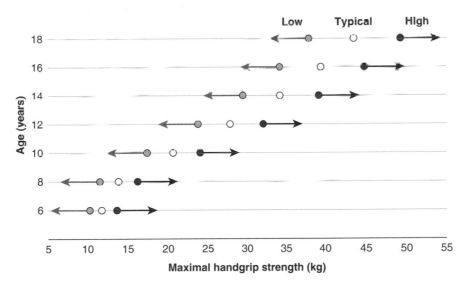

Figure 8.19 Maximal handgrip strength classifications in boys: high—75th percentile; typical—50th percentile; low—25th percentile.

Data from (26).

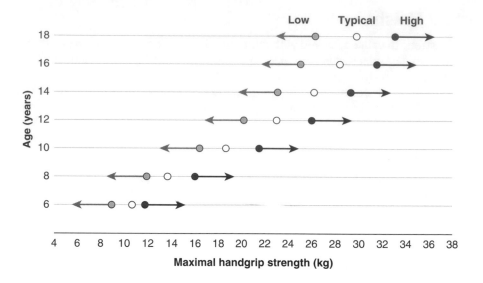

Figure 8.20 Maximal handgrip strength classifications in girls: high—75th percentile; typical—50th percentile; low—25th percentile.

Data from (26).

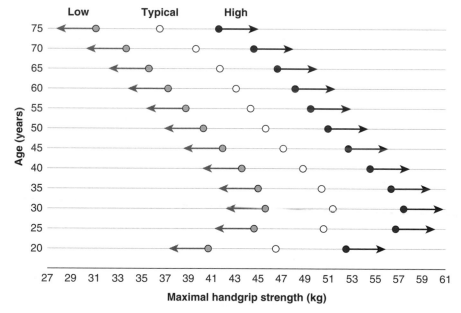

Figure 8.21 Maximal handgrip strength classifications in men: high—75th percentile; typical—50th percentile; low—25th percentile.

Data from (26).

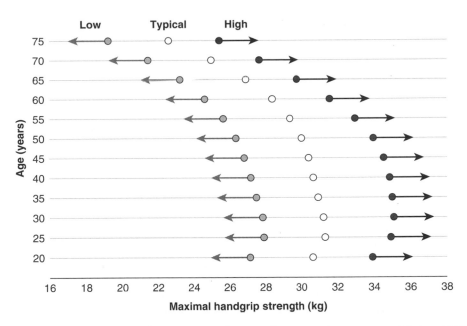

Figure 8.22 Maximal handgrip strength classifications in women: high—75th percentile; typical—50th percentile; low—25th percentile.

Data from (26).

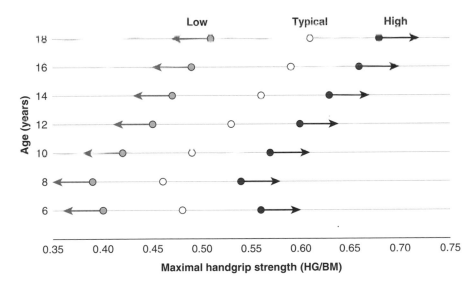

Figure 8.23 Maximal handgrip (HG) strength classifications relative to body mass (BM) in boys: high—75th percentile; typical—50th percentile; low—25th percentile.

Data from (26).

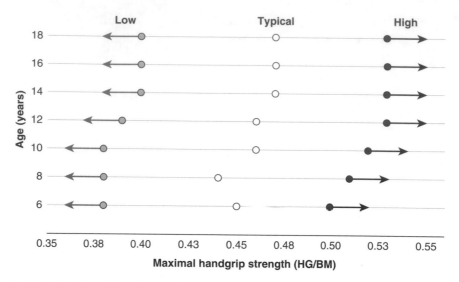

Figure 8.24 Maximal handgrip (HG) strength classifications relative to body mass (BM) in girls: high—75th percentile; typical—50th percentile; low—25th percentile.
Data from (26).

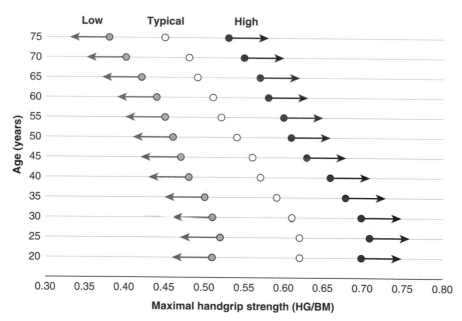

Figure 8.25 Maximal handgrip (HG) strength classifications relative to body mass (BM) in men: high—75th percentile; typical—50th percentile; low—25th percentile.
Data from (26).

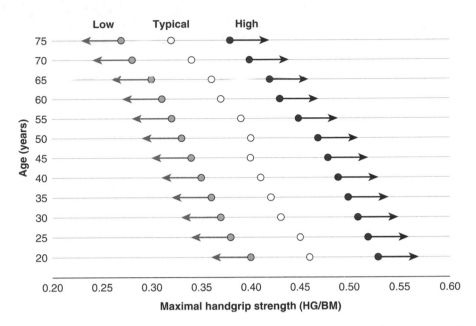

Figure 8.26 Maximal handgrip (HG) strength classifications relative to body mass (BM) in women: high—75th percentile; typical—50th percentile; low—25th percentile.

Data from (26).

STATIC MUSCULAR ENDURANCE TESTS

Purpose

Static muscular endurance tests measure the ability of specific muscle groups to maintain the body in the required position for an extended period of time.

Outcomes

Accumulated time, in seconds, until the client or athlete is unable to hold the required position

Equipment Needed

Stopwatch or timing device; pull-up bar and spotter for the flexed/bent arm hang test

Before You Begin

A standardized warm-up should be conducted prior to beginning the assessment.

Protocol

1. Begin the procedure by saying to the client or athlete: *"We are going to measure how long you can hold your body in certain positions. Are you ready to begin?"*

2. Next, select and describe the required position from one of the following scripts:

   - Plank (or prone bridge): *"Please lie face-down on the ground. When I say 'Begin,' get into a plank position with your body propped up by just your elbows and forearms and your toes. Your elbows should be shoulder-width apart, your feet should be close but not touching, and keep your legs, trunk, and neck in a straight line. I will tell you if you begin to get out of position and the test will end if you cannot correct your position after two warnings"* (see figure 8.27).

   - Half-squat (or wall-sit): *"Stand with your feet parallel and shoulder-width apart and place the back of your head flat against the wall. Squat down and adjust your body to be in a sitting, half-squat position with your ankles, knees, and hips at right angles (90°). Allow your arms to hang down at your sides and keep the back of your shoulders and arms (down to the palms of your hands) in contact with the wall. After you are in the correct the position, I will say 'Begin' and start the test"* (see figure 8.28).

   - Flexed-arm hang (or bent-arm hang): *"With the assistance of a spotter to lift you up to the bar, reach up and grasp the bar with both hands wider than your shoulders a comfortable distance apart with your palms facing forward and thumbs wrapped around the bar. Pull your body high enough so that your chin is above the bar and then hold that position. After you are motionless, the spotter will step back and I will say 'Begin' and start the test"* (see figure 8.29).

3. Say to the client or athlete: *"Please continue breathing normally throughout the test and maintain this position for as long as possible."*

4. Verbally signal the client or athlete *"Begin,"* and record the time until the client or athlete can no longer maintain the required position.

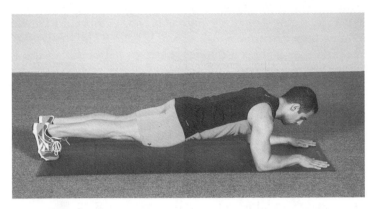

Figure 8.27   Prone bridge (or plank).

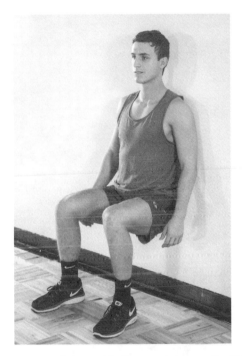

Figure 8.28   Half-squat (or wall-sit).

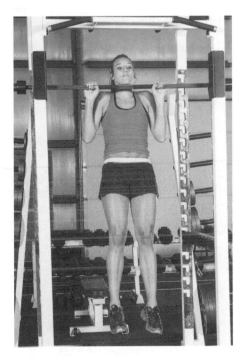

Figure 8.29   Flexed-arm hang (or bent-arm hang).

Alternatives or Modifications

The lumbar stability tests as described in chapter 5 are also assessments of static muscular endurance. Endurance time during the flexed-arm hang test has also been recorded until the client or athlete can no longer hold the elbow joint at a specific angle (i.e., 90°).

After You Finish

The length of time the client or athlete is able to hold the required position is the final result.

Research Notes

The relevance for static muscular endurance varies depending on the sport or activity of interest. Elite standup paddle boarders (approximately 184 seconds) demonstrate greater plank endurance time than recreational boarders (approximately 96 seconds) and sedentary individuals (approximately 88 seconds) (33), while plank and half-squat endurance reportedly correlates to the time needed to complete the pack hike test (3 miles [4.83 km] while wearing a 45-pound [20.4 kg] weight vest) in firefighters (27). Half-squat endurance may be predictive of injury in collegiate American football players with a cutoff value of less than 88 seconds differentiating between athletes who became injured and those who did not (43). As might be expected, more experienced climbers perform better during the flexed-arm hang test compared to their less experienced counterparts (3). Interestingly, military personnel with increasing numbers of health risk factors also show decreasing flexed-arm hang endurance values (approximately 60 seconds for those with no risk factors compared to approximately 28 seconds in those with three risk factors) (20).

Normative Data

Static muscular endurance classification values are provided for the plank in figure 8.30, flexed-arm hang for boys in figure 8.31, flexed-arm hang for girls in figure 8.32, half-squat for adult men in figure 8.33, and half-squat for adult women in figure 8.34.

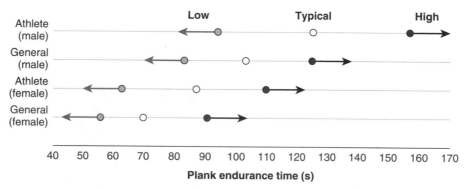

Figure 8.30   Plank endurance time in adult men and women: high—70th percentile; typical—50th percentile; low—30th percentile.

Data from (37a).

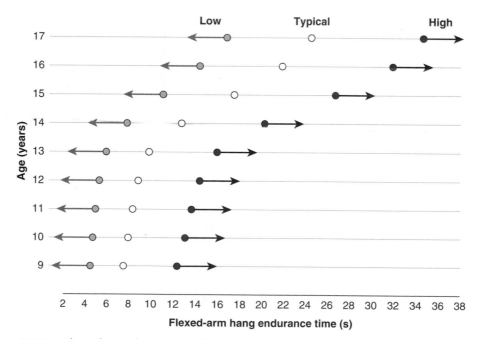

Figure 8.31   Flexed-arm hang classifications in boys: high—70th percentile; typical—50th percentile; low—30th percentile.

Data from (39).

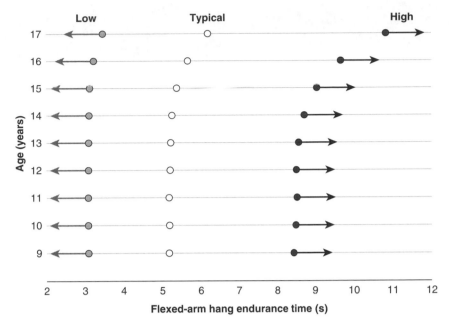

Figure 8.32 Flexed-arm hang classifications in girls: high—70th percentile; typical—50th percentile; low—30th percentile.

Data from (39).

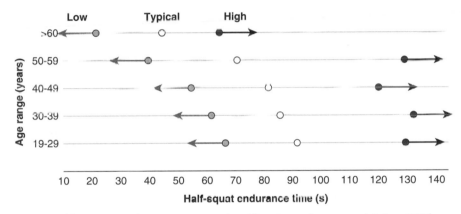

Figure 8.33 Half-squat endurance time classifications for men: high—75th percentile; typical—50th percentile; low—25th percentile.

Data from (22).

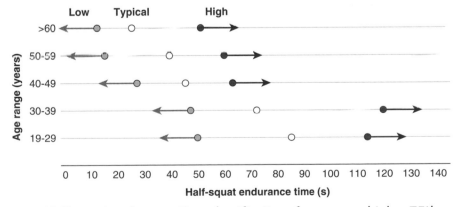

Figure 8.34 Half-squat endurance time classifications for women: high—75th percentile; typical—50th percentile; low—25th percentile.

Data from (22).

DYNAMIC MUSCULAR ENDURANCE TESTS

Purpose

Dynamic muscular endurance tests measure the ability of specific muscle groups to perform repetitive movements for an extended period of time.

Outcomes

Number of repetitions that the client or athlete is able to complete while maintaining the required movement pattern or within a given time period

Equipment Needed

Stopwatch or timing device; metronome, measuring tape, and adhesive tape for the curl-up test; pull-up bar for the pull-up test

Before You Begin

Determine the required movement pattern and if the repetitions will be counted over a given time period (typically between 30 sec and 2 min) or until there is a breakdown in form and technique. For the partial curl-up test, place two strips of adhesive tape parallel to each other on the floor separated by 10 centimeters (4 in.) and set a metronome to 40 beats per minute for a pace of 20 repetitions per minute (see figure 8.35).

Protocol

1. Begin the procedure by saying to the client or athlete: *"We are going to measure how many times you can complete certain movement patterns. Are you ready to begin?"*

2. Next, select and describe the required position from one of the following scripts:

   - Partial curl-ups: *"Lie flat on your back with your arms directly at your side. Adjust your body so that your fingers are touching the first of the two strips of adhesive tape on the floor and your feet so that your knees are at a right angle (90°). Keep your feet on the ground and close together but not touching. When I say 'Begin,' curl your trunk and back up so that your fingers will move from the starting position along the floor to the second strip of tape. Slowly uncurl your torso so that your fingers return to the starting position and continue to go back and forth so that the strip of tape is reached with each of the audible beeps provided by the metronome"* (see figure 8.35).

   - Push-ups: *"Lie flat on the ground with your chest facing downward and your ____ (feet typically for men; knees typically for women) next to each other. Then place the palms of your hands on the ground just wider than your shoulders. Next, push your body up until just your hands and ____ (toes typically for men; knees typically for women) are touching the ground to assume the starting positions. When I say 'Begin,' bend your elbows until your upper arms are parallel to the ground and then return to the starting position while keeping your legs, trunk, and neck in a straight line"* (see figure 8.36 for men and figure 8.37 for women).

   - Squats: *"In a standing position with your feet parallel and shoulder-width apart, place your hands behind your head or cross your arms against your chest. When I say 'Begin,' bend your knees and hips to lower your body into a half-squat sitting position with your ankles, knees, and hips at right angles (90°). Keep your back straight and your eyes facing forward throughout the movement. Once your thighs are parallel to the ground, stop the downward movement and extend your knees and hips to stand back up to the starting position"* (see figure 8.38).

- Pull-ups: *"Reach up and grasp the bar a comfortable distance outside your shoulders with both hands so that your palms are facing forward and thumbs are wrapped around the bar. While maintaining your grip, let your body hang down with your elbows fully extended. When I say 'Begin,' pull your body up to the bar until your chin is above the bar and then lower back down to the starting position. Continue this up-and-down movement and minimize excessive motion or swinging of your body"* (see figure 8.39).

3. Say: *"Please continue breathing normally throughout the test and complete as many repetitions as possible while maintaining the required movement pattern (or until the test ends)."*

4. Verbally signal the client or athlete *"Begin,"* and record the number of full repetitions that are completed with good technique or until the predetermined time has elapsed.

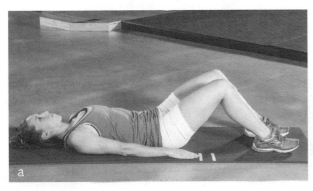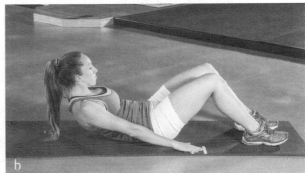

Figure 8.35 Partial curl-up.

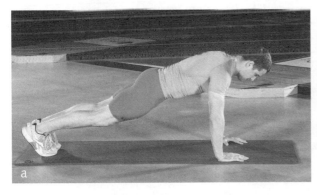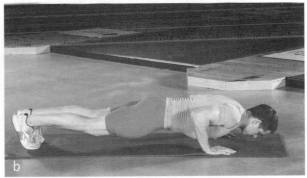

Figure 8.36 Push-up.

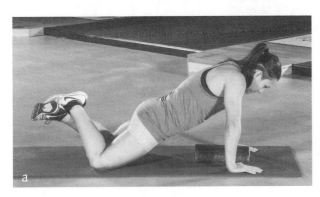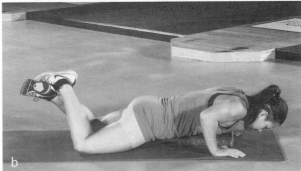

Figure 8.37 Modified push-up.

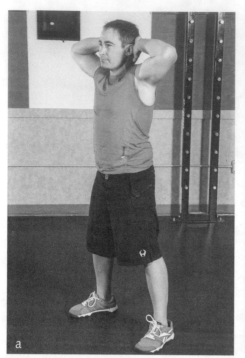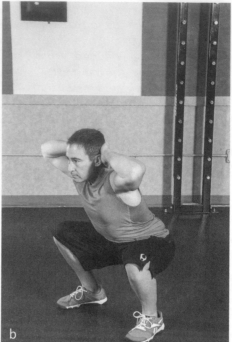

Figure 8.38 Squat.

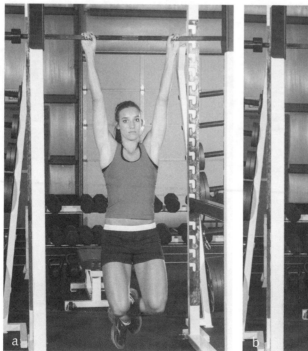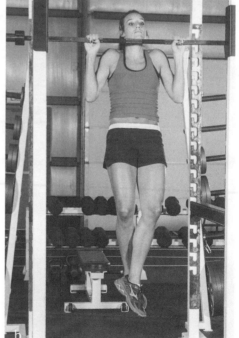

Figure 8.39 Pull-up.

Alternatives or Modifications

The verification of an appropriate push-up varies between protocols, including the client's or athlete's chest making contact with the evaluator's fist or a relatively soft object approximately 7 centimeters (3 in.) high for each repetition, or the client's or athlete's chin making contact with the ground.

A common alternative for evaluating the muscular endurance of the abdominal muscles is to use bent-knee sit-ups with the same position of the lower body as partial curl-ups but with the hands placed behind the head or the arms placed across the chest instead. In these versions, a partner typically anchors the feet and the repetitions are counted when the elbows make contact with the thighs (see figure 8.40).

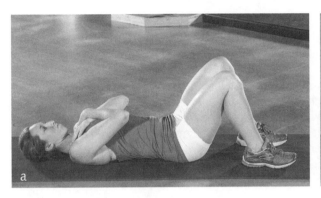
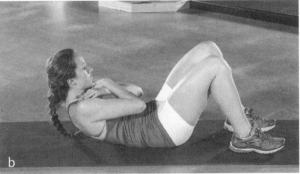

Figure 8.40   Bent-knee sit-up.

Many clients or athletes may have difficulty completing a single pull-up (which would make the test one that measures muscular strength instead of endurance), so a modified pull-up may be used. The modified pull-up uses a bar placed 2.5 to 5 centimeters (1 to 2 in.) above the client's or athlete's outstretched arms and fingers while lying flat on the back. The tested movement requires the client or athlete to support his or her body weight with the heels while holding the bar and pulling his or her body from a position roughly parallel to the floor until the chest makes contact with an elastic band placed 18 to 20 centimeters (7 to 8 in.) below the bar (see figure 8.41).

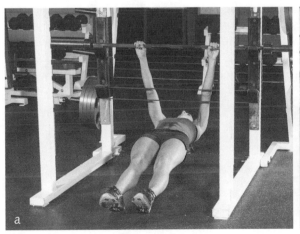
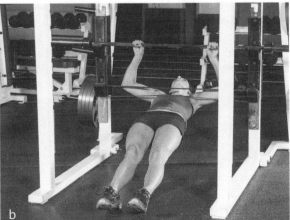

Figure 8.41   Modified pull-up.

An appropriately sized chair or plyometric box may be used as a reference (and an extra safety precaution) during the squat test. The chair or box should be less than the height of the bottom of the client's or athlete's thighs at the bottom of the squat when they are parallel to the ground (10 to 20 in. [25-50 cm] with 0.5-in. [1.3 cm] mats available to make slight adjustments). The squat test for muscular endurance can involve counting the number of repetitions completed before there is a breakdown in the required technique or the number of repetitions completed within a specific time period (e.g., 1 or 2 min).

After You Finish

The number of full repetitions completed for the required movement pattern is the final result.

Research Notes

Similar to static strength tests, dynamic muscular endurance is typically indicative of the muscle groups used by a client or athlete. For example, youth athletes engaged in martial arts and grappling sports were able to complete more curl-ups in 30 seconds and 60 seconds than those involved in team sports and nonathletes (16) because their sport routinely trains the trunk musculature. Testing completed during military-related training demonstrated that the number of push-ups completed in 60 seconds moderately correlated to upper-body maximal strength, while the number of squats completed in 60 seconds was more strongly related to aerobic capacity than lower-body maximal strength (41). Furthermore, differences in dynamic muscular endurance were reported between military personnel with less than one week of sick leave (on average, approximately 35 push-ups, 37 sit-ups, and 55 squats in 60 seconds) and more than one week of sick leave (on average, approximately 32 push-ups, 35 sit-ups, and 53 squats in 60 seconds) (19).

Normative Data

Push-up classification values are provided for boys in figure 8.42, for girls in figure 8.43, for adult men in figure 8.44, and for adult women in figure 8.45. Partial curl-up classification values are provided for men in figure 8.46 and women in figure 8.47. Bent-knee sit-up classification values are provided for boys (completed in 30 seconds) in figure 8.48, for girls (completed in 30 seconds) in figure 8.49, for boys (completed in one minute) in figure 8.50, and for girls (completed in one minute) in figure 8.51.

Muscular endurance classifications from the United States Navy Physical Readiness Test are provided for push-ups completed in two minutes for men in figure 8.52 and for women in figure 8.53, and for sit-ups completed in two minutes for men in figure 8.54 and for women in figure 8.55. Muscular endurance classifications for the number of sit-up, push-up, and squat repetitions completed before a breakdown in the required technique for adult men and women are provided in figure 8.56. Due to difficulties related to upper-body strength relative to body mass, limited normative data are available for the pull-up and none are included in this chapter. Coaches or fitness professionals are encouraged to track and maintain their own database of pull-up scores.

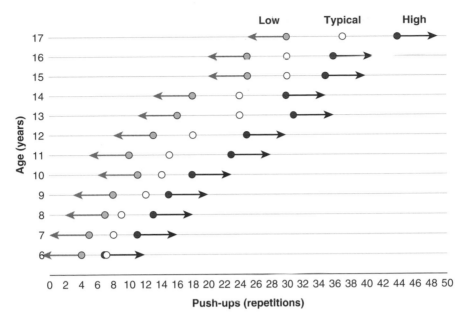

Figure 8.42 Push-up classifications in boys (completed at a set pace of 20 repetitions per minute until a breakdown in form): high—70th percentile; typical—50th percentile; low—30th percentile.

Data from (13).

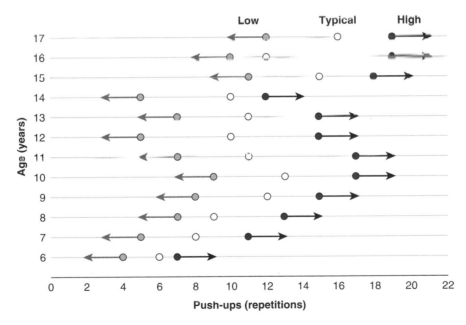

Figure 8.43 Push-up classifications in girls (completed at a set pace of 20 repetitions per minute until a breakdown in form): high—70th percentile; typical—50th percentile; low—30th percentile.

Data from (13).

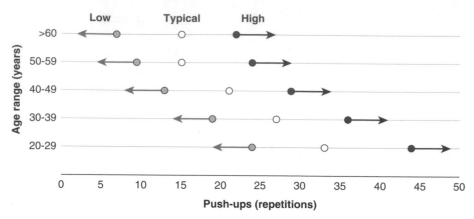

Figure 8.44 Push-up classifications in adult men: high—75th percentile; typical—50th percentile; low—25th percentile.

Data from (24).

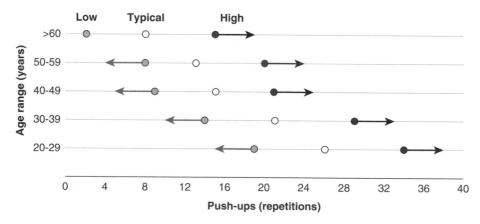

Figure 8.45 Push-up classifications in adult women: high—75th percentile; typical—50th percentile; low—25th percentile.

Data from (24).

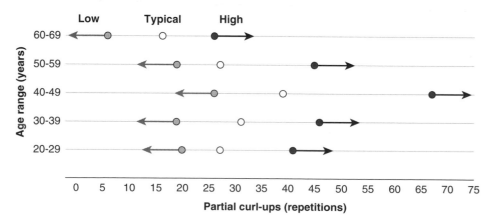

Figure 8.46 Partial curl-up classifications in men (with a maximum of 75 repetitions): high—70th percentile; typical—50th percentile; low—30th percentile.

Data from (1).

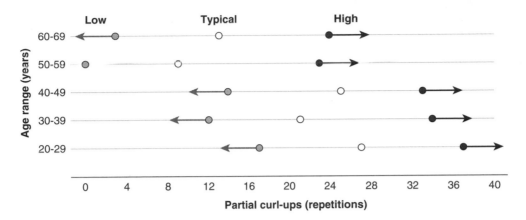

Figure 8.47 Partial curl-up classifications in women (with a maximum of 75 repetitions): high—70th percentile; typical—50th percentile; low—30th percentile.

Data from (1).

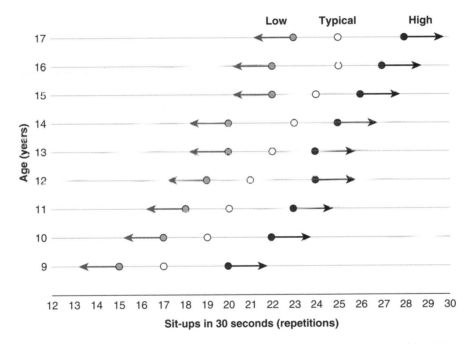

Figure 8.48 Sit-up classifications in boys (full repetitions completed in 30 seconds; hands held behind head with partner holding feet): high—70th percentile; typical—50th percentile; low—30th percentile.

Data from (39).

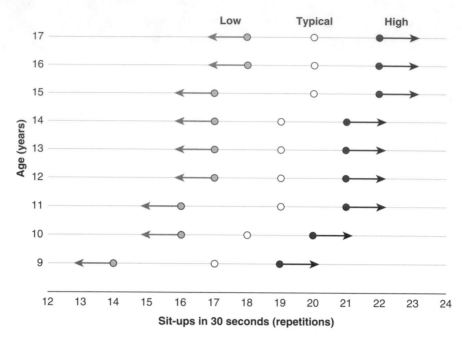

Figure 8.49   Sit-up classifications in girls (full repetitions completed in 30 seconds; hands held behind head with partner holding feet): high—70th percentile; typical—50th percentile; low—30th percentile.

Data from (39).

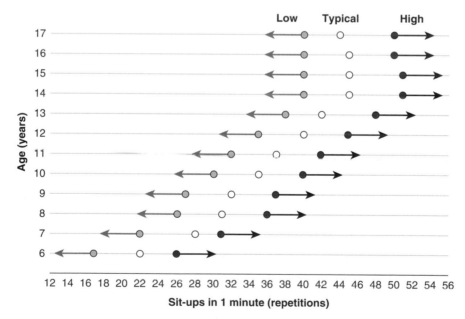

Figure 8.50   Sit-up classifications in boys (full repetitions completed in one minute; arms across chest with partner holding feet): high—70th percentile; typical—50th percentile; low—30th percentile.

Data from (13).

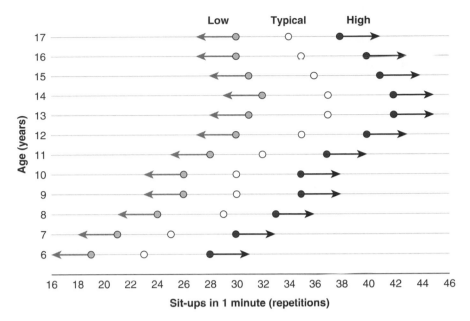

Figure 8.51 Sit-up classifications in girls (full repetitions completed in one minute; arms across chest with partner holding feet): high—70th percentile; typical—50th percentile; low—30th percentile.

Data from (13).

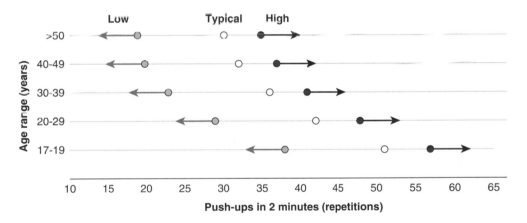

Figure 8.52 Navy Physical Readiness Test push-up classifications in men (full repetitions completed in two minutes): high—80th percentile; typical—50th percentile; low—20th percentile.

Data from (12).

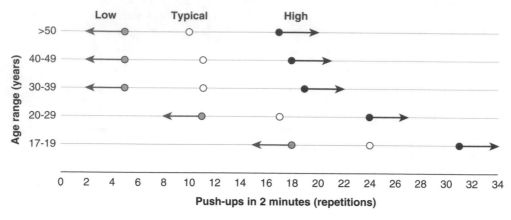

Figure 8.53 Navy Physical Readiness Test push-up classifications in women (full repetitions completed in two minutes): high—80th percentile; typical—50th percentile; low—20th percentile.

Data from (12).

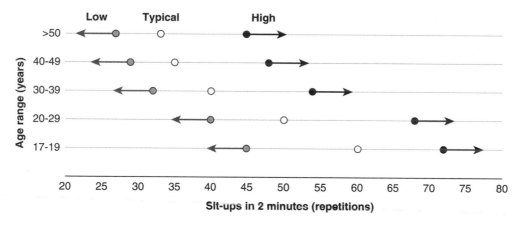

Figure 8.54 Navy Physical Readiness Test sit-up classifications in men (full repetitions completed in two minutes; arms across chest with partner holding feet): high—80th percentile; typical—50th percentile; low—20th percentile.

Data from (12).

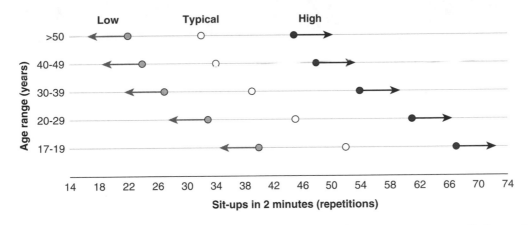

Figure 8.55 Navy Physical Readiness Test sit-up classifications in women (full repetitions completed in two minutes; arms across chest with partner holding feet): high—80th percentile; typical—50th percentile; low—20th percentile.

Data from (12).

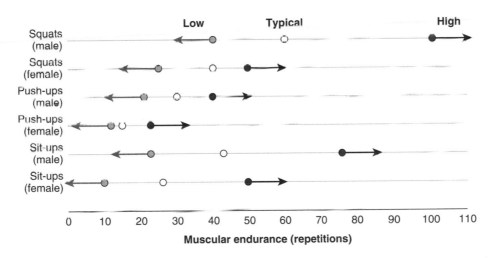

Figure 8.56 Sit-up, push-up, and squat performance in adults (number completed before a breakdown in form): high—75th percentile; typical—50th percentile; low—25th percentile.

Data from (4).

YMCA BENCH PRESS TEST

Purpose

The YMCA bench press test measures upper-body muscular endurance.

Outcomes

Maximum number of repetitions completed; estimated one-repetition maximum strength

Equipment Needed

Rack or stands; flat bench; barbell; safety locks; weight plates; spotter; metronome

Before You Begin

Review the basic elements of the bench press (preferably during a familiarization session prior to testing) with the client or athlete and spotter as outlined in table 8.3 and figure 8.3. A standardized warm-up should be conducted prior to beginning the assessment. Load a barbell to a total of 80 pounds (36.3 kg) for men or 35 pounds (15.9 kg) for women. Set a metronome to 60 beats per minute for a pace of 30 repetitions per minute.

Protocol

1. Begin the procedure by saying the following to the client or athlete: *"We are going to measure your upper-body muscular endurance during the bench press. Are you ready to begin? If so, please get into the starting position for the bench press"* (see figure 8.57).

2. Direct the client or athlete *"Remove the barbell from the rack and begin performing repetitions in a smooth, controlled manner with the highest and lowest points of the movements in cadence with an audible beep of the metronome."*

3. Next, request that he or she: *"Please continue breathing normally throughout the test and complete as many bench press repetitions as possible while maintaining good technique and keeping up with 30 repetitions per minute."* The spotter must be prepared to assist the client or athlete upon completion of the test.

4. Record the number of full repetitions that the client or athlete completes with good technique or until the pace set by the metronome can no longer be maintained.

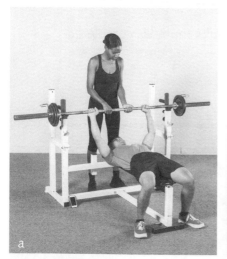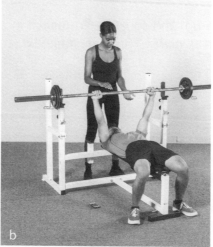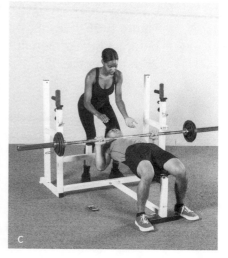

Figure 8.57   YMCA bench press test.

Alternatives or Modifications

An alternative to the YMCA bench press test for male athletes uses a standardized weight of 132 pounds (60 kg) without a set pace (i.e., no metronome) (2). This version of the test is complete when the athlete or client can no longer maintain good technique or requires a rest (pause) between repetitions.

After You Finish

The number of repetitions completed throughout the test is the final result. The coach or fitness professional may also wish to estimate the client's or athlete's one-repetition maximum (1RM) bench press strength from this result using the following formulas (17):

Men; in kilograms

$$\text{Predicted 1RM (kg)} = (1.55 \times \text{bench press repetitions}) + 37.9$$

Women; in kilograms

$$\text{Predicted 1RM (kg)} = (0.31 \times \text{bench press repetitions}) + 19.2$$

The calculation of 1RM strength can also be facilitated by use of the conversion nomograms provided in figure 8.58.

Research Notes

Muscular endurance typically declines following childbirth; however, a 12-week, 3-sessions-per-week exercise training program combining low-impact aerobic training, resistance training, and stretching has been shown to improve YMCA bench press test performance in women 4 to 6 weeks postpartum with no adverse effects on lactation (45).

The alternative version that uses a 132-pound (60 kg) load demonstrated differences in the number of repetitions completed between professional rugby league players (approximately 33 repetitions) and those in a lower-tier competitive division (approximately 24 repetitions), while results from the test were related to 1RM bench press strength and the individual athlete's competitive level (2).

Normative Data

YMCA bench press test classification values are provided for men in figure 8.59 and for women in figure 8.60.

Figure 8.58 Conversion nomograms for estimating one-repetition maximum (1RM) strength from the number of repetitions completed during the YMCA bench press test.

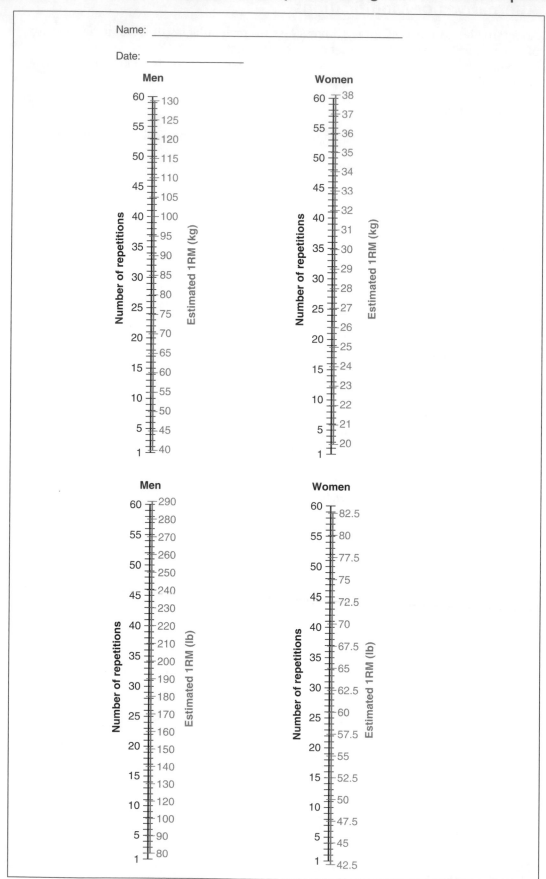

From D. Fukuda, *Assessments for Sport and Athletic Performance*. (Champaign, IL: Human Kinetics, 2019). Using Kim (17) formulas.

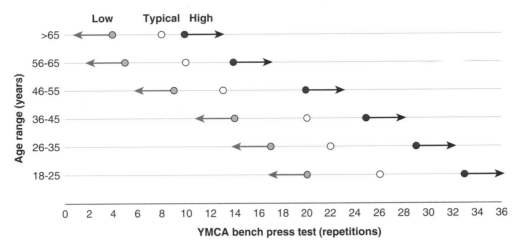

Figure 8.59 YMCA bench press test repetitions across the lifespan in men: high—70th percentile; typical—50th percentile; low—30th percentile.

Data from (21).

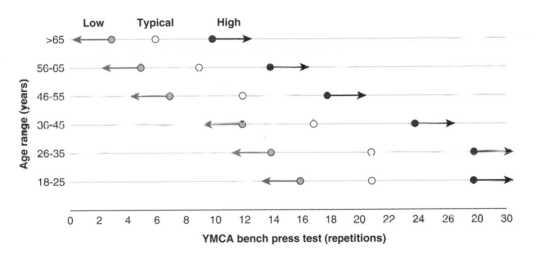

Figure 8.60 YMCA bench press test repetitions across the lifespan in women: high—70th percentile; typical—50th percentile; low—30th percentile.

Data from (21).

CHAPTER 9

Cardiorespiratory Fitness

"If we have data, let's look at data. If all we have are opinions, let's go with mine."

Jim Barksdale, former Netscape CEO

Although cardiorespiratory fitness provides a general indication of health and the ability of the heart, lungs, and muscles to use oxygen, it is also related to an individual's aerobic endurance performance and the ability to recover after a bout of high-intensity exercise. The typical gold standard or criterion measure for cardiorespiratory fitness is *maximal aerobic capacity* (also called *maximal oxygen uptake* or *$\dot{V}O_2max$*) that is measured using gas-exchange analysis. That type of assessment requires expensive equipment, working knowledge of the cardiovascular system by the evaluator, and maximal exertion by the client or athlete in a controlled environment such as a research laboratory or hospital. Fortunately, there are maximal and submaximal field tests that are based on the relationship between exercise intensity and the body's response to physical exertion (e.g., exercise heart rate).

Maximal cardiorespiratory fitness tests evaluate exercise performance with increasing intensities up to a maximal effort and, therefore, are suited for active, healthy individuals. Submaximal tests are based on heart rate responses to steady-state aerobic exercise that is monitored by asking the athlete or client to maintain a certain intensity (e.g., a walking or running pace).

The selection of a specific cardiorespiratory fitness test is based on the type of activity the athlete or client will do in the subsequent training program, the length of the test (with longer durations or distances giving a better indicator of aerobic endurance), whether the test is continuous or intermittent, and the training status of the person being tested. The assessments covered in this chapter are as follows:

- 20-meter multi-stage shuttle run (or PACER or beep test) (31, 55, 59)
- Yo-Yo intermittent recovery test (6, 59)
- Distance-based walk and run tests (19, 21)
- Time-based walk or run tests (12-minute test) (19, 21)
- Submaximal step test (or Queens College or YMCA step test) (20, 21)
- Submaximal rowing ergometer test (21)
- 45-second squat test (or Ruffier-Dickson test) (51)

20-METER MULTI-STAGE SHUTTLE RUN

Purpose

The 20-meter multi-stage shuttle run (or PACER or beep test) provides a running-based measure of cardiorespiratory fitness using a continuous change-of-direction protocol with increasing intensity leading to maximal effort.

Outcomes

Final stage and number of 20-meter shuttles completed; distance covered; estimated maximal aerobic capacity

Equipment Needed

Two cones or markers, adhesive tape, or field paint; measuring tape; mobile app or prerecorded audio file (various options available online); device to play the audio file; audio system or speakers

Before You Begin

Draw two lines or place two cones or markers 20 meters (65.6 ft) apart, with one line or cone designated as the start line and the other as the turn line (see figure 9.1). A data collection sheet for a commonly used version of the 20-meter multi-stage shuttle run is provided in table 9.1 (see the "Alternatives or Modifications" section for additional options); however, coaches or fitness professionals should take care to verify the specific protocol for the audio recording, software, or app.

A standardized warm-up followed by three to five minutes of rest and recovery should be conducted prior to beginning the assessment.

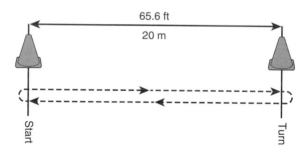

Figure 9.1   Setup for the 20-meter multi-stage shuttle run.

Protocol

1. Begin the procedure by saying to the athlete or client: *"We are going to measure how long you can continue jogging, running, and eventually sprinting laps between the cones. Are you ready to begin? If so, please stand behind the start line."*

2. Next, explain to the athlete or client: *"When the audio recording indicates the start of the test, jog forward to the turn line, aiming to arrive in time with the first beep, then turn back and jog in the opposite direction to the start line in time with the next beep. As the test progresses past seven laps, the beeps will come closer together so you will have to run faster to make it to the lines in time. For a lap to count, you will need to step at least one foot on or over the lines. Continue going back and forth until you cannot reach the opposite line in time with the beep two times in a row. If that happens, the test is over."*

3. An evaluator will be positioned at each line, marker, or cone. The evaluators will verify that at least one of the athlete's or client's feet has reached the line in time with the beep and give a verbal warning if unable to do so. A tally system or counting device should be used to accurately count the number of laps completed. If the athlete or client does not reach the next line in time with the beep, the test is finished and the final stage completed and total number of laps completed (including the last two attempts) are recorded.

Table 9.1 Data Collection Sheet for the 20-meter Multi-stage Shuttle Run

Stage	Speed (kph)	Pace (min/km)	Speed (mph)	Pace (min/mi)	Time per 20-meter lap(s)	Number of 20-meter laps	Stage completed?	Laps completed
S1	8.5	7.1	5.3	11.3	8.5	① ② ③ ④ ⑤ ⑥ ⑦		___ / 7
S2	9	6.7	5.6	10.7	8.0	① ② ③ ④ ⑤ ⑥ ⑦ ⑧		___ / 8
S3	9.5	6.3	5.9	10.2	7.6	① ② ③ ④ ⑤ ⑥ ⑦ ⑧		___ / 8
S4	10	6.0	6.2	9.7	7.2	① ② ③ ④ ⑤ ⑥ ⑦ ⑧ ⑨		___ / 9
S5	10.5	5.7	6.5	9.2	6.9	① ② ③ ④ ⑤ ⑥ ⑦ ⑧ ⑨		___ / 9
S6	11	5.5	6.8	8.8	6.5	① ② ③ ④ ⑤ ⑥ ⑦ ⑧ ⑨ ⑩		___ / 10
S7	11.5	5.2	7.1	8.5	6.3	① ② ③ ④ ⑤ ⑥ ⑦ ⑧ ⑨ ⑩		___ / 10
S8	12	5.0	7.5	8.0	6.0	① ② ③ ④ ⑤ ⑥ ⑦ ⑧ ⑨ ⑩ ⑪		___ / 11
S9	12.5	4.8	7.8	7.7	5.8	① ② ③ ④ ⑤ ⑥ ⑦ ⑧ ⑨ ⑩ ⑪		___ / 11
S10	13	4.6	8.1	7.4	5.5	① ② ③ ④ ⑤ ⑥ ⑦ ⑧ ⑨ ⑩ ⑪		___ / 11
S11	13.5	4.4	8.4	7.1	5.3	① ② ③ ④ ⑤ ⑥ ⑦ ⑧ ⑨ ⑩ ⑪ ⑫		___ / 12
S12	14	4.3	8.7	6.9	5.1	① ② ③ ④ ⑤ ⑥ ⑦ ⑧ ⑨ ⑩ ⑪ ⑫		___ / 12
S13	14.5	4.1	9.0	6.7	5.0	① ② ③ ④ ⑤ ⑥ ⑦ ⑧ ⑨ ⑩ ⑪ ⑫ ⑬		___ / 13
S14	15	4.0	9.3	6.5	4.8	① ② ③ ④ ⑤ ⑥ ⑦ ⑧ ⑨ ⑩ ⑪ ⑫ ⑬		___ / 13
S15	15.5	3.9	9.6	6.3	4.6	① ② ③ ④ ⑤ ⑥ ⑦ ⑧ ⑨ ⑩ ⑪ ⑫ ⑬		___ / 13
S16	16	3.8	9.9	6.1	4.5	① ② ③ ④ ⑤ ⑥ ⑦ ⑧ ⑨ ⑩ ⑪ ⑫ ⑬ ⑭		___ / 14
S17	16.5	3.6	10.3	5.8	4.4	① ② ③ ④ ⑤ ⑥ ⑦ ⑧ ⑨ ⑩ ⑪ ⑫ ⑬ ⑭		___ / 14
S18	17	3.5	10.6	5.7	4.2	① ② ③ ④ ⑤ ⑥ ⑦ ⑧ ⑨ ⑩ ⑪ ⑫ ⑬ ⑭ ⑮		___ / 15
S19	17.5	3.4	10.9	5.5	4.1	① ② ③ ④ ⑤ ⑥ ⑦ ⑧ ⑨ ⑩ ⑪ ⑫ ⑬ ⑭ ⑮		___ / 15
S20	18	3.3	11.2	5.4	4.0	① ② ③ ④ ⑤ ⑥ ⑦ ⑧ ⑨ ⑩ ⑪ ⑫ ⑬ ⑭ ⑮ ⑯		___ / 16
S21	18.5	3.2	11.5	5.2	3.9	① ② ③ ④ ⑤ ⑥ ⑦ ⑧ ⑨ ⑩ ⑪ ⑫ ⑬ ⑭ ⑮ ⑯		___ / 16
							Total laps	

From D. Fukuda, *Assessments for Sport and Athletic Performance* (Champaign, IL: Human Kinetics, 2019).

Alternatives or Modifications

The 20-meter multi-stage shuttle run can be used to assess small groups of athletes or clients in a single session. This approach requires enough space between those being tested (i.e., at least 2 m [6.6 ft]) and additional evaluators to record the final results. If the measurement of maximal heart rate is desired, the coach or fitness professional should measure the athlete's or client's heart rate immediately after completing the test using one of the methods described in chapter 10.

Various versions of the 20-meter multi-stage shuttle run protocol exist with slight differences in the initial speed or the number of shuttles completed at a given speed in order to keep each stage at approximately one minute (55). For example, the first stage during the Eurofit and PACER tests is completed at a speed of 8 kilometers per hour (7.5 min/km) or approximately 5 miles per hour (12 min/mi) with 9 seconds per 20-meter lap and the rest of the protocol being identical to the 20-meter multi-stage shuttle run protocol (55).

When the availability of space is an issue, a modified 15-meter multi-stage shuttle run with a greater number of laps and shuttles per stage is an option (37). However, if this version is used, the conversion nomogram provided in the next section will not be accurate.

After You Finish

The last completed stage and the total number of laps completed (including the final two attempts) are the final result. From the example data provided in table 9.2, the athlete or client completed stage 6 and 6 laps in stage 7 for a total of 57 laps.

The last completed stage and the athlete's or client's age can be used to estimate maximal aerobic capacity using the conversion nomogram provided in figure 9.2. If the athlete or client from the previous example is 14 years old, the estimated maximal aerobic capacity is 44.8 ml/kg/min.

Research Notes

In support of its inclusion in several youth physical fitness testing batteries, results from the 20-meter multi-stage shuttle run have been shown to be highly related to cardiorespiratory fitness assessed using laboratory-based maximal aerobic capacity measures (34). Cutoff values for boys (stage 4 for 10- to 12-year-olds, stage 5 for 13-year-olds, stage 6 for 14- to 15-year-olds, stage 7 for 16- to 17-year-olds, stage 8 for 18-year-olds) and girls (stage 3 for 10- to 12-year-olds and stage 4 for 13- to 18-year-olds) have been established with those youth failing to achieve the proposed stages having 3 to 4 times greater odds of having risk factors associated with metabolic syndrome (52). Interestingly, results from studies using the 20-meter multi-stage shuttle run in adults may provide an even better indicator of cardiorespiratory fitness than in children (34).

Normative Data

Twenty-meter multi-stage shuttle run classification values for laps completed are provided for boys in figure 9.3 and for girls in figure 9.4. Twenty-meter multi-stage shuttle run classification values for maximal aerobic capacity are provided for boys in figure 9.5 and for girls in figure 9.6. Descriptive values for the 20-meter multi-stage shuttle run in various athletic populations are provided in figure 9.7. General maximal aerobic capacity classification values are provided for men in figure 9.8 and for women in figure 9.9.

Table 9.2 Example Data for the 20-meter Multi-stage Shuttle Run

Stage	Speed (kph)	Pace (min/km)	Speed (mph)	Pace (min/mi)	Time per 20-meter lap (s)	Number of 20-meter laps	Stage Completed?	Laps Completed
S1	8.5	7.1	5.3	11.3	8.5	①②③④⑤⑥✗	✓	**7** / 7
S2	9	6.7	5.6	10.7	8.0	①②③④⑤⑥⑦✗	✓	**8** / 8
S3	9.5	6.3	5.9	10.2	7.6	①②③④⑤⑥⑦✗	✓	**8** / 8
S4	10	6.0	6.2	9.7	7.2	①②③④⑤⑥⑦⑧✗	✓	**9** / 9
S5	10.5	5.7	6.5	9.2	6.9	①②③④⑤⑥⑦⑧✗	✓	**9** / 9
S6	11	5.5	6.8	8.8	6.5	①②③④⑤⑥⑦⑧⑨✗	✓	**10** / 10
S7	11.5	5.2	7.1	8.5	6.3	①②③④⑤✗⑦⑧⑨⑩		**6** / 10
S8	12	5.0	7.5	8.0	6.0	①②③④⑤⑥⑦⑧⑨⑩⑪		____ / 11
S9	12.5	4.8	7.8	7.7	5.8	①②③④⑤⑥⑦⑧⑨⑩⑪		____ / 11
S10	13	4.6	8.1	7.4	5.5	①②③④⑤⑥⑦⑧⑨⑩⑪		____ / 11
S11	13.5	4.4	8.4	7.1	5.3	①②③④⑤⑥⑦⑧⑨⑩⑪⑫		____ / 12
S12	14	4.3	8.7	6.9	5.1	①②③④⑤⑥⑦⑧⑨⑩⑪⑫		____ / 12
S13	14.5	4.1	9.0	6.7	5.0	①②③④⑤⑥⑦⑧⑨⑩⑪⑫⑬		____ / 13
S14	15	4.0	9.3	6.5	4.8	①②③④⑤⑥⑦⑧⑨⑩⑪⑫⑬		____ / 13
S15	15.5	3.9	9.6	6.3	4.6	①②③④⑤⑥⑦⑧⑨⑩⑪⑫⑬		____ / 13
S16	16	3.8	9.9	6.1	4.5	①②③④⑤⑥⑦⑧⑨⑩⑪⑫⑬⑭		____ / 14
S17	16.5	3.6	10.3	5.8	4.4	①②③④⑤⑥⑦⑧⑨⑩⑪⑫⑬⑭		____ / 14
S18	17	3.5	10.6	5.7	4.2	①②③④⑤⑥⑦⑧⑨⑩⑪⑫⑬⑭⑮		____ / 15
S19	17.5	3.4	10.9	5.5	4.1	①②③④⑤⑥⑦⑧⑨⑩⑪⑫⑬⑭⑮		____ / 15
S20	18	3.3	11.2	5.4	4.0	①②③④⑤⑥⑦⑧⑨⑩⑪⑫⑬⑭⑮⑯		____ / 16
S21	18.5	3.2	11.5	5.2	3.9	①②③④⑤⑥⑦⑧⑨⑩⑪⑫⑬⑭⑮⑯		____ / 16
							Total laps	**57**

Figure 9.2 Conversion nomogram for estimated maximal aerobic capacity using the last stage completed during the 20-meter multi-stage shuttle run and athlete or client age

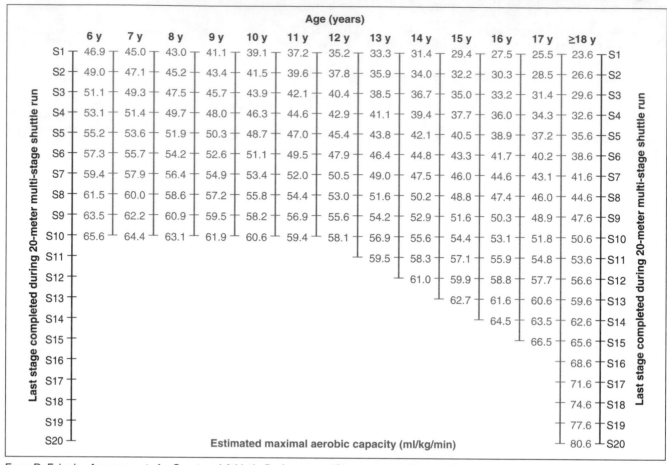

Age (years)

	6 y	7 y	8 y	9 y	10 y	11 y	12 y	13 y	14 y	15 y	16 y	17 y	≥18 y	
S1	46.9	45.0	43.0	41.1	39.1	37.2	35.2	33.3	31.4	29.4	27.5	25.5	23.6	S1
S2	49.0	47.1	45.2	43.4	41.5	39.6	37.8	35.9	34.0	32.2	30.3	28.5	26.6	S2
S3	51.1	49.3	47.5	45.7	43.9	42.1	40.4	38.5	36.7	35.0	33.2	31.4	29.6	S3
S4	53.1	51.4	49.7	48.0	46.3	44.6	42.9	41.1	39.4	37.7	36.0	34.3	32.6	S4
S5	55.2	53.6	51.9	50.3	48.7	47.0	45.4	43.8	42.1	40.5	38.9	37.2	35.6	S5
S6	57.3	55.7	54.2	52.6	51.1	49.5	47.9	46.4	44.8	43.3	41.7	40.2	38.6	S6
S7	59.4	57.9	56.4	54.9	53.4	52.0	50.5	49.0	47.5	46.0	44.6	43.1	41.6	S7
S8	61.5	60.0	58.6	57.2	55.8	54.4	53.0	51.6	50.2	48.8	47.4	46.0	44.6	S8
S9	63.5	62.2	60.9	59.5	58.2	56.9	55.6	54.2	52.9	51.6	50.3	48.9	47.6	S9
S10	65.6	64.4	63.1	61.9	60.6	59.4	58.1	56.9	55.6	54.4	53.1	51.8	50.6	S10
S11								59.5	58.3	57.1	55.9	54.8	53.6	S11
S12								61.0	59.9	58.8	57.7	56.6	S12
S13									62.7	61.6	60.6	59.6	S13
S14									64.5	63.5	62.6	S14
S15									66.5	65.6	S15
S16										68.6	S16
S17										71.6	S17
S18										74.6	S18
S19										77.6	S19
S20										80.6	S20

Last stage completed during 20-meter multi-stage shuttle run

Estimated maximal aerobic capacity (ml/kg/min)

From D. Fukuda, *Assessments for Sport and Athletic Performance* (Champaign, IL: Human Kinetics, 2019). Adapted from L.A. Léger, D. Mercier, C. Gadoury, and J. Lambert, "The Multistage 20 Metre Shuttle Run Test for Aerobic Fitness," *Journal of Sports Sciences* 6 (1988): 93-101.

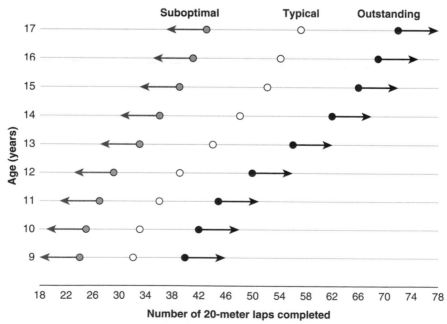

Figure 9.3 Twenty-meter multi-stage shuttle run laps classifications in boys: outstanding—70th percentile; typical—50th percentile; suboptimal—30th percentile.

Data from (54).

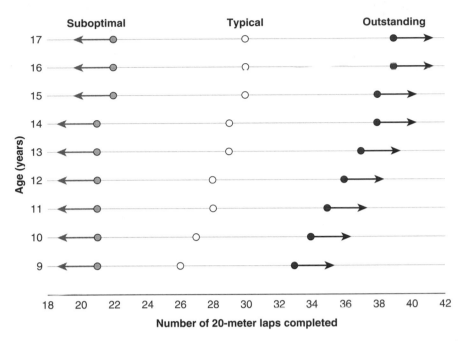

Figure 9.4 Twenty-meter multi-stage shuttle run laps classifications in girls: outstanding—70th percentile; typical—50th percentile; suboptimal—30th percentile.

Data from (54).

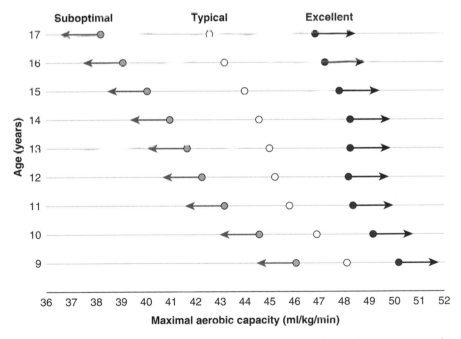

Figure 9.5 Twenty-meter multi-stage shuttle run maximal aerobic capacity classifications in boys: outstanding—70th percentile; typical—50th percentile; suboptimal—30th percentile.

Data from (54).

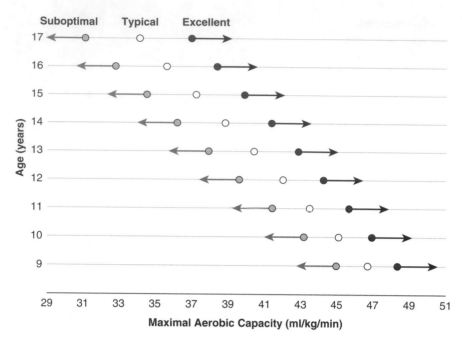

Figure 9.6 Twenty-meter multi-stage shuttle run maximal aerobic capacity classifications in girls: outstanding—70th percentile; typical—50th percentile; suboptimal—30th percentile.

Data from (54).

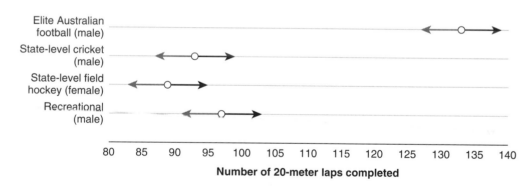

Figure 9.7 Descriptive values for the 20-meter multi-stage shuttle run in various athletic populations.

Data from (61).

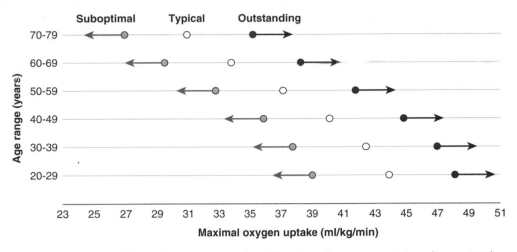

Figure 9.8 Maximal aerobic capacity classifications in men: outstanding—75th percentile; typical—50th percentile; suboptimal—25th percentile.

Data from (4).

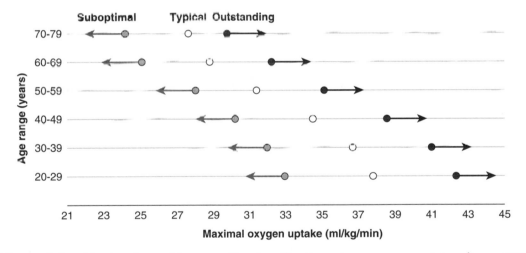

Figure 9.9 Maximal aerobic capacity classifications in women: outstanding—75th percentile; typical—50th percentile; suboptimal—25th percentile.

Data from (4).

YO-YO INTERMITTENT RECOVERY TEST

Purpose

The Yo-Yo intermittent recovery tests provide a running-based measure of cardiorespiratory fitness using intermittent change-of-direction protocols with increasing intensity leading to maximal effort.

Outcomes

Number of 20-meter shuttle runs completed; distance covered; estimated maximal aerobic capacity

Equipment Needed

Three cones or markers, adhesive tape, or field paint; measuring tape; mobile app or prerecorded audio file (various options available online); device to play the audio file; audio system or speakers

Before You Begin

Draw two lines or place two cones or markers 20 meters (65.6 ft) apart, with one line or cone designated as the start line and the other as the turn line (see figure 9.10). Place an additional cone or marker, designated as the recovery line, 5 meters (16.4 ft) past the start line (outside of the 20-meter distance between the start and turn lines).

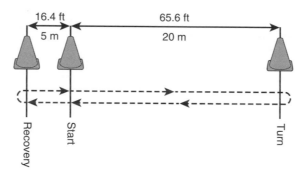

Figure 9.10 Set-up for the Yo-Yo intermittent recovery test.

The coach or fitness professional can decide between two versions of the Yo-Yo intermittent recovery test: level 1 (Yo-Yo IR1) or level 2 (Yo-Yo IR2). While both versions feature 10-second periods of active recovery between shuttles, the Yo-Yo IR1 test starts at a lower speed, and the Yo-Yo IR2 test increases in speed more quickly. The Yo-Yo IR2 test may be more appropriate for athletes who perform intermittent bouts of high-intensity exercise (i.e., most team sports and strength or power athletes), while the Yo-Yo IR1 test may be more appropriate for aerobic endurance athletes or less-trained individuals engaged in intermittent bouts of high-intensity exercise. If an individual can complete the entire Yo-Yo IR1 test protocol, the Yo-Yo IR2 protocol should be used for future testing purposes. A data collection sheet for the Yo-Yo IR1 test is provided in table 9.3 and for the Yo-Yo IR2 test in table 9.4 (see the "Alternatives or Modifications" section for additional options); however, coaches or fitness professionals should take care to verify the specific protocol for the audio recording, software, or app. A standardized warm-up followed by three to five minutes of rest and recovery should be conducted prior to beginning the assessment.

Protocol

1. Begin the procedure by saying to the athlete or client: *"We are going to measure how long you can continue jogging, running, and eventually sprinting laps between the cones. You will have a 10-second recovery period after each shuttle. Are you ready to begin? If so, please stand behind the start line."*

2. Next, explain: *"When the audio recording indicates the start of the test, jog forward to the turn line, aiming to arrive in time with the first beep, then turn back and jog in the opposite direction to the start line in time with the next beep. When you reach the start line, slow down until you reach the recovery line, then immediately return to the start line and stand still until the next beep indicates the start of the next shuttle. As the test progresses, the beeps will come closer together so you will have to run faster to make it to the lines in time. For a shuttle to count, you will need to step at least one foot on or over the start line. Continue going back and forth with the 10-second recovery periods in between shuttles until you cannot return to the start line in time with the beep two times in a row. If that happens, the test is over."*

3. An evaluator will be positioned at each line, marker, or cone. The evaluators will verify that at least one of the athlete's or client's feet has reached the start line in time with the beep and provide a warning if the athlete or client was unable to do so. A tally system or counting device should be used to accurately count the number of laps completed. If the athlete or client does not return to the start line in time with the beep, the test is finished and the total number of shuttles completed (including the last two incomplete attempts) are recorded.

4. If the measurement of maximal heart rate is desired, the coach or fitness professional should measure the athlete's or client's heart rate immediately after completing the test using one of the methods described in chapter 10.

Table 9.3 Data Collection Sheet for the Yo-Yo Intermittent Recovery Test Level 1 (IR1)

Stage	Speed (km/h)	Pace (min/km)	Speed (mph)	Pace (min/mi)	Time per 20 m lap (sec)	Number of shuttles (2 × 20 m laps)	Shuttles completed
S1	10	6.0	6.2	9.7	7.20	①	
S2	11.5	5.2	7.1	8.5	6.26	①	
S3	13	4.6	8.1	7.4	5.54	①②	
S4	13.5	4.4	8.4	7.1	5.33	①②③	
S5	14	4.3	8.7	6.9	5.14	①②③④	
S6	14.5	4.1	9.0	6.7	4.97	①②③④⑤⑥⑦⑧	
S7	15	4.0	9.3	6.5	4.80	①②③④⑤⑥⑦⑧	
S8	15.5	3.9	9.6	6.3	4.65	①②③④⑤⑥⑦⑧	
S9	16	3.8	9.9	6.1	4.50	①②③④⑤⑥⑦⑧	
S10	16.5	3.6	10.3	5.8	4.36	①②③④⑤⑥⑦⑧	
S11	17	3.5	10.6	5.7	4.24	①②③④⑤⑥⑦⑧	
S12	17.5	3.4	10.9	5.5	4.11	①②③④⑤⑥⑦⑧	
S13	18	3.3	11.2	5.4	4.00	①②③④⑤⑥⑦⑧	
S14	18.5	3.24	11.5	5.2	3.89	①②③④⑤⑥⑦⑧	
S15	19	3.16	11.8	5.1	3.79	①②③④⑤⑥⑦⑧	
						Total shuttles	

From D. Fukuda, *Assessments for Sport and Athletic Performance* (Champaign, IL: Human Kinetics, 2019).

Table 9.4 Data Collection Sheet for the Yo-Yo Intermittent Recovery Test Level 2 (IR2)

Stage	Speed (km/h)	Pace (min/km)	Speed (mph)	Pace (min/mi)	Time per 20 meter lap (sec)	Number of shuttles (2 × 20 meter laps)	Shuttles completed
S1	13	4.6	8.1	7.4	5.54	①	
S2	15	4.0	9.3	6.5	4.80	①	
S3	16	3.8	9.9	6.1	4.50	①②	
S4	16.5	3.6	10.3	5.8	4.36	①②③	
S5	17	3.5	10.6	5.7	4.24	①②③④	
S6	17.5	3.4	10.9	5.5	4.11	①②③④⑤⑥⑦⑧	
S7	18	3.3	11.2	5.4	4.00	①②③④⑤⑥⑦⑧	
S8	18.5	3.2	11.5	5.2	3.89	①②③④⑤⑥⑦⑧	
S9	19	3.2	11.8	5.1	3.79	①②③④⑤⑥⑦⑧	
S10	19.5	3.1	12.1	5.0	3.69	①②③④⑤⑥⑦⑧	
S11	20	3.0	12.4	4.8	3.60	①②③④⑤⑥⑦⑧	
S12	20.5	2.93	12.7	4.7	3.51	①②③④⑤⑥⑦⑧	
S13	21	2.86	13.0	4.6	3.43	①②③④⑤⑥⑦⑧	
S14	21.5	2.8	13.4	4.5	3.35	①②③④⑤⑥⑦⑧	
S15	22	2.7	13.7	4.4	3.27	①②③④⑤⑥⑦⑧	
						Total shuttles	

From D. Fukuda, *Assessments for Sport and Athletic Performance* (Champaign, IL: Human Kinetics, 2019).

Alternatives or Modifications

The Yo-Yo intermittent recovery tests can be used to assess small groups of athletes or clients in a single session. This approach requires enough spacing between those being tested (i.e., at least 2 meters [6.6 ft]) and additional evaluators to record the final results. If the measurement of maximal heart rate is desired, the coach or fitness professional should measure the athlete's or client's heart rate immediately after completing the test using one of the methods described in chapter 10.

The Yo-Yo IR1 test can be modified for children (6 to 10 years old) by decreasing the laps to 16 meters (52.5 ft) and the recovery distance to 4 meters (13.1 ft), which has been shown to allow most children to complete at least three minutes of the test (7). Submaximal versions of the Yo-Yo IR1 and IR2 tests are a recommended tool for athlete monitoring (see chapter 10) (42, 57).

Aerobic endurance-based versions of these tests—Yo-Yo intermittent endurance test level 1 (Yo-Yo IE1) and level 2 (Yo-Yo IE2)—have also been developed with the same 20-meter (65.6 ft) shuttle distance but with a 5-second active recovery period conducted over a 2.5-meter (8.2 ft) distance. The Yo-Yo IE1 test (with speeds between 8 and 14.5 km/h [5 to 9 mph]) has been primarily used in nonelite and youth athletes (11, 58), whereas the Yo-Yo IE2 test (with speeds between 11.5 and 18 km/h [7 to 11.2 mph]) has been primarily used in female soccer athletes (10).

After You Finish

The total number of shuttles completed (including the final two attempts) is the final result. The total number of shuttles can be multiplied by 40 meters per shuttle to calculate the total distance covered during the test.

From the example data provided in table 9.5, the athlete or client completed a total of 24 shuttles during the Yo-Yo IR1 test for a total distance covered of 960 meters (24 shuttles × 40 meters per shuttle). The total distance covered can also be used to estimate maximal aerobic capacity using the following formulas (6):

Yo-Yo IR1 test; in ml/kg/min

$$\dot{V}O_2 \text{ max} = (IR1 \text{ distance in m} \times 0.0084) + 36.4$$

Yo-Yo IR2 test; in ml/kg/min

$$\dot{V}O_2 \text{ max} = (IR2 \text{ distance in m} \times 0.0136) + 45.3$$

From the example data provided in table 9.5, the athlete or client with a total distance covered of 1,000 meters (25 shuttles × 40 meters per shuttle) during the Yo-Yo IR1 test has an estimated maximal aerobic capacity of:

$$\dot{V}O_2 \text{ max} = (1000 \text{ m} \times 0.0084) + 36.4 = 44.8 \text{ ml/kg/min}$$

Or, instead of using the formulas, conversion nomograms provided in figure 9.11 can be used to estimate maximal aerobic capacity.

Table 9.5 Sample Data Collection Sheet for the Yo-Yo Intermittent Recovery Test Level 1 (IR1)

Stage	Speed (km/h)	Pace (min/km)	Speed (mph)	Pace (min/mi)	Time per 20-meter lap (sec)	Number of shuttles (2 × 20 meter laps)	Shuttles completed
S1	10	6.0	6.2	9.7	7.20	⊗	1/1
S2	11.5	5.2	7.1	8.5	6.26	⊗	1/1
S3	13	4.6	8.1	7.4	5.54	①⊗	2/2
S4	13.5	4.4	8.4	7.1	5.33	①②⊗	3/3
S5	14	4.3	8.7	6.9	5.14	①②③⊗	4/4
S6	14.5	4.1	9.0	6.7	4.97	①②③④⑤⑥⑦⊗	8/8
S7	15	4.0	9.3	6.5	4.80	①②③④⑤⊗⑦⑧	6/8
S8	15.5	3.9	9.6	6.3	4.65	①②③④⑤⑥⑦⑧	_/8
S9	16	3.8	9.9	6.1	4.50	①②③④⑤⑥⑦⑧	_/8
S10	16.5	3.6	10.3	5.8	4.36	①②③④⑤⑥⑦⑧	_/8
S11	17	3.5	10.6	5.7	4.24	①②③④⑤⑥⑦⑧	_/8
S12	17.5	3.4	10.9	5.5	4.11	①②③④⑤⑥⑦⑧	_/8
S13	18	3.3	11.2	5.4	4.00	①②③④⑤⑥⑦⑧	_/8
S14	18.5	3.24	11.5	5.2	3.89	①②③④⑤⑥⑦⑧	_/8
S15	19	3.16	11.8	5.1	3.79	①②③④⑤⑥⑦⑧	_/8
						Total shuttles	25

Figure 9.11 Conversion nomograms for estimating maximal aerobic capacity from the Yo-Yo intermittent recovery test level 1 (IR1) and level 2 (IR2)

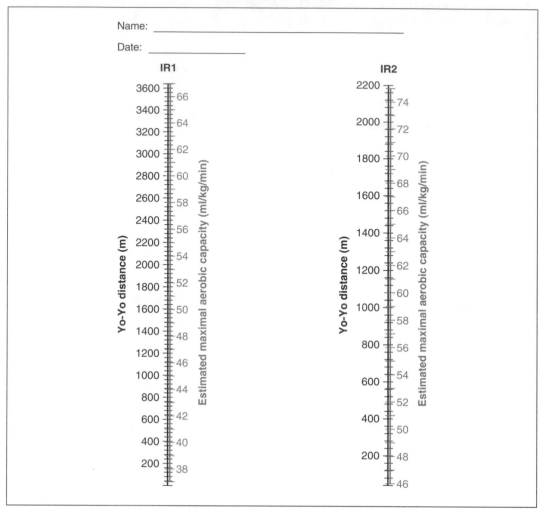

From D. Fukuda, *Assessments for Sport and Athletic Performance* (Champaign, IL: Human Kinetics, 2019). Using formulas from (6).

Research Notes

Yo-Yo IR1 performance has shown to be related to high-intensity running by both athletes and referees during soccer matches (6). Twelve weeks of high-intensity interval training in soccer referees resulted in a 23-percent increase in high-intensity running during a match (before: 1,690 m; after: 2,060 m), primarily in the second half, coupled with a 31-percent increase in the Yo-Yo IR1 distance covered (before: 1,345 m; after: 1,763 m) (26). Yo-Yo IR2 performance has shown to distinguish between playing positions and competitive level in soccer (28), while being related to the greatest distance covered while running at high intensities within a five-minute period during a match.

In other sports, Yo-Yo IR1 performance in basketball players was reportedly related to decreased line drill times following a game (12), and rugby league players with higher Yo-Yo IR2 scores, indicating better high-intensity running ability, were less fatigued 24 hours and 48 hours following a match compared to players with lower scores (24).

Normative Data

Descriptive values for the Yo-Yo intermittent recovery test in various populations are provided in figure 9.12 through figure 9.16. Typical maximal aerobic capacity values for various athletes are provided in table 9.6.

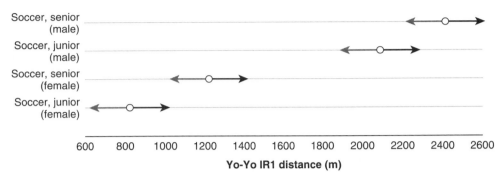

Figure 9.12 Descriptive data for Yo-Yo intermittent recovery test level 1 (IR1) in male and female soccer players.

Data from (41).

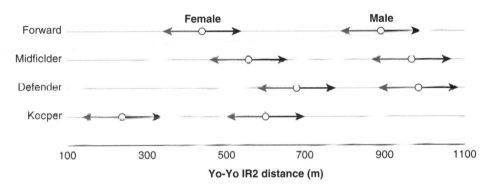

Figure 9.13 Descriptive data for Yo-Yo intermittent recovery test level 2 (IR2) distance in elite male and collegiate female soccer players by position.

Data from (28, 32).

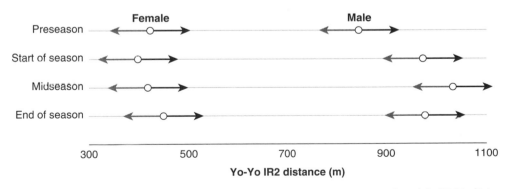

Figure 9.14 Descriptive data for Yo-Yo intermittent recovery test level 2 (IR2) distance in elite male and female soccer players over the course of a season.

Data from (33, 40).

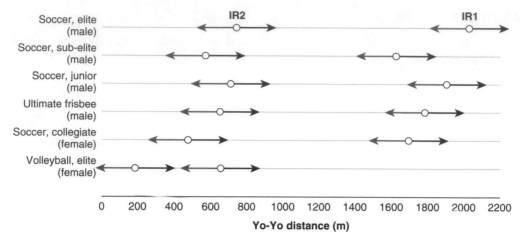

Figure 9.15 Descriptive data for Yo-Yo intermittent recovery test level 1 (IR1) and level 2 (IR2) in various populations.

Data from (15, 23, 27, 32, 45).

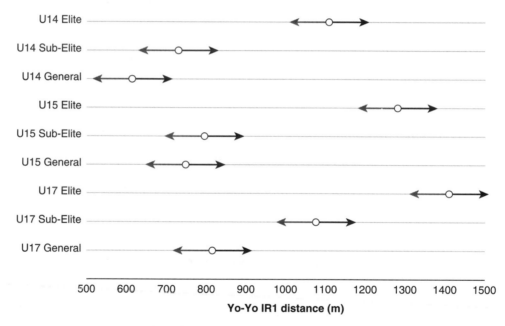

Figure 9.16 Descriptive data for Yo-Yo intermittent recovery test level 1 (IR1) distance in elite basketball players, subelite basketball players, and age-matched nonathletes (general).

Data from (56).

Table 9.6 Typical Maximal Aerobic Capacity ($\dot{V}O_2$max) Values for Various Athletes

| Classification | $\dot{V}O_2$max (ml/kg/min) | | Sport |
	Males	Females	
Extremely high	70+	60+	Cross-country skiing Middle-distance running Long-distance running
Very high	63-69	54-59	Bicycling Rowing Race walking
High	57-62	49-53	Soccer Middle-distance swimming Canoe racing Handball Racquetball Speed skating Figure skating Downhill skiing Wrestling
Above average	52-56	44-48	Basketball Ballet dancing American football (offensive/defensive backs) Gymnastics Hockey Horse racing (jockey) Sprint swimming Tennis Sprint running Jumping
Average	44-51	35-43	Baseball Softball American football (linemen, quarterbacks) Shotput Discus throw Olympic-style weightlifting Bodybuilding

Reprinted by permission from M. McGuigan, "Administration, Scoring, and Interpretation of Selected Tests." In *Essentials of Strength Training and Conditioning,* 4th ed., edited by G.G. Haff and N.T. Triplett for the National Strength and Conditioning Association (Champaign, IL: Human Kinetics, 2016), 308.

DISTANCE-BASED WALK AND RUN TESTS

Purpose

Distance-based walk and run tests provide measures of cardiorespiratory fitness using continuous fixed-distance protocols.

Outcomes

Time, in seconds, needed to cover the intended distance; estimated maximal aerobic capacity

Equipment Needed

Track or measured course; cones or markers; measuring tape; stopwatch or timing device

Before You Begin

Place the markers the selected distance apart (1.5 miles [2.4 km] will be used for this explanation), clearly designating a measured course and a starting line. If a 400-meter (437.5 yd) track is used instead of a 440-yard track (see figure 9.17), remember to account for the 2.3-meter (2.5 yd) difference for each lap to be completed. For example, the 1.5-mile run/walk requires the athlete or client to complete 6 full laps on a 440 yd track, or 6 full laps and an additional 13.8 meters (2.3 meters × 6 laps) on a 400-meter (437.5 yd) track.

A standardized warm-up followed by three to five minutes of rest and recovery should be conducted prior to beginning the assessment.

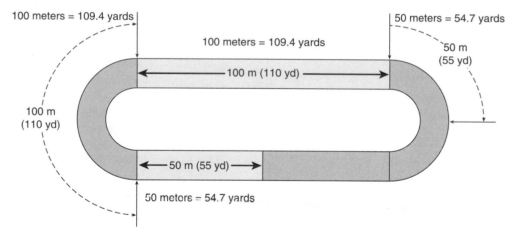

Figure 9.17 A 400-meter (437.5 yd) track.

Protocol

1. Begin the procedure by saying to the athlete or client: *"We are going to measure how quickly you can run or walk 1.5 miles (2.4 km). Are you ready to begin? If so, please stand behind the starting line."*

2. Next, explain: *"When I say 'Go,' run (or walk or jog as needed) as fast as possible to complete the test."*

3. Verbally signal the athlete or client *"3, 2, 1, go,"* and record how much time is required, to the nearest second, to cover the intended distance. A tally system or counting device should be used to accurately count the number of laps completed.

Alternatives or Modifications

For the 1-mile (1.6 km) Rockport walk test, a 15-second pulse count is taken after completing the distance. That number, along with the athlete's or client's age, sex, and body weight, are used to estimate maximal aerobic capacity.

After You Finish

The time required to cover the selected distance is the final result. To determine time in minutes from seconds, divide the number of seconds by 60. The following distance-specific formulas can be used to estimate maximal aerobic capacity ($\dot{V}O_2$max; in ml/kg/min):

One-mile (1.6 km) run/walk formulas; developed using 18- to 25-year-olds (14):

Males

$$\dot{V}O_2\text{max} = (-9.06 \times \text{time in min}) + (0.38 \times (\text{time in min})^2) + 98.49$$

Females

$$\dot{V}O_2\text{max} = (-6.04 \times \text{time in min}) + (0.22 \times (\text{time in min})^2) + 82.2$$

As an example, a woman who takes 9 minutes (540 seconds divided by 60) to cover 1 mile (1.6 km) has an estimated maximal aerobic capacity of:

$$\dot{V}O_2\text{max} = (-6.04 \times 9 \text{ min}) + (0.22 \times (9 \text{ min})^2) + 82.2$$

$$\dot{V}O_2\text{max} = -54.36 + (0.22 \times 81) + 82.2$$

$$\dot{V}O_2\text{max} = -54.36 + 17.82 + 82.2 = 45.7 \text{ ml/kg/min}$$

Or, instead of using the formulas, conversion nomograms for the 1-mile (1.6 km) run/walk test provided in figure 9.18 can be used to estimate maximal aerobic capacity (14).

Formulas for 1.5-mile (2.4 km) run/walk; developed using 18- to 29-year-olds (16):

Males

$$\dot{V}O_2\text{max} = 91.736 - (0.1656 \times \text{wt in kg}) - (2.767 \times \text{time in min})$$

Females

$$\dot{V}O_2\text{max} = 88.020 - (0.1656 \times \text{wt in kg}) - (2.767 \times \text{time in min})$$

As an example, a man who weighs 70 kilograms (154 lbs) and takes 11.5 minutes (690 seconds divided by 60) to cover 1.5 miles (2.4 km) has an estimated maximal aerobic capacity of:

$$\dot{V}O_2\text{max} = 91.736 - (0.1656 \times 70 \text{ kg}) - (2.767 \times 11.5 \text{ min})$$

$$\dot{V}O_2\text{max} = 91.736 - 11.592 - 31.821 = 48.3 \text{ ml/kg/min}$$

Or, instead of using the formulas, conversion nomograms for the 1.5-mile (2.4 km) run/walk test provided in figure 9.19 can be used to estimate maximal aerobic capacity (16).

Formulas for 2-mile (3.2 km) run/walk; developed using 20- to 37-year-olds (39):

Males

$$\dot{V}O_2\text{max} = 99.7 - (3.35 \times \text{time in min})$$

Females

$$\dot{V}O_2\text{max} = 72.9 - (1.77 \times \text{time in min})$$

As an example, a woman who takes 14.75 minutes (885 seconds divided by 60) to cover 2 miles (3.2 km) has an estimated maximal aerobic capacity of:

$$\dot{V}O_2max = 72.9 - (1.77 \times 14.75 \text{ min})$$

$$\dot{V}O_2max = 72.9 - 26.1 = 46.8 \text{ ml/kg/min}$$

Or, instead of using the formulas, conversion nomograms for the 2-mile (3.2 km) run/walk test provided in figure 9.20 can be used to estimate maximal aerobic capacity (39).

Figure 9.18   Conversion nomograms for estimating maximal aerobic capacity from 1-mile (1.6 km) run/walk times in men and women

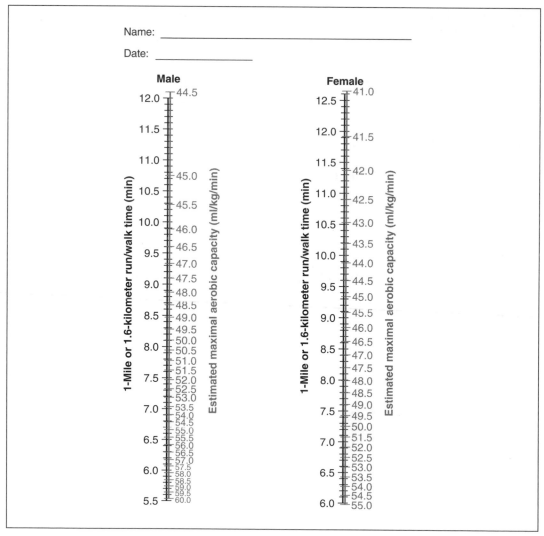

From D. Fukuda, *Assessments for Sport and Athletic Performance* (Champaign, IL: Human Kinetics, 2019). Using formulas from (14).

Research Notes

Distance-based run/walk tests are typical components of military physical fitness tests, such as the 1.5-mile (2.4 km) test used by the U.S. Navy and the 2-mile (3.2 km) test used by the U.S. Army, because the resultant scores are related to gold standard measures of cardiorespiratory fitness (i.e., $\dot{V}O_2$max) and can be conducted easily on a large scale (30).

Children with higher levels of cardiorespiratory fitness typically demonstrate better academic performance than those with lower levels of cardiorespiratory fitness (50). One research study reported that each additional minute needed to complete the 1-mile (1.6 km) run/walk test was associated with a 1.9-point decline in math scores and a 1.1-point decline in reading scores on standardized tests in 10- to 16-year-olds (48).

A review of 123 research studies examining cardiorespiratory fitness assessments suggested that the 1.5-mile (2.4 km) run/walk test demonstrated the best relationship with maximal aerobic capacity among the commonly used distance-based field tests (35).

Figure 9.19   Conversion nomograms for estimating maximal aerobic capacity from 1.5-mile (2.4 km) run/walk times in men and women

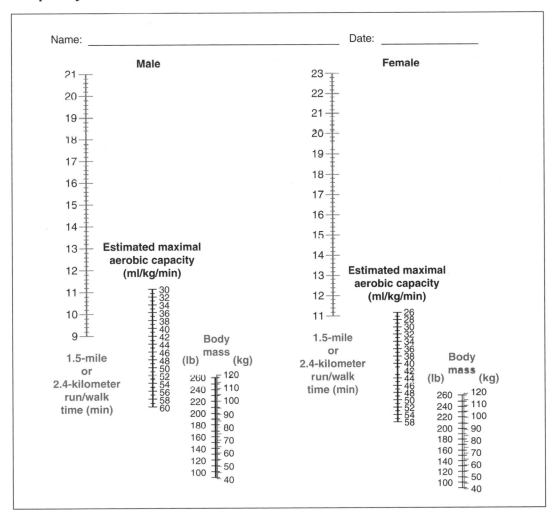

From D. Fukuda, *Assessments for Sport and Athletic Performance* (Champaign, IL: Human Kinetics, 2019). Using formulas from (16).

Normative Data

Time classification values for the 1-mile (1.6 km) run/walk test are provided in figure 9.21 (boys) and figure 9.22 (girls), for the 1.5-mile (2.4 km) run/walk test in figure 9.23 (men) and figure 9.24 (women), and for the 2-mile (3.2 km) run/walk test in figure 9.25 (men) and figure 9.26 (women).

Figure 9.20 Conversion nomograms for estimating maximal aerobic capacity from 2-mile (3.2 km) run/walk times in men and women

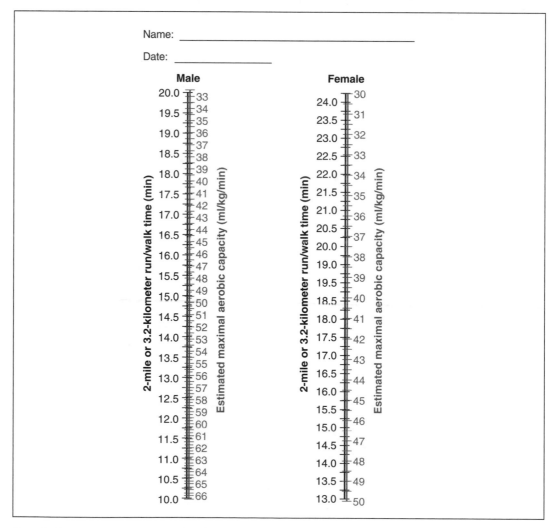

From D. Fukuda, *Assessments for Sport and Athletic Performance* (Champaign, IL: Human Kinetics, 2019). Using formulas from (39).

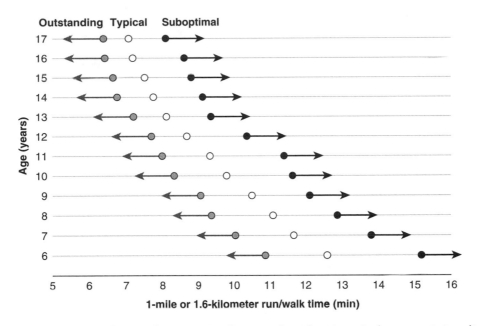

Figure 9.21 One-mile (1.6 km) run/walk time classifications in boys: outstanding—75th percentile; typical—50th percentile; suboptimal—25th percentile.

Data from (46).

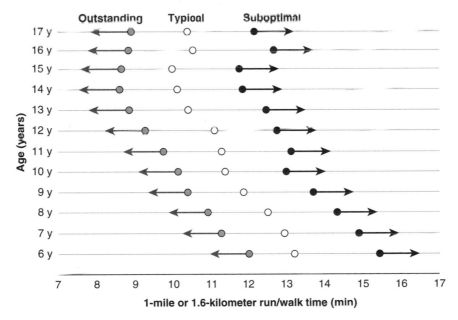

Figure 9.22 One-mile (1.6 km) run/walk time classifications in girls: outstanding—75th percentile; typical—50th percentile; suboptimal—25th percentile.

Data from (46).

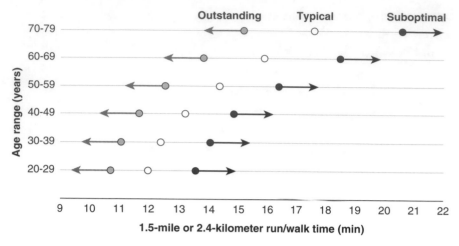

Figure 9.23 Time classifications for 1.5-mile (2.4 km) run/walk in men: outstanding—75th percentile; typical—50th percentile; suboptimal—25th percentile.
Data from (4).

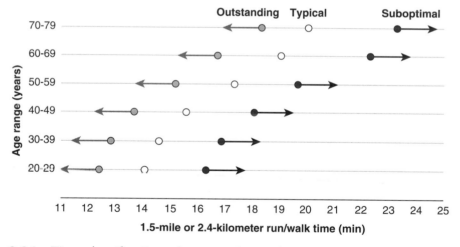

Figure 9.24 Time classifications for 1.5-mile (2.4 km) run/walk in women: outstanding—75th percentile; typical—50th percentile; suboptimal—25th percentile.
Data from (4).

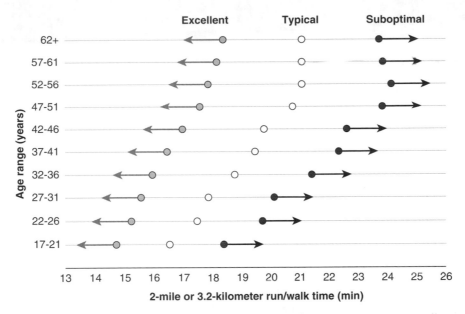

Figure 9.25 Two-mile (3.2 km) run/walk time classifications in men: excellent—75th percentile; typical—50th percentile; suboptimal—25th percentile.

Data from (1).

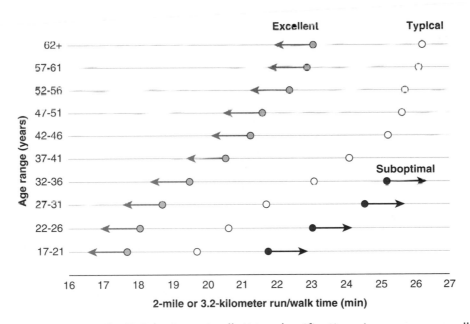

Figure 9.26 Two-mile (3.2 km) run/walk time classifications in women: excellent—75th percentile; typical—50th percentile; suboptimal—25th percentile (unavailable for 37+ yr).

Data from (1).

TIME-BASED WALK OR RUN TESTS

Purpose

Time-based walk or run tests provide measures of cardiorespiratory fitness using a continuous fixed-time protocol.

Outcomes

Distance covered, in miles (or yards) or kilometers (or meters), within the selected time frame; estimated maximal aerobic capacity

Equipment Needed

Track or measured course; cones or markers; measuring tape; stopwatch or timing device

Before You Begin

Determine the selected time frame (12 minutes will be used for this explanation), which will likely be influenced by the space available and the training status of the athlete or client, with longer distances being better tolerated by trained individuals than less trained individuals. Clearly designate a measured course and use cones or markers to identify evenly spaced interval distances.

A standardized warm-up followed by three to five minutes of rest and recovery should be conducted prior to beginning the assessment.

Protocol

1. Begin the procedure by saying to the athlete or client: "*We are going to measure how far you can run or walk in 12 minutes. Are you ready to begin? If so, please stand behind the starting line.*"
2. Next, explain: "*When I say 'Go,' run (or walk or jog as needed) as far as possible for 12 minutes to complete the test.*"
3. Verbally signal the athlete or client "*3, 2, 1, go,*" and record the distance covered, to the nearest 50 meters (55 yd) within the selected time frame. A tally system or counting device should be used to accurately count the number of laps completed.

Alternatives or Modifications

Tests that determine the distance covered in 9 minutes or in 15 minutes are also commonly used for time-based field assessments of cardiorespiratory fitness. In addition, the 6-minute walk test is part of the Senior Fitness Test (47) and consists of completing as many 50-yard (45.7 m) laps around a 20- x 5-yard (18.3- by 4.6-m) course within 6 minutes.

After You Finish

The total distance covered within the selected time frame is the final result. To convert the distance covered from meters to kilometers, divide the number of meters by 1,000, or to convert the distance covered from yards to miles, divide the number of yards by 1,760. The following formulas can be used to estimate maximal aerobic capacity ($\dot{V}O_2max$; in ml /kg/min):

12-minute run/walk formulas (13)

$$\dot{V}O_2max = (22.35 \times \text{distance in km}) - 11.28$$

$$\dot{V}O_2max = (35.97 \times \text{distance in mi}) - 11.28$$

For example, an athlete or client who covers 2.75 kilometers (2,750 meters divided by 1,000) during the 12-minute run/walk test has an estimated maximal aerobic capacity of:

$$\dot{V}O_2max = (22.35 \times 2.75 \text{ km}) - 11.28$$

$$\dot{V}O_2max = 61.46 - 11.28 = 50.18 \text{ ml/kg/min}$$

Or, instead of using the formula, conversion nomograms for the 12-minute run/walk test provided in figure 9.27 can be used to estimate maximal aerobic capacity (13).

Research Notes

Relative age effects are characterized by a greater representation of individuals born during a specific part of the year. Potentially due to the selection process and various other factors in competitive sports, there may be a larger number of relatively older athletes who are born just after an age group cutoff (i.e., January) compared to relatively younger athletes who are born

Figure 9.27 Conversion nomograms for estimating maximal aerobic capacity from 12-minute run/walk distance

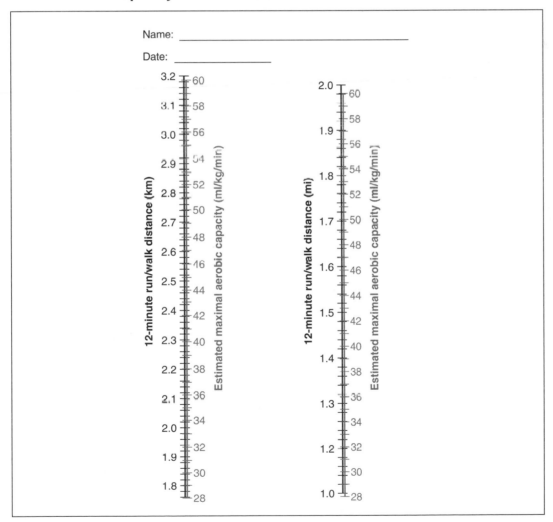

From D. Fukuda, *Assessments for Sport and Athletic Performance* (Champaign, IL: Human Kinetics, 2019). Using formulas from (13).

closer to the end of a particular birth year (i.e., December). For example, a greater number of youth alpine skiers were reportedly born January through March (28 to 34%) than October through December (18 to 21%) (18).

Correspondingly, 13- to 14-year-old skiers born later in the year covered less distance during the 12-minute run/walk test than those born earlier in the year. Additionally, differences in distance covered during the 12-minute run/walk test have been shown between under-21-year-old alpine skiers who were selected to the national squad and those were not selected (17).

A review of 123 research studies examining cardiorespiratory fitness assessments suggested that the 12-minute run/walk test demonstrated the best relationship with maximal aerobic capacity among the commonly used time-based field tests (35).

Normative Data

Distance classification values for the 12-minute run/walk test are provided in figure 9.28 (men) and figure 9.29 (women). Descriptive values for the 12-minute run/walk test in youth alpine skiers are provided in figure 9.30 (boys) and figure 9.31 (girls).

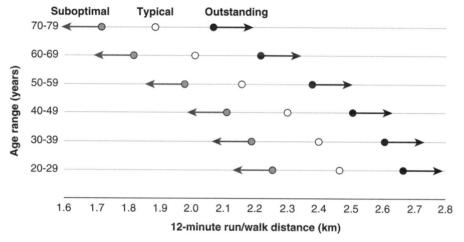

Figure 9.28 Twelve-minute run/walk distance classifications in men: outstanding—75th percentile; typical—50th percentile; suboptimal—25th percentile.
Data from (4).

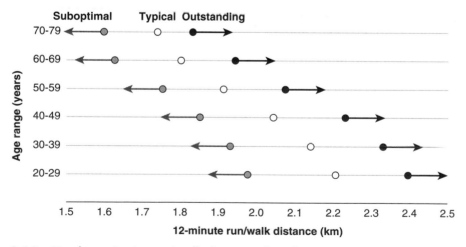

Figure 9.29 Twelve-minute run/walk distance classifications in women: outstanding—75th percentile; typical—50th percentile; suboptimal—25th percentile.
Data from (4).

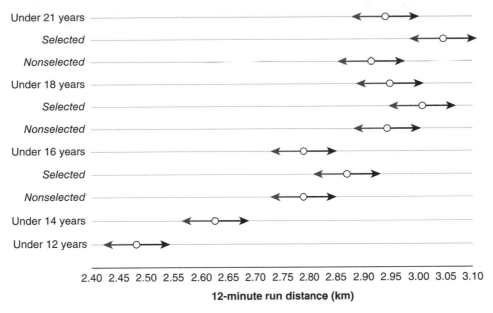

Figure 9.30 Descriptive values from male youth alpine skiers.
Data from (17).

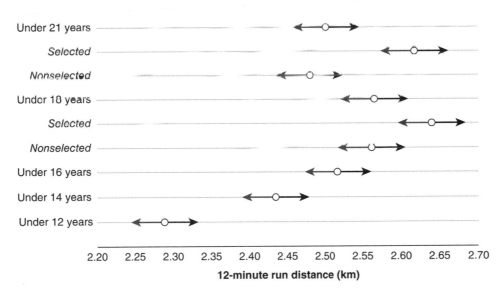

Figure 9.31 Descriptive values from female youth alpine skiers.
Data from (17).

SUBMAXIMAL STEP TEST

Purpose

The submaximal step test (or Queens College or YMCA step test) provides a measure of cardio-respiratory fitness using a continuous fixed-cadence protocol.

Outcomes

Recovery heart rate in beats per minute; estimated maximal aerobic capacity

Equipment Needed

A sturdy bench, step, or box with a height of 16.25 inches (41.3 cm); timing device; metronome; heart rate monitor (if available)

Before You Begin

Review the heart rate measurement guidelines provided in chapter 10. Set a metronome to either 88 beats per minute (a pace of 22 steps per minute) for women or 96 beats per minute (a pace of 24 steps per minute) for men.

Protocol

1. Begin the procedure by saying to the athlete or client: *"We are going to measure your heart rate after you complete a three-minute step test. Are you ready to begin? If so, please stand in front of the bench."*

2. Next, explain: *"When I say 'Go,' start by stepping up with one foot followed by the other foot and then stepping down in the reverse order. You may start with either foot as the lead foot, and if that leg becomes tired, feel free to change to the other foot as the lead foot. Do your best to make each step in time with the audible signal provided by the metronome. I will let you know after three minutes that the test is over. Please stay in the standing position with both feet on the ground while I measure your heart rate by placing my fingers on your neck or wrist."* (See figure 9.32.)

3. Verbally signal the athlete or client *"3, 2, 1, go,"* and monitor that the athlete or client can safely keep up with the metronome pace. If the athlete or client cannot maintain the required pace following encouragement, stop the test and consider an alternative assessment. Approximately 5 seconds after the test is finished, measure and record the 15-second pulse count.

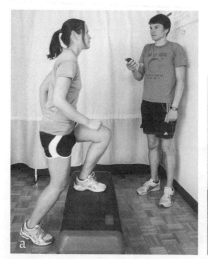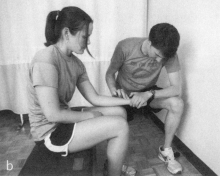

Figure 9.32 *(a)* Submaximal step test and *(b)* recovery heart rate measurement. Note: the recovery heart rate is measured in the standing position for the Queens College step test and in the seated position for the YMCA step test.

Alternatives or Modifications

The YMCA step test uses the same protocol but with a 13-inch (33 cm) bench with a heart rate measurement that is conducted one minute after the test with the athlete or client in a seated position (60).

The Forestry step test uses different bench heights for men (40 cm [15.75 in.]) and women (33 cm [13 in.]), a step rate of 22.5 steps per minute (90 beats per minute), a testing period of 5 minutes, and a recovery heart rate measurement that begins 15 seconds after the test (2).

For older adults, an alternative version of the test lasts for two minutes and does not involve an actual step. Rather, the individual steps in place (similar to marching) with the lead leg raised to a point that is at least level with the midway point between the kneecap and the top of the hip bone (47).

After You Finish

The 15-second pulse count measured at the end of the test is the final result. Multiply this value by four to calculate heart rate in beats per minute (bpm), which can be used to estimate maximal aerobic capacity. See the following formulas that were developed in healthy, young adults (36):

Women; in ml/kg/min

$$\dot{V}O_2max = 65.81 - (0.1847 \times \text{heart rate in bpm})$$

Women; in ml/kg/min

$$\dot{V}O_2max = 111.33 - (0.42 \times \text{heart rate in bpm})$$

For example, a woman who completes the submaximal step test with an immediate postexercise heart rate of 120 beats per minute (a 15-second pulse count multiplied by 4) has an estimated maximal aerobic capacity of:

$$\dot{V}O_2max = 65.81 - (0.1847 \times 120 \text{ bpm})$$

$$\dot{V}O_2max = 65.81 - 22.16 = 43.65 \text{ ml/kg/min}$$

Or, instead of using the formula, conversion nomograms for the submaximal step test provided in figure 9.33 can be used to estimate maximal aerobic capacity (36).

Research Notes

While step tests can be easily conducted in most settings and have been shown to be related to cardiorespiratory fitness in generally healthy adults (8), they may not be feasible for all individuals. One research study reported that 73 percent of 189 individuals were only able to complete 2 minutes or less of the YMCA step test with age (>50 years old), sex (females), height (shorter individuals), and health (greater number of self-reported risk factors) likely playing a role (9).

Due to their similarities with the work-related tasks, step tests are often used to evaluate cardiorespiratory fitness in firefighters. Approximately an 18-percent decrease in estimated maximal aerobic capacity as measured by the Queens College step test has been demonstrated when firefighters are wearing personal protective gear and a self-contained breathing apparatus compared to standard athletic clothing (43). Furthermore, 13 percent of the firefighters were not able to complete the test with the additional safety equipment.

Figure 9.33 Conversion nomograms for estimating maximum aerobic capacity from recovery heart rate measured five seconds after completing the step test

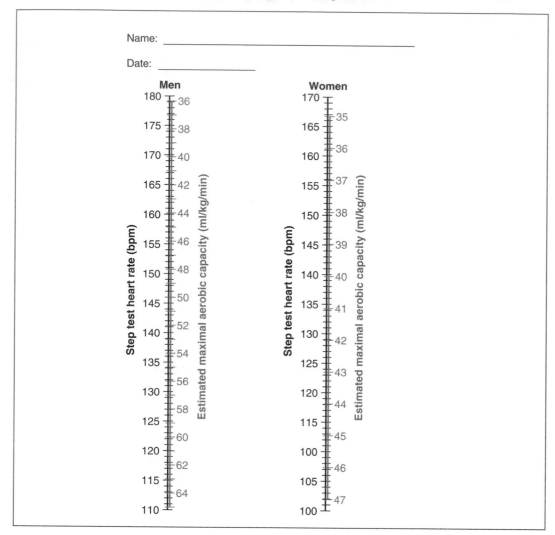

From D. Fukuda, *Assessments for Sport and Athletic Performance* (Champaign, IL: Human Kinetics, 2019). Using formulas from (36).

Normative Data

Step test recovery heart rate classification values after five seconds are provided in figure 9.34, and after one minute in figure 9.35 (men) and figure 9.36 (women).

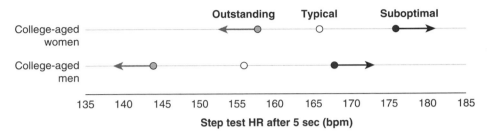

Figure 9.34 Submaximal step test recovery heart rate (HR; after 5 sec) classifications in young, untrained men and women. Women: outstanding–75th percentile; typical –50th percentile; suboptimal–25th percentile. Using a 16.25-inch (41.3 cm) bench.

Data from (36).

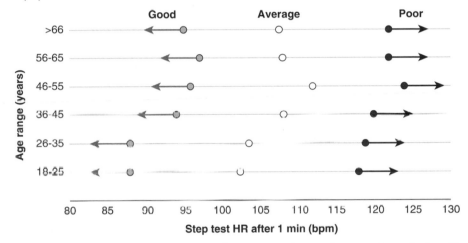

Figure 9.35 YMCA step test recovery heart rate (HR; after 1 minute) classifications in men across the lifespan. Using a 13-inch (33 cm) bench.

Data from (40a).

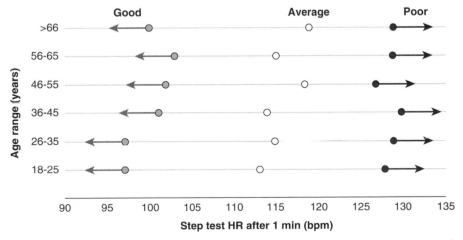

Figure 9.36 YMCA step test recovery heart rate (HR; after 1 minute) classifications in women across the lifespan. Using a 13-inch (33 cm) bench.

Data from (40a).

SUBMAXIMAL ROWING ERGOMETER TEST

Purpose

The submaximal rowing ergometer test provides an indicator of cardiorespiratory fitness using a continuous fixed-cadence protocol.

Outcomes

Recovery heart rate in beats per minute; estimated maximal aerobic capacity

Equipment Needed

Concept2 rowing ergometer; timing device; heart rate monitor (if available)

Before You Begin

Review the basic elements of a rowing stroke (preferably during a familiarization session prior to testing) with the athlete or client as outlined in table 7.1. See the heart rate measurement guidelines provided in chapter 10. Follow the procedures outlined in chapter 4 to record the athlete's or client's body weight in kilograms or pounds. Set the adjustable resistance level to the highest setting (10) and the on-board computer to display watts and strokes per minute (and heart rate if a heart rate monitor is being used). A standardized warm-up followed by three to five minutes of rest and recovery should be conducted prior to beginning the assessment.

Protocol

1. Begin the procedure by saying to the athlete or client: *"We are going to measure your heart rate while you exercise on the rowing ergometer at a comfortable intensity. Are you ready to begin? If so, please have a seat on the rowing ergometer, tighten the foot plate straps around your feet, and grasp the handle with both hands."*

2. Next, explain: *"When I say 'Go,' start pulling on the handle while going completely through the start, drive, finish, and recovery phases at an intensity that you think you can maintain for 5 to 10 minutes. Do not attempt to perform at a maximal level. We will check your heart rate after each minute of exercise until it appears to level off, which will signal the end of the test."*

3. Position yourself so that you can clearly view the performance monitor. Verbally signal the athlete or client *"3, 2, 1, go,"* and verify that the athlete or client performs at a consistent submaximal intensity and stroke rate with a heart rate below 170 beats per minute. If a heart rate monitor is being used, the heart rate values should be visible on the performance monitor; however, if a heart rate monitor is not being used, the coach or fitness professional will need to ask the athlete or client to briefly pause in the starting position with hands remaining on the handle while his or her heart rate is measured.

4. When the athlete's or client's heart rate appears to stabilize for a period of two minutes, record this value, as well as the power output (in watts), and stop the test.

After You Finish

The stabilized heart rate measured during the final two minutes of the test is the final result. Use the nomogram in figure 9.37, which was developed in healthy, young, untrained rowers, to determine the estimated absolute maximal aerobic capacity (in L/min). Then, convert the absolute value to the estimated relative maximal aerobic capacity (in ml/kg/min) using one of the following formulas:

$$\dot{V}O_2\text{max in ml/kg/min} = \frac{\dot{V}O_2\text{max in L/min}}{\text{body weight in kg}} \times 1,000$$

$$\dot{V}O_2max \text{ in ml/kg/min} = \frac{\dot{V}O_2max \text{ in L/min}}{\text{body weight in lb} \div 2.2} \times 1,000$$

As an example, a 160-pound (72.6 kg) man whose heart rate is 146 beats per minute after completing two minutes of rowing at a power output of 225 watts has an absolute $\dot{V}O_2max$ of 3.5 L/min. Relative $\dot{V}O_2max$ is calculated as follows:

$$\dot{V}O_2max \text{ in ml/kg/min} = \frac{3.5 \text{ L/min}}{160 \div 2.2} \times 1,000$$

$$\dot{V}O_2max \text{ in ml/kg/min} = \frac{3.5 \text{ L/min}}{72.7 \text{ kg}} \times 1,000$$

$$\dot{V}O_2max \text{ in ml/kg/min} = 0.04814 \times 1,000 = 48.14 \text{ ml/kg/min}$$

Figure 9.37 Nomogram for estimating maximal aerobic capacity from power output and heart rate during the submaximal rowing ergometer test

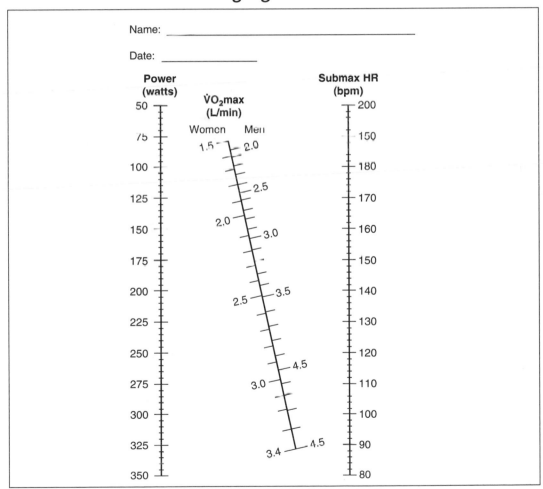

From D. Fukuda, Assessments for Sport and Athletic Performance (Champaign, IL: Human Kinetics, 2019). From *Concept II Rowing Ergometer Nomogram for Prediction of Maximal Oxygen Consumption,* by Dr. Fritz Hagerman, Ohio University, Athens, OH. The nomogram is not appropriate for use with non-Concept2 rowing ergometers and is designed to be used by noncompetitive or unskilled rowers participating in aerobic conditioning programs. Adapted by permission of Concept2, Inc., 105 Industrial Park Drive, Morrisville, VT 05661 (800) 245-5676.

Research Notes

Because it contains elements of both aerobic endurance and resistance training, rowing training yields exceptional cardiorespiratory fitness and musculoskeletal adaptations (5). Furthermore, rowing is a non-weight-bearing activity that engages a large percentage of the muscles in the body: an estimated 50 percent of the power generated during a rowing stroke comes from the trunk, 40 percent from the legs, and 10 percent from the arms (53). Therefore, recommendations for rowing training have been made for improvements in both sport performance and health across the lifespan (5, 25).

These features of rowing provide an alternative to the primarily running-based options available for assessing cardiorespiratory fitness in the field. In support of the assessment protocol provided in this section, the exercise intensity and heart rate response to submaximal rowing has been shown to be predictive of cardiorespiratory fitness in both trained and untrained rowers (29).

Normative Data

Estimated maximal aerobic capacity values from the submaximal rowing ergometer can be compared to the normative data provided in figure 9.38 for men and figure 9.39 for women.

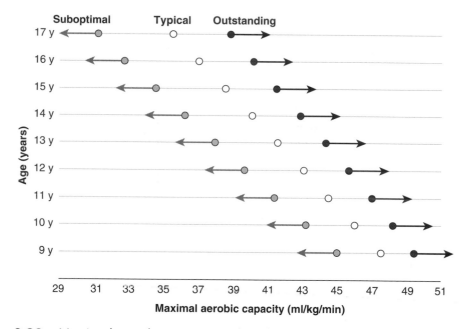

Figure 9.38 Maximal aerobic capacity classifications in men: outstanding—75th percentile; typical—50th percentile; suboptimal—25th percentile.

Data from (4).

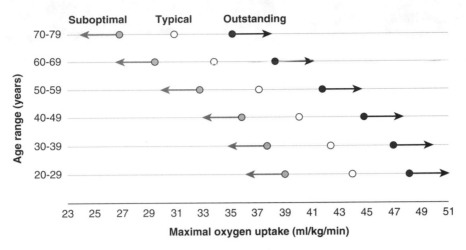

Figure 9.39 Maximal aerobic capacity classifications in women: outstanding—75th percentile; typical—50th percentile; suboptimal—25th percentile.

Data from (4).

45-SECOND SQUAT TEST

Purpose

The 45-second squat test (or Ruffier-Dickson test) provides measure of cardiorespiratory fitness using heart rate recovery following a fixed cadence protocol.

Outcomes

Heart rate recovery values; Ruffier-Dickson index; estimated maximal aerobic capacity

Equipment Needed

Sturdy training table; timing device; metronome; heart rate monitor (if available)

Before You Begin

Follow the procedures outlined in chapter 4 to record the athlete's or client's height. See the heart rate measurement guidelines provided in chapter 10. Set a metronome to 80 beats per minute, at a pace of 40 squats per minute.

Protocol

1. Begin the procedure by saying to the athlete or client: *"We are going to measure your heart rate before and after you complete 30 body-weight squats. You will squat down and stand back up again in sync with the beeps of a metronome. At the rate that the metronome is set, you will do 30 squats in 45 seconds. Are you ready to begin? If so, please lie down on the training table for the next five minutes so that we can determine your resting heart rate."*

2. At the end of the resting period, either record the reading displayed by the heart rate monitor or say, *"I'm now going to measure your heart rate by placing my fingers on your neck or wrist."*

3. Next, direct the athlete or client: *"Please stand up with your arms either crossed or extended in front of your chest with your feet parallel and shoulder width apart. When I say 'Go,' start bending your knees and hips to lower your body into a squatted position until your ankles, knees, and hips are at right angles (90°). Keep your back straight and your eyes facing forward throughout the movement. Squat down quickly enough to reach the bottom position at the same time as when you hear the beep. Then extend your knees and hips to return to the starting position in time with the next beep"* (see figure 9.40).

4. Request: *"Focus on breathing normally throughout the test, and squat with the metronome for the duration of the 45 seconds. After you've completed the 30 squats, I will have you lie back down on the table so that I can measure your heart rate."*

5. Position yourself so that you can clearly view the squatting movements. Verbally signal the athlete or client *"3, 2, 1, go,"* and verify that the athlete or client performs at the required pace while tracking the time.

6. After 45 seconds, direct the athlete or client: *"Please lie back down on the training table so that I can measure your heart rate."*

7. Record a heart rate value as soon as possible (within 15 seconds) after the athlete or client lies down and once again after resting for one minute (within 75 seconds).

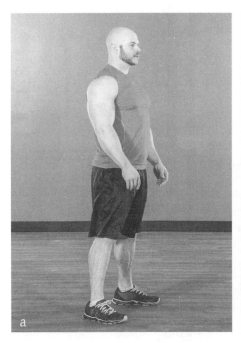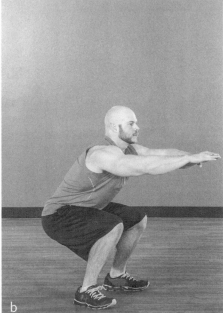

Figure 9.40   Body-weight squat.

Alternatives or Modifications

The original version of the 45-second squat test required the athlete or client to complete a full squat movement with the heels close to the buttocks, but the test can be modified to a 90-degree bend at the knees to account for those individuals with limited range of motion in the lower body.

After You Finish

The heart rate values recorded at rest (HR_{rest}), within 15 seconds after exercise (HR_{15s}), and 1 minute after exercise (HR_{75s}) are used to calculate the Ruffier-Dickson Index (RDI) as follows:

$$RDI = \frac{(HR_{15s} - 70) + 2(HR_{75s} - HR_{rest})}{10}$$

For example, an athlete or client with a HR_{rest} of 47 beats per minute, a HR_{15s} of 121 beats per minute, and a HR_{75s} of 50 beats per minute has an RDI of:

$$RDI = \frac{(120 \text{ bpm} - 70) + 2(55 \text{ bpm} - 47 \text{ bpm})}{10}$$

$$RDI = \frac{55 + 2(8)}{10} = \frac{51 + 16}{10} = \frac{67}{10} = 6.7$$

The RDI can be used to evaluate general cardiorespiratory fitness or, when combined with age and height, to estimate absolute maximal aerobic capacity (in L/min) with the following formulas:

Men

$$\dot{V}O_2max$$

$$= (-0.0309 \times \text{age in yr}) + (4.533 \times \frac{\text{height in cm}}{100})$$
$$- (0.0864 \times \text{RDI}) - 3.228$$

$$\dot{V}O_2max = (-0.0309 \times \text{age in yr}) + (4.533 \times \text{height in in.} \times 0.0254)$$
$$- (0.0864 \times \text{RDI}) - 3.228$$

Women

$$\dot{V}O_2max$$

$$= (-0.0309 \times \text{age in yr}) + (4.533 \times \frac{\text{height in cm}}{100})$$
$$- (0.0864 \times \text{RDI}) - 3.788$$

$$\dot{V}O_2max = (-0.0309 \times \text{age in yr}) + (4.533 \times \text{height in in.} \times 0.0254)$$
$$- (0.0864 \times \text{RDI}) - 3.788$$

For example, a 28–year–old man with an RDI of 6.7 and who is 68 inches tall has an estimated maximal aerobic capacity of:

$$\dot{V}O_2max = (-0.0309 \times 28 \text{ yr}) + (4.533 \times 68 \text{ in.} \times 0.0254) - (0.0864 \times 6.7) - 3.228$$

$$\dot{V}O_2max = -0.865 + 7.829 - 0.579 - 3.228 = 3.94 \text{ L/min}$$

The absolute value can then be converted to estimated relative maximal aerobic capacity (in ml/kg/min) using one of the following formulas:

$$\dot{V}O_2max \text{ in ml/kg/min} = \frac{\dot{V}O_2max \text{ in L/min}}{\text{body weight in kg}} \times 1000$$

$$\dot{V}O_2max \text{ in ml/kg/min} = \frac{\dot{V}O_2max \text{ in L/min}}{\text{body weight in lb} \div 2.2} \times 1{,}000$$

For example, a 175–pound (79.4 kg) man with an absolute $\dot{V}O_2max$ of 3.94 L/min has a relative $\dot{V}O_2max$ as follows:

$$\dot{V}O_2max \text{ in ml/kg/min} = \frac{3.94 \text{ L/min}}{175 \text{ lb} \div 2.2} \times 1{,}000$$

$$\dot{V}O_2max \text{ in ml/kg/min} = \frac{3.94 \text{ L/min}}{79.5 \text{ kg}} \times 1{,}000$$

$$\dot{V}O_2max \text{ in ml/kg/min} = 0.04956 \times 1{,}000 = 49.56 \text{ ml/kg/min}$$

Research Notes

Direct measurement of oxygen consumption during the 45-second squat test has shown to result in approximately 6 times greater energy expenditure than resting values. This corresponds to vigorous exercise intensity in less fit individuals and moderate exercise intensity in more fit individuals (51). RDI values have shown to correlate to maximal aerobic capacity in healthy individuals (51) and blood flow during recovery from the 45-second squat test in rugby athletes (44). While low RDI values have been reported in athletes (e.g., 2.5 in male rugby players), the ability to estimate cardiorespiratory fitness from RDI may be limited because of overestimations in less fit individuals and underestimations in highly fit individuals (3, 44, 51).

A research study examining three different two-week physical activity interventions reported decreased RDI values (potentially indicating improved cardiorespiratory fitness) in individuals using a mobile-based step-count application as well as both mobile-based training and gym-based supervised training sessions (49).

Normative Data

Generally speaking, lower RDI values represent better cardiorespiratory fitness, while higher values represent lower cardiorespiratory fitness. Recommendations (51) suggest that RDI values less than or equal to 5 are considered good cardiorespiratory fitness, values between 6 and 10 are considered fair, and values greater than or equal to 11 are considered poor. If estimated maximal aerobic capacity values are calculated, the normative data provided in figure 9.41 for men and figure 9.42 for women can be used.

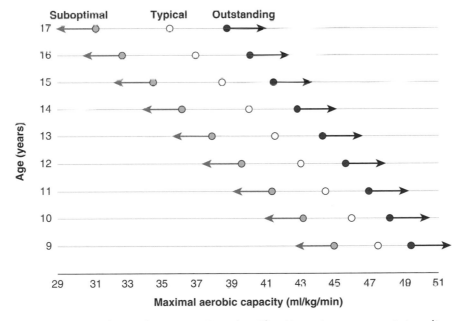

Figure 9.41 Maximal aerobic capacity classifications in men: outstanding—75th percentile; typical—50th percentile; suboptimal—25th percentile.

Data from (4).

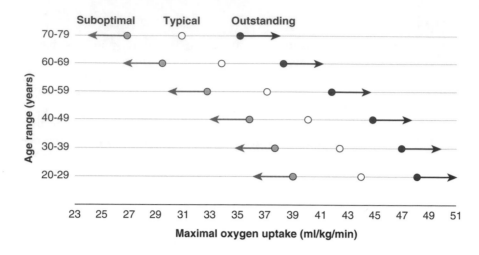

Figure 9.42 Maximal aerobic capacity classifications in women: outstanding—75th percentile; typical—50th percentile; suboptimal—25th percentile.

Data from (4).

CHAPTER 10

Monitoring Training

> *Continuous effort—not strength or intelligence—is the key to unlocking our potential.*
>
> Liane Cordes, Author

The majority of the assessments in part II are intended to be used as part of a baseline evaluation or as a periodic follow-up (retest) to determine the effectiveness of a training program or other intervention. Performing a full-scale battery of tests is time-consuming and very fatiguing, so it may not be realistic to test more frequently than once every few months. However, coaches and fitness professionals are required to constantly observe their athletes and clients and make adjustments to their training on a daily or weekly basis to maximize their performance and minimize risk of injury—a process called *monitoring*. Training monitoring tools allow coaches and fitness professionals to evaluate trends by comparing test results to a common value or a certain threshold (such as more than a 5 to 10% change from a previous test or a baseline) that would indicate a stable period of training or a positive or negative training adaptation.

For example, heart rate measurements can be used as indicators of exercise intensity and a means of evaluating the athlete's or client's response to exercise, both of which may be particularly useful for monitoring training. Body weight maintenance, hydration status, and fluid loss recovery are additional factors that could be monitored before and after a training session.

Beyond those physiological factors, monitoring training load and physical readiness can reveal valuable insight about an athlete's or client's training adaptive status. Training load is influenced by a balance of *external training loads* (the training activities completed by the athlete or client), and *internal training loads* (the athlete's or client's response to the training activities) (21, 37). A decision matrix for the balance between external and internal training loads is provided in figure 10.1. Notably, an imbalance in the types of training load likely signals positive (high external training load with low internal training load) or negative adaptations (low external training load with high internal training load) (21). Low values in both categories indicate a need for more aggressive training progression, and high values in both categories indicate a need for less aggressive training progression.

Physical readiness is described as the athlete's or client's ability to engage in the training activities on a particular day (21, 37). Both training load and physical readiness must be considered with respect to how well the training process is being tolerated by the athlete or client, which is termed *perceptual well-being* (21, 37).

Decision matrices for the balance between perceptual well-being and physical readiness, and between perceptual well-being and the training load, are provided in figure 10.2. An imbalance between the training load and perceptual well-being scores likely signals the need to alter the training program, high values in both categories indicate

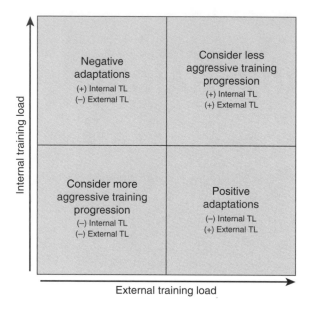

Figure 10.1 Decision matrix for the balance between external and internal training loads.

Adapted from T.J. Gabbett, G.P. Nassis, E. Oetter, et al., "The Athlete Monitoring Cycle: A Practical Guide to Interpreting and Applying Training Monitoring Data," *British Journal of Sports Medicine* 51 (2017): 1451-1452.

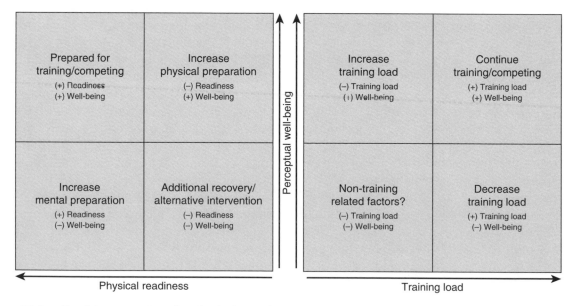

Figure 10.2 Decision matrices for the balance between perceptual well-being and physical readiness and between perceptual well-being and training load.

Adapted from T.J. Gabbett, G.P. Nassis, E. Oetter, et al., "The Athlete Monitoring Cycle: A Practical Guide to Interpreting and Applying Training Monitoring Data," *British Journal of Sports Medicine* 51 (2017): 1451-1452.

a stable training environment, and low values in both categories may indicate issues outside the training program (21). An imbalance between physical readiness and perceptual well-being scores likely signals the need for either additional physical preparation (due to high perceptual well-being and low physical readiness) or mental preparation (caused by low perceptual well-being and high physical readiness). High values in both categories indicate a stable training environment, and low values in both categories may indicate the need for additional recovery or an alternative intervention (21).

The sections of information provided within the decision matrices are simply suggestions that must be guided by the intuition, professional preparation, and sport- or activity-specific knowledge of the coach or fitness professional.

In addition to physical measures, assessments of external training load, internal training load, perceptual well-being, and physical readiness are provided within this chapter, and much of the training monitoring data can be collected using training logs.

The assessments covered in this chapter are as follows:

- Heart rate measurement (26)
- Body weight maintenance and hydration status (1)
- Fluid loss evaluation (36)
- External training load (21, 34, 37)
- Internal training load (21, 37)
- Perceptual well-being (21, 37)
- Physical readiness (21, 37)

HEART RATE MEASUREMENT

Purpose

Heart rate (HR) provides a measure of the balance of numerous physiological systems and the current state of the body, including its ability to recover from and respond to exercise.

Background and Approach

HR values are highly individualized, with resting values typically ranging between 60 and 80 beats per minute. Women and children under 12 years old usually have greater resting HR values compared to men and adults, respectively. To minimize day-to-day fluctuations in HR that are not related to training, standardized testing conditions are needed because many environmental, dietary, physical, and psychological factors can affect resting values. Also, some medications directly or indirectly affect resting and exercise HR.

Use the middle finger and index finger together to locate the athlete's or client's pulse by applying slight pressure near the desired artery. The radial artery is located in the wrist at the intersection of the thumb and palm (see figure 10.3a), while the carotid artery is located in the neck along the side of the throat below the jaw line (see figure 10.3b). The thumb has its own pulse and should not be used for HR measurement.

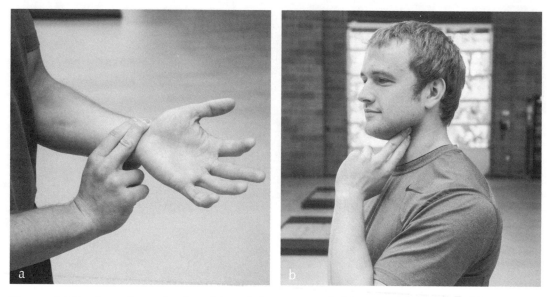

Figure 10.3 Locations for the (a) radial artery and (b) carotid artery.

After locating the pulse, count the number of heartbeats felt during a predetermined period (between 15 and 60 seconds for resting values and less than 15 seconds for exercise or postexercise values to get a real-time snapshot). When starting the timing device, count the first beat as zero; however, if a timing device that is currently running is used (i.e., a round or lap timer or a wall-mounted clock), count the first beat as one.

Resting HR measurements should be completed in a seated position or lying down after a rest period of 5 to 10 minutes. Exercise and postexercise HR measurements should be completed as close to the end of the exercise session as possible or during a specified time point to minimize the influence of recovery. The pulse count can be used to calculate HR using the formulas provided in table 10.1.

Table 10.1   Pulse Count Conversion Formulas to Determine Heart Rate (HR) in Beats per Minute (bpm) at Rest and During Exercise

Exercise		6 sec pulse count	×	10	=	HR in bpm
		10 sec pulse count	×	6	=	HR in bpm
	Rest	15 sec pulse count	×	4	=	HR in bpm
		30 sec pulse count	×	2	=	HR in bpm
		60 sec pulse count	×	1	=	HR in bpm

Alternatives or Modifications

A variety of HR monitors are available that use a chest strap or arm- or wrist-based devices to measure HR continuously while transmitting the data to a watch or mobile app.

Knowledge of an athlete's or client's maximum HR allows for a more informed assessment of exercise intensity and gives an indication of when a particular assessment is reaching an appropriate stopping point (e.g., approximately 85% of maximum HR during a submaximal test). While the actual measurement of maximum HR is preferred during assessments with gradual increases in exercise resulting in maximal exertion, such as the 20-meter multi-stage shuttle run or the Yo-Yo intermittent recovery test presented in chapter 9, the calculation of age-predicted values can be completed using one of the following formulas (56a):

$$\text{Age-predicted maximum HR in bpm} = 220 - \text{age in yr}$$

$$\text{Age-predicted maximum HR in bpm} = 208 - (0.7 \times \text{age in yr})$$

Research Notes

The rate that HR returns to its resting level after exercise improves following training, and the recovery rate is faster in trained versus untrained individuals (4, 14). The usefulness of HR as a monitoring tool during training may be dictated by the length of the training program and how it is measured (7). Changes in resting HR may be noticeable over shorter training periods (<2 wk), while changes in submaximal exercise HR may be noticeable over longer training periods (>2 wk), and changes in maximal exercise HR could occur as a response to both shorter and longer training periods. Furthermore, it is recommended that HR measures be used in conjunction with other monitoring tools to give a coach or fitness professional better insight into how the athlete or client is handling the stress of the training program (8).

Applied Examples

Following are two applied examples:

Scenario 1
Determine, in beats per minute, the resting HR and age-predicted maximum HR (using both formulas) for a 30-year-old with a resting 30-second pulse count of 27 beats:

$$\text{Resting HR} = 27 \text{ beats} \times 2 = 54 \text{ bpm}$$

$$\text{Age-predicted maximum HR} = 220 - 30 \text{ yr} = 190 \text{ bpm}$$

$$\text{Age-predicted maximum HR} = 208 - (0.7 \times 30 \text{ yr}) = 187 \text{ bpm}$$

Scenario 2
Determine, in beats per minute, the exercise HR and age-predicted maximum HR (using both formulas) for a 22-year-old with an exercise 10-second pulse count of 25 beats:

$$\text{Exercise HR} = 25 \text{ beats} \times 6 = 150 \text{ bpm}$$

$$\text{Age-predicted maximum HR} = 220 - 22 \text{ yr} = 198 \text{ bpm}$$

$$\text{Age-predicted maximum HR} = 208 - (0.7 \times 22 \text{ yr}) = 193 \text{ bpm}$$

BODY WEIGHT MAINTENANCE AND HYDRATION STATUS

Purpose

Body weight maintenance provides a measure of hydration status.

Background and Approach

Striking a balance between the fluid lost during exercise and fluid intake is a key consideration for training and competition. Accordingly, dehydration, which may accumulate over time, has been shown to negatively affect performance and cognitive function (32, 39). The most straightforward method of determining hydration status is by frequent body weight measurements when the athlete or client is not purposely losing or gaining weight and when there is a consistent fluid intake. Stable or normal weight can be determined by averaging three consecutive body weight measurements using the protocol outlined in chapter 4. Subsequently, day-to-day variations in body weight should differ by no more than 1 percent; it is concerning if this variation is greater than 2 percent specifically due to dehydration (1, 12). The following formula can be used to determine the percent change in body weight between measurements (or compared to stable, normal weight):

$$\text{Percent change in body weight} = \frac{\text{day 2 BW} - \text{day 1 BW}}{\text{day 1 BW}} \times 100$$

$$\text{Percent change in body weight} = \frac{\text{measured BW} - \text{normal BW}}{\text{normal BW}} \times 100$$

Hydration status can also be determined by examining the color of urine. This simple assessment can be completed by the athlete or client by collecting a sample of urine in a clear container and comparing its color against a white background to a commercially available color chart (1). Urine that is associated with ratings of one through three indicate a well-hydrated state (closer to very pale yellow); colors associated with ratings of seven through eight (closer to green) indicate extreme dehydration. If the urine color is found to be darker on several occasions throughout the day, the athlete or client should focus on drinking more water periodically over the course of the next day until the urine returns to a pale yellow color. However, the fluid intake should not be excessive or consumed all at once because severe complications can occur as a result of not having enough sodium relative to body fluids—a state that is termed *hyponatremia*—which can result in several health problems and may require hospitalization. Some fruits and vegetables, vitamins, and medications, as well as intense exercise sessions can also cause urine to change color, so recent changes in the athlete's or client's diet or training regimen need to be considered when evaluating hydration status.

Alternatives or Modifications

To further simplify the process of evaluating hydration status without the hassle of purchasing a container and handling urine, the athlete or client can also estimate the color directly from the urine stream (28) or potentially from the toilet bowl after urination. However, these approaches may be less precise.

Research Notes

Dehydration is a major issue in sports that are divided by weight categories for competitive events. It is common for athletes to lose 2 to 5 percent or possibly up to 10 percent of their body weight during preparation for competition (19). An evaluation of wrestling, taekwondo, and boxing athletes noted significant differences in urine color between adequately hydrated athletes and severely dehydrated athletes (17).

The importance of hydration status is apparent in most sport settings. For example, a study examining low-handicap golfers under typically hydrated (with a urine color rating of 2) and dehydrated (with a urine color rating of 4) conditions showed impairments in both shot distance and accuracy using a variety of clubs (5-, 7-, and 9-irons) following fluid restriction that caused a 1.5 percent decrease in body weight (55).

Applied Examples

Following are two applied examples:

Scenario 1

Determine the percent change in body weight for an athlete or client who weighs 76.5 kilograms and has a stable or normal body weight of 78 kilograms.

$$\text{Percent change in body weight} = \frac{76.5 \text{ kg} - 78 \text{ kg}}{78 \text{ kg}} \times 100 = -1.92\%$$

Scenario 2

Determine the percent change in body weight for an athlete or client who weighs 112 pounds today and weighed 112.5 pounds yesterday.

$$\text{Percent change in body weight} = \frac{112 \text{ lb} - 112.5 \text{ lb}}{112.5 \text{ lb}} \times 100 = -0.44\%$$

FLUID LOSS EVALUATION

Purpose

Fluid loss evaluation provides a measure of the hydration needs in response to a training session.

Background and Approach

Varying amounts of fluid may be lost during a training session with individual rates of sweating, exercise duration, exercise intensity, and environmental factors (i.e., heat and humidity) increasing the need for rehydration. Therefore, the coach or fitness professional may choose to track an athlete's or client's fluid intake and sweat loss while establishing guidelines for rehydration.

Prior to a training session, request that the athlete or client use the restroom and, if possible, to refrain from using it again until after the postexercise measurements are completed. Follow the procedures outlined in chapter 4 to record the athlete's or client's initial body weight (in pounds or kilograms). Record the initial volume (in ounces or milliliters) of any beverages that may be consumed during the training session. Proceed with the training session and ensure that the athlete or client only drinks from the premeasured beverage container. Following the training session, request that the athlete or client dries off any sweat from the skin and record the postexercise body weight (in pounds or kilograms). Subtract the volume of the unconsumed beverage from the initial volume to determine the amount that was consumed during the training session. Fluid loss can then be calculated using one of the following formulas:

$$\text{Fluid loss in milliliters (mL)} = [(\text{initial BW in kg} - \text{final BW in kg}) \times 1000] + \text{initial beverage volume in mL} - \text{final beverage volume in mL}$$

$$\text{Fluid loss in ounces (oz)} = [(\text{initial BW in lb} - \text{final BW in lb}) \times 15.34] + \text{initial beverage volume in oz} - \text{final beverage volume in oz}$$

Over the course of the next 8 to 12 hours, the athlete or client should aim to drink 1 to 1.5 times the calculated fluid loss during the training session. More simply, 1.5 liters (53 fl oz) of fluid should be consumed for each kilogram (2.2 lb) of body weight lost.

Alternatives or Modifications

The fluid loss calculation can be simplified to only consider the difference between the initial and final body weight values if the athlete or client does not intend to drink during a short-duration training session. For extended-duration training sessions, urine volume may need to be tracked and subtracted from the fluid loss formulas.

If the duration of the training session is measured, an athlete's or client's sweat rate is calculated using the following formula:

$$\text{Sweat rate in mL/min or oz/min} = \frac{\text{fluid loss in mL or oz}}{\text{training session duration in min}}$$

Because sweat rate is specific to the individual athlete or client, this value can be used to customize approximately how much fluid should be consumed during training sessions of varying length. This simply requires multiplying sweat rate by the intended length of the training session.

It is difficult to specify sweat rates for a given sport because a combination of factors influence fluid balance and the risk for dehydration, including the frequency of high-intensity efforts, fluid availability and drinking opportunities, and environmental conditions (43). Despite this, figure 10.4 provides a range of sweat rates for team sport athletes. Note that the sweat rate calculated in mL/min must be multiplied by 60 minutes and divided by 1000 mL to compare with sweat rate reported as L/h, or multiplied by 60 minutes and divided by body weight (in kilograms) to compare with sweat rate reported as ml/kg/h.

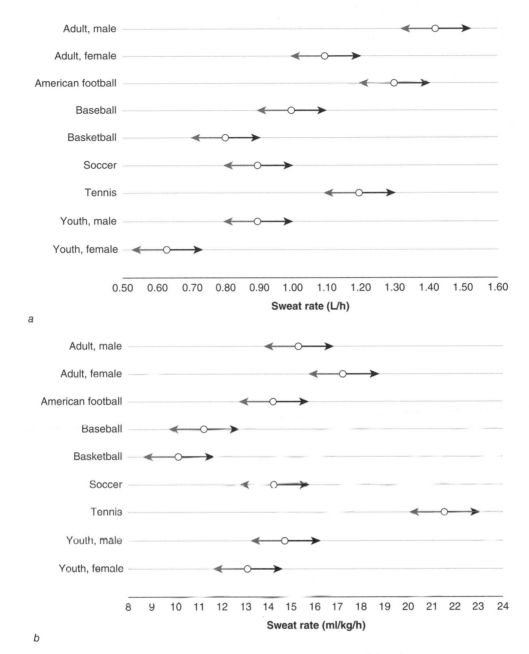

Figure 10.4 Sweat rates for athletes in *(a)* L/h and *(b)* ml/kg/h.

Data from (1a).

Research Notes

Hot and humid environments require additional consideration for fluid balance. Following a typical 90-minute training session in tropical conditions (85.1 °F [29.5 °C] and relative humidity of 78%), male and female youth judo athletes lost between 600 milliliters (21 fl oz) and 1,200 milliliters (42 fl oz) despite maintaining their usual fluid intake habits (50). Sweat rates between 6.7 and 13.3 mL/min (0.24 and 0.47 oz/min) were reported. Most of the athletes regained the body weight lost during training within 24 hours; however, some symptoms of dehydration, such as thirst and headaches, were still reported during this period.

Fluid balance is also an issue in milder climates. Following 90-minute training sessions in a cool environment (49.6 °F [9.8 °C] and relative humidity of 63%), female youth soccer players lost 0.84 percent of their body weight (fluid loss of approximately 1,150 mL [40 fl oz]) with a sweat rate of 11.5 mL/min (0.40 oz/min), providing evidence that not enough fluid was consumed and mild dehydration occurred (23). The researchers also noted that the weight loss during training was highly variable, with some players losing greater than 2 percent of their body weight (thereby raising the risk of more frequent and more serious dehydration-related symptoms over sequential training sessions).

Applied Examples

Following are two applied examples:

Scenario 1

The athlete or client weighed 73 kilograms prior to the training session and 72 kilograms after the training session. During the 90-minute training session, he drank 300 milliliters of a 500-milliliter beverage. His fluid loss is calculated as follows:

$$\text{Fluid loss in mL} = [(73 \text{ kg} - 72 \text{ kg}) \times 1{,}000] + (500 \text{ mL} - 300 \text{ mL}) = 1{,}200 \text{ mL}$$

The athlete or client should aim to drink 1,200 to 1,800 milliliters of fluid in the next 8 to 12 hours. His sweat rate is calculated as follows:

$$\text{Sweat rate in mL/min} = \frac{1{,}200 \text{ mL}}{90 \text{ min}} = 13.3 \text{ mL/min}$$

If a future training session, conducted under similar environmental conditions, lasts only 60 minutes, the athlete or client might plan to drink 798 milliliters of fluid (60 min × 13.3 mL/min) while exercising to maintain his preexercise body weight.

Scenario 2

The athlete or client weighed 120 pounds prior to the training session and 118.5 pounds after the training session. During the 45-minute training session, she drank 30 ounces of a 32-ounce beverage. Her fluid loss is calculated as follows:

$$\text{Fluid loss in oz} = [(120 \text{ lb} - 118.5 \text{ lb}) \times 15.34] + (32 \text{ oz} - 28 \text{ oz}) = 25 \text{ oz}$$

The athlete or client should aim to drink 25 to 38 ounces of fluid in the next 8 to 12 hours. Her sweat rate is calculated as follows:

$$\text{Sweat rate in oz/min} = \frac{25 \text{ oz}}{45 \text{ min}} = 0.56 \text{ oz/min}$$

If a future training session, conducted under similar environmental conditions, lasts 75 minutes, the athlete or client might plan to drink 42 ounces of fluid (75 min × 0.56 oz/min) while exercising to maintain her preexercise body weight.

EXTERNAL TRAINING LOAD

Purpose

External training load provides a measure of the physical stress of a training session.

Background and Approach

The evaluation of external training load is dictated by the athlete's or client's sport or activity, and it is typically gauged by training volume, intensity, or both. Training volume is simply calculated as the number of repetitions completed (lifts, sprints, intervals, jumps, etc.), distance covered, or duration of the training session. For the purposes of this discussion, definitions and calculations are based on resistance training.

Training volume is determined as the total number of repetitions completed during a resistance training session:

$$\text{Volume (in repetitions)} = \text{sets} \times \text{repetitions}$$

However, to get a clearer indication of the true external training load, volume load (VL) is often calculated by multiplying the total number of repetitions by the weight lifted for a particular exercise (35).

$$\text{VL (in kg or lb)} = \text{sets} \times \text{repetitions} \times \text{load (in kg or lb)}$$

If several different exercises are incorporated into a training session (with a unique number of sets, repetitions, and loads), VL is separately calculated for each exercise and then added together with the sum representing the total VL of the session.

$$\text{Total VL (in kg or lb)} = \text{VL for exercise A (in kg or lb)} + \text{VL for exercise B (in kg or lb)}$$

Training intensity can be quantified as the percentage of an individual's maximum intensity as indicated by HR, speed, strength, or power values. During a resistance training session, this can also be calculated as the average weight lifted per repetition (56) using the following formula:

$$\text{Training intensity (in kg/repetition or lb/repetition)} = \frac{\text{total VL (in kg or lb)}}{\text{total repetitions}}$$

Another method to measure the intensity of a training session is based on the amount of rest between bouts of work. This is called *exercise density* (34). Continuing with the examples from resistance training, exercise density is calculated by dividing VL by the total amount of rest between sets. (Note: the rest period following the last set of the last exercise is not counted.) This calculation provides a distinction between two training sessions with similar VL values but results in a larger exercise density for a session with shorter rest periods and smaller exercise density for a session with longer rest periods.

$$\text{Exercise density (in kg/sec or lb/sec)} = \frac{\text{total VL (in kg or lb)}}{\text{total rest between sets (in sec)}}$$

Alternatives or Modifications

Real-time HR monitoring and global positioning system (GPS) data from wearable technology can help measure external training load by providing feedback throughout an entire training session. Specifically, this information can be used to determine how long an athlete or client trains within specific intensity zones (e.g., ranges of percentages of maximal HR, speed, or power output). Many commercial HR and GPS devices also provide their own measures of external training load. Commercial devices and mobile applications can be used to determine total work and the speed of the barbell during a specific lifting motion (or the movement velocity of the body or almost any implement) to compare with maximal values or normative data.

Research Notes

Volume load during a nine-week, three-sessions-per-week resistance training program has been shown to be greater when individuals are given the option to select their own exercises as opposed to being given specific exercises (49). This may have important implications for changes in muscular strength and size that may be related to VL during resistance training programs (47).

A comparison of a resistance training program aimed at increasing muscular strength (5 sets of 5 repetitions with a 5-repetition maximum load and 180 seconds of rest between sets) and another aimed at increasing muscular size (3 sets of 10 repetitions with a 10-repetition maximum load and 60 seconds of rest between sets) revealed a difference in the number of repetitions completed but no differences in the VL (34). Interestingly, training intensity was greater during the muscular strength program, but exercise density was greater during the muscular size program. However, only exercise density and the number of repetitions completed were related to the overall metabolic stress caused by the workouts.

Applied Examples

Following are two applied examples:

Scenario 1

The athlete or client completed a training session consisting of 5 sets of 5 repetitions using a 150-pound load for the back squat exercise and a 110-pound load for the bench press exercise. The rest period between sets was 180 seconds. Various measures of external load are calculated as follows:

$$\text{Back squat VL} = 5 \text{ sets} \times 5 \text{ repetitions} \times 150 \text{ lb} = 3{,}750 \text{ lb}$$

$$\text{Bench press VL} = 5 \text{ sets} \times 5 \text{ repetitions} \times 110 \text{ lb} = 2{,}750 \text{ lb}$$

$$\text{Total VL} = 3{,}750 \text{ lb (back squat VL)} + 2{,}750 \text{ lb (bench press VL)} = 6{,}500 \text{ lb}$$

$$\text{Training intensity} = \frac{6{,}500 \text{ lb (total VL)}}{25 \text{ reps (back squat)} + 25 \text{ reps (bench press)}} = 130 \text{ lb/rep}$$

$$\text{Exercise density} = \frac{6{,}500 \text{ lb (total VL)}}{9 \text{ total rest periods} \times 180 \text{ sec}} = 4.5 \text{ lb/sec}$$

Scenario 2

The athlete or client completed a training session consisting of 3 sets of 10 repetitions using an 80-kilogram load for the back squat exercise and a 60-kilogram load for the bench press exercise. The rest period between sets was 60 seconds. Various measures of external load are calculated as follows:

$$\text{Back squat VL} = 3 \text{ sets} \times 10 \text{ repetitions} \times 80 \text{ kg} = 2{,}400 \text{ kg}$$

$$\text{Bench press VL} = 3 \text{ sets} \times 10 \text{ repetitions} \times 60 \text{ kg} = 1{,}800 \text{ kg}$$

$$\text{Total VL} = 2{,}400 \text{ kg (back squat VL)} + 1{,}800 \text{ kg (bench press VL)} = 4{,}200 \text{ kg}$$

$$\text{Training intensity} = \frac{4{,}200 \text{ kg (total VL)}}{30 \text{ reps (back squat)} + 30 \text{ reps (bench press)}} = 70 \text{ kg/rep}$$

$$\text{Exercise density} = \frac{4{,}200 \text{ kg (total VL)}}{5 \text{ total rest periods} \times 60 \text{ sec}} = 140 \text{ kg/sec}$$

INTERNAL TRAINING LOAD

Purpose

Internal training load provides a measure of the response to a training session.

Background and Approach

The athlete's or client's subjective perception of a training session provides a noninvasive way to measure internal training load that would otherwise require advanced wearable technology, blood samples, or an analysis of oxygen consumption.

When subjectively measuring internal training load, it is important that the athlete or client clearly understands the measurement scale, including its definition, rating system, meaning of the highest and lowest anchor values, and enough detail about the rest of the ratings to allow the athlete or client to accurately differentiate (and then choose) the values across the scale. It is also important that the athlete or client knows that there are no correct or incorrect responses because the information is specific to the individual. Furthermore, the athlete or client should be encouraged and be made comfortable to provide a truthful description of the internal training load.

Rating of perceived exertion (RPE) scales are commonly used to subjectively evaluate effort during a training session (16). The RPE is generally used to estimate the effort of the entire body that results from a combination of physiological (i.e., the lungs and the involved muscles) and psychological components. Several variations of RPE scales exist, but most use a rating of 0 or 1 to indicate no effort or doing nothing at all, and the highest rating, which varies depending on the scale, as maximum effort or unable to continue exercising. An example of a 10-point RPE scale is provided in figure 10.5.

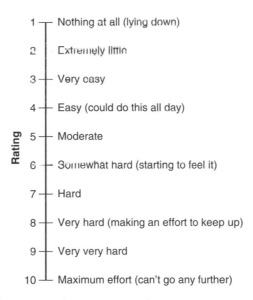

Rating

1 — Nothing at all (lying down)

2 — Extremely little

3 — Very easy

4 — Easy (could do this all day)

5 — Moderate

6 — Somewhat hard (starting to feel it)

7 — Hard

8 — Very hard (making an effort to keep up)

9 — Very very hard

10 — Maximum effort (can't go any further)

Figure 10.5 Rating of perceived exertion scale.

RPE values can be recorded within a training session at logical intervals, such as between drills or sets. Whenever possible, RPE should be used in conjunction with exercise HR to provide a multidimensional view of internal training load as they provide both subjective and objective feedback. Further, a comparison between the intended RPE designed into a training program by a coach or fitness professional and the actual RPE provided by the athlete or client during a training session is an effective monitoring tool that can help guide adjustments.

The coach or fitness professional can also ask the athlete or client to provide an RPE value that describes the overall training session or competition (called the *session RPE*) that can be multiplied by the duration of the activity or number of repetitions completed to determine the session load (18) as follows:

$$\text{Session load (in arbitrary units)} = \text{session RPE} \times \text{activity duration in min}$$

$$\text{Session load (in arbitrary units)} = \text{session RPE} \times \text{number of repetitions}$$

Calculating session load allows for comparisons to be made between longer and shorter training sessions or workouts that contain greater or fewer repetitions in which an athlete or client reports similar session RPE values.

Although RPE was originally intended to estimate the effort of the entire body, it can also be used to identify the effort of different muscle groups or regions of the body. One approach is to provide the athlete or client with an anatomical diagram and ask him or her to provide an RPE for specific muscles to determine the perceived requirements of the training activity or competition (42). A labeled anatomical diagram is provided in figure 10.6 along with a blank muscle group RPE template in figure 10.7.

When it is important to monitor recovery within a session, a perceived readiness scale may be used to indicate how ready the athlete or client feels to continue training (15). Perceived readiness can be recorded between sets of repetitions or intervals, with the lowest rating of 1 described as "fully recovered" and "able to exercise at maximal intensity" and the highest rating of 7 described as "exhausted" and "unable to exercise" (see figure 10.8). Taken together, RPE and perceived readiness provide information that the coach or fitness professional can use to assign appropriate work-to-rest ratios during a training session.

Alternatives or Modifications

The original RPE scale proposed by Borg featured a 6 to 20 rating system (6) that corresponded to the typical HR response during exercise when multiplied by 10 (i.e., $6 \times 10 = 60$ bpm indicating resting values and $20 \times 10 = 200$ bpm indicating maximal values). The 10-point RPE scale has also been expanded to a 100-point scale (5) that may be more intuitive because it can be presented as a percentage of maximal effort.

Research Notes

The use of RPE scales during resistance training has been shown to be related to load intensity (i.e., percentage of one-repetition maximum strength), while session RPE has been recommended to monitor training for a variety of activities and sports (24, 54).

Throughout a competitive season, elite soccer players reported significantly higher session load during matches (approximately 600 arbitrary units) compared to training after match day (<50 arbitrary units), which consisted of recovery interventions, as well as normal training days (approximately 200 to 300 arbitrary units) (57). As an indication of the tapering regimen, the session load progressively decreased by approximately 60 arbitrary units per day during the 3-day lead-up to a match (57). In contrast, elite male fencers reported higher session loads during training consisting of footwork (approximately 93 arbitrary units) and sparring (approximately 525 arbitrary units) as compared to competitions consisting of preliminary or poule rounds (approximately 31 arbitrary units) and elimination or knockout rounds (approximately 137 arbitrary units) (59).

Greco-Roman wrestlers at the world championships reported an average overall RPE of 13.8 (using the Borg 6 to 20 scale) during matches and the highest muscle group RPE values in the forearm flexors, deltoids, and biceps brachii that are consistent with the sport's demand on the upper body (42). Comparatively, individuals who completed 12 sessions of slackline training (consisting of maintaining balance on an elevated polyester band anchored on both ends) over 6 weeks stated an average overall RPE of 8.3 (using the Borg 6 to 20 scale) and the highest muscle group RPE values in the gastrocnemius, hamstrings, soleus, quadriceps, lumbar extensors, and tibialis anterior. This is consistent with the importance of the lower-body and postural muscles during this type of activity (51).

Division I collegiate hockey players completed a repeated sprint assessment on a nonmotorized treadmill consisting of five 45-second sprints designed to mimic line shifts, which were separated by 90-second recovery periods during pre- and postseason testing (30). The athletes reported lower perceived readiness ratings prior to sprints four and five along with decreased RPE following sprints three, four, and five at postseason compared to preseason testing (30). Both the perceived readiness and RPE ratings were shown to be related to performance variables, including average power and percent decline, during the repeated sprint assessment (30).

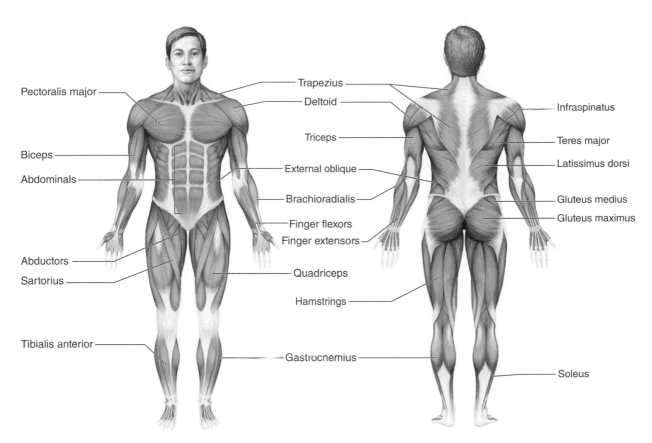

Figure 10.6 Labeled anatomical diagram featuring specific muscle groups.

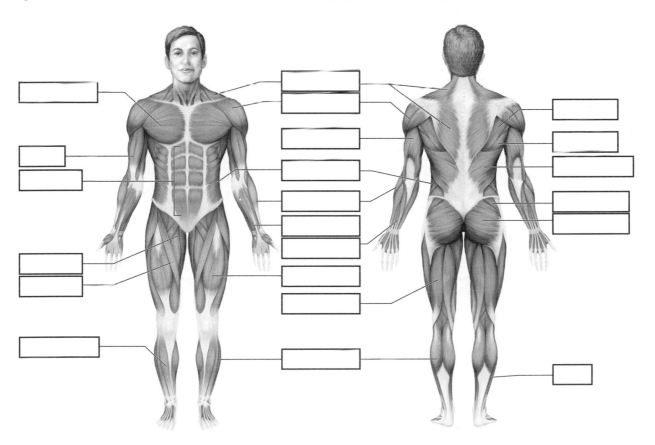

Figure 10.7 Anatomical diagram for determining muscle group rating of perceived exertion (RPE).

From D. Fukuda, *Assessments for Sport and Athletic Performance* (Champaign, IL: Human Kinetics, 2019).

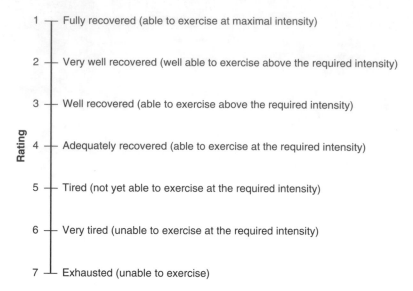

Rating	
1 —	Fully recovered (able to exercise at maximal intensity)
2 —	Very well recovered (well able to exercise above the required intensity)
3 —	Well recovered (able to exercise above the required intensity)
4 —	Adequately recovered (able to exercise at the required intensity)
5 —	Tired (not yet able to exercise at the required intensity)
6 —	Very tired (unable to exercise at the required intensity)
7 —	Exhausted (unable to exercise)

Figure 10.8 Perceived readiness scale.

Applied Examples

Following are three applied examples:

Scenario 1

Determine the session load for a soccer athlete reporting a session RPE of 4 (on a 1 to 10 scale) following a 90-minute training session:

$$\text{Session load} = \text{session RPE of } 4 \times 90 \text{ min} = 360 \text{ arbitrary units}$$

Scenario 2

Determine the session load for a judo athlete reporting a session RPE of 8 (on a 1 to 10 scale) following a 5-minute match:

$$\text{Session load} = \text{session RPE of } 8 \times 5 \text{ min} = 40 \text{ arbitrary units}$$

Scenario 3

Determine the session load for an athlete or client reporting a session RPE of 7 following a training session comprised of 50 total repetitions:

$$\text{Session load} = \text{session RPE of } 7 \times 50 \text{ repetitions} = 350 \text{ arbitrary units}$$

PERCEPTUAL WELL-BEING

Purpose

Perceptual well-being measures provide an indication of how the training process is tolerated by the athlete or client.

Background and Approach

Although perceptual well-being and internal training load are both subjective measurements provided by the athlete or client, perceptual well-being aims to determine the broader impact of training activities on the life of the athlete or client rather than just the activities completed during a given training session.

Perceptual well-being measures can range from a single focused measure, such as soreness or recovery, to a wellness inventory spanning several different aspects of the athlete's or client's life. One approach sums the individual ratings from the athlete or client's subjective evaluation of overall sleep quality, muscle soreness, stress, and fatigue to determine a single index (referred to as the *Hooper index* when a 1 to 7 rating scale is used) (27). Figure 10.9 provides an example of a wellness inventory questionnaire with lower ratings describing worse perceptual well-being and higher ratings describing better perceptual well-being. The value of this approach is that the coach or fitness professional can review both the individual contributions of the selected categories as well as the overall rating that can also be compared with other monitored factors to support or modify the current training program.

A single perceptual well-being measurement tool has been developed to evaluate an individual's perceived recovery status (following a brief warm-up) to determine his or her performance potential during an upcoming training session (31). Figure 10.10 provides the perceived recovery status scale with 0 representing very poorly recovered or extremely tired and 10 representing very well recovered or highly energetic (31). Accordingly, athletes or clients reporting values between 1 and 3 might expect a decline in performance, those with values between 3 and 7 might expect similar performance, and those with values between 7 and 10 might expect improved performance due to low, average, and high levels of recovery, respectively.

In addition to standardized numeric rating scales, visual analog scales (VAS) are sometimes used to record perceptual measures. A VAS is represented by a line with a predetermined length (100 mm, for example) with one end identified as the lowest possible rating and the opposite end as the highest possible rating (44). Soreness from delayed-onset muscle soreness

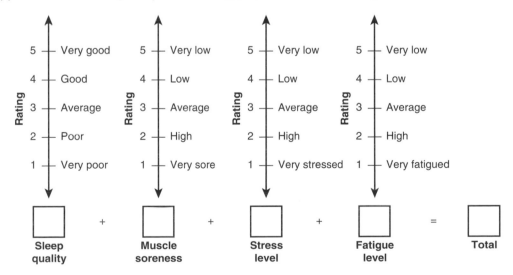

Figure 10.9 Wellness inventory for sleep quality, muscle soreness, stress level, and fatigue level.

From D. Fukuda, *Assessments for Sport and Athletic Performance* (Champaign, IL: Human Kinetics, 2019).

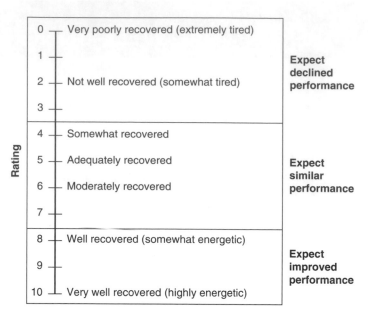

Figure 10.10 Perceived recovery status scale.

(DOMS) can be monitored in this manner, with the left side of the scale representing no pain and the right side of the scale representing unbearable pain (29). The athlete or client is asked to make a mark along the VAS that identifies the current level of overall soreness. Then, the reported level of soreness is calculated as the distance (in mm) along the VAS relative to the total length of the line or is simply compared from one training session to the next. Figure 10.11 shows a VAS with numbered ratings and pictorial references for muscle soreness. The VAS approach for soreness can also be extended to evaluate the lingering effects of previous training sessions on individual muscle groups in a similar way as providing specific ratings of perceived exertion of different muscle groups or body regions.

Alternatives or Modifications

Perceptual well-being measures can be expanded to a variety of different categories. For example, the total quality recovery scale covers the areas of self-reported nutrition and hydration, sleep and rest, relaxation and emotional support, and stretching and active rest. Figure 10.12 features a 0 to 10 rating system with 0 indicating very, very poor recovery, 5 indicating reasonable recovery, and 10 indicating very, very good recovery (37).

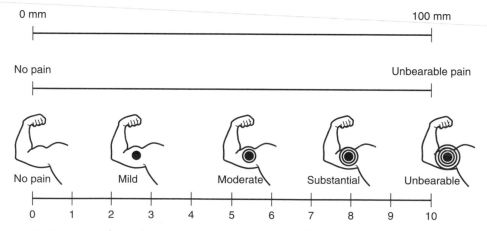

Figure 10.11 Visual analog scale (VAS) and modified scale with numbered ratings and pictorial references for muscle soreness.

Adapted by permission from M. McGuigan, *Monitoring Training and Performance in Athletes* (Champaign, IL: Human Kinetics, 2017), 92.

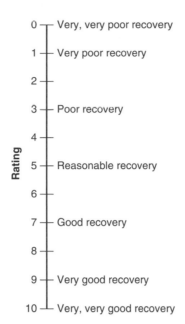

Figure 10.12 Total quality recovery scale.

Research Notes

Subjective measures of well-being have been shown to reflect changes in both short-term and long-term training progressions (52). Decreased wellness ratings, consisting of self-reported measures of muscular soreness, sleep quality, fatigue, stress, and energy level, were reported to result in decreased external training load variables, including total high-speed distance and number of runs at maximal velocity during training in elite soccer players (33). Furthermore, well-being ratings were greatest on match days and appeared to drastically decrease for two days after matches, followed by increases until the next match (33).

Perceived recovery status has shown to be related to changes in the time needed to complete a series of high-intensity intermittent sprints and to be indicative of an individual's ability to predict improvements or declines in subsequent performance (31). With respect to a high-volume resistance training session, perceived recovery status reportedly declined after 48 hours (from 8.6 to 4.2 on a 0 to 10 scale) and was significantly related to creatine kinase, a blood marker of muscle damage (53). Interestingly, elite soccer players reported lower perceived recovery scores (using a 0 to 6 scale, with 0 being not recovered at all and 6 being fully recovered) following night matches (score of approximately 1.9) compared to day matches (score of approximately 3.5) and training days (score of approximately 4.5) (20).

Soreness ratings using a VAS have been shown to differ during recovery from different types of resistance training sessions. A high-volume workout (8 sets of 3 repetitions at 90% of 1-repetition maximum back squat) resulted in minimal changes from baseline (3). On the other hand, a high-intensity workout (8 sets of 10 repetitions at 70% of 1-repetition maximum back squat) resulted in significant values for three days postexercise in previously trained men (3).

Applied Examples

Following are two applied examples:

Scenario 1

Determine the wellness index for an athlete or client with potentially suboptimal values.

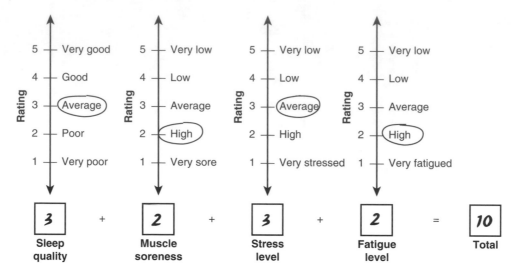

Figure 10.13 Sample wellness index: suboptimal values.

Determine the wellness index for an athlete or client with potentially optimal values.

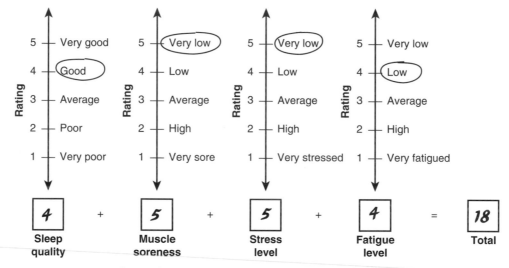

Figure 10.14 Sample wellness index: optimal values.

Scenario 2
VAS score reported the day after training session A:

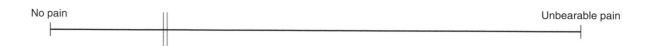

No pain   Unbearable pain

VAS score reported the day after training session B:

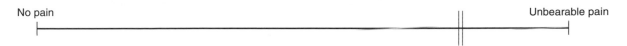

Comparing VAS scores for soreness following different training sessions:

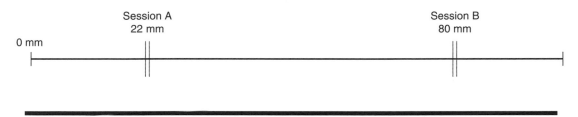

PHYSICAL READINESS

Purpose

Physical readiness provides a measure of how prepared the athlete or client is to perform in an upcoming training session.

Background and Approach

Physical readiness assessments are typically nonfatiguing tests that can be performed quickly before a training session. The selected assessments should be standardized so the results can be easily compared to the athlete's or client's previous results or a group of athletes or clients. Furthermore, coaches or fitness professionals may need to rely on their own expertise and perception to determine how large of a change in day-to-day physical readiness requires an alteration in the training program. The two approaches in this section include preworkout power or speed testing (with a comparison to typical values) and the athlete's or client's HR response to submaximal exercise.

Using power or speed testing to determine physical readiness is based on a comparison of an athlete's or client's preworkout maximal power or speed to his or her previously tested power or speed to evaluate the percentage of typical capacity. The formula for interpreting physical readiness will differ depending on if higher or lower values are considered optimal performance. For jump height or power, where decreased capacity would be indicated by lower values, the following formula is used:

$$\text{Percentage of typical capacity} = \frac{\text{measured jump}}{\text{typical jump}} \times 100$$

For sprint speed where decreased capacity would be indicated by longer sprint times, the following formula is used:

$$\text{Percentage of typical capacity} = \frac{\text{typical sprint}}{\text{measured sprint}} \times 100$$

In general, measured daily values that are close to typical capacity indicate a more physically ready athlete who is well prepared for the upcoming training session.

A variety of power assessments are provided in chapter 7. While most power tests may be adapted for the purpose of evaluating physical readiness, the most straightforward are probably distance-based assessments such as vertical jump, broad jump, or medicine ball throws. Similarly, short-distance (typically ≥30 m [or yd]) sprint times using the straight-line sprint testing protocol provided in chapter 6 may yield additional insight into daily variations in physical readiness (22, 40).

Submaximal HR response testing requires the completion of a standardized training activity from which a typical HR response for an athlete or client is already known. The evaluation could also serve as a warm-up routine prior to a training session. This can be as simple as having the athlete or client run for 5 minutes at a set submaximal speed such as 9 km/h (5.6 mph) with a seated HR assessment immediately after the test and again at 60 seconds during the recovery (9). The absolute HR recovery can then be calculated using the following formula:

$$\text{Absolute HR recovery in bpm} = \text{HR immediately after the test} - \text{recovery HR}$$

If the athlete's or client's maximal HR is known, it could be used as a reference and the minute five HR (i.e., the HR immediately after a five-minute submaximal run) can be divided by this value to determine the percentage of the individual's typical maximum HR (10), as follows:

$$\text{Postexercise HR as \% of max} = \frac{\text{min 5 HR}}{\text{maximum HR}}$$

The running speed during the five-minute submaximal run can be set using a series of prerecorded beeps or a timing system indicating that the athlete or client has covered a specific distance within a given time frame using the following values:

For 9 kilometers per hour
20 meters every 8 seconds
50 meters every 20 seconds
100 meters every 40 seconds

For 5.6 miles per hour
20 yards every 7.3 seconds
50 yards every 18.3 seconds
100 yards every 36.5 seconds

Alternatively, a treadmill can be used by setting the desired speed. Also, a cycling protocol has been developed with the athlete biking for 5 minutes on a stationary bike at 130 watts while pedaling at 85 revolutions per minute (58).

A few submaximal tests in chapter 9 involve measuring exercise HR during the assessment, such as the 45-second squat test and submaximal rowing ergometer test; however, most standardized activities may be modified to determine physical readiness. A common approach is to use submaximal versions of the Yo-Yo intermittent running level one (IR1) and level two (IR2) tests. The submaximal versions of the Yo-Yo IR1 consist of completing just the first 6 minutes of the protocol (following stage 6 at 14.5 km/h) and measuring the individual's HR while in a standing position immediately after finishing the test and again at 90 seconds or 120 seconds of recovery (46). The HR recovery percentage can then be calculated using the following formula:

$$\text{HR recovery \%} = \frac{\text{min 6 HR} - \text{recovery HR}}{\text{min 6 HR}} \times 100$$

If the athlete's or client's typical maximal HR is known, it can be used as a reference, and the minute six HR can be divided by this value to determine the percentage of the individual's maximum HR (38), as follows:

$$\text{Postexercise HR as \% of max} = \frac{\text{min 6 HR}}{\text{maximum HR}} \times 100$$

The submaximal version of the Yo-Yo IR2 consists of 18-meter laps rather the standard 20-meter laps and completing just the first 4 minutes of the protocol with the individual's standing HR taken immediately after finishing the test and again at 120 seconds or 180 seconds of recovery (60). The HR recovery percentage can then be calculated using the following formula:

$$\text{HR recovery \%} = \frac{\text{min 4} - \text{recovery HR}}{\text{min 4 HR}} \times 100$$

Research Notes

Countermovement jump height can be used to monitor neuromuscular function throughout periods of training (13). (Note, though, that the coach or fitness professional should use the average of several jumps rather than a single best jump from a single testing session (13).) For example, countermovement jump height has been shown to decrease in response to both separate six-day strength training (approximately 93.6% of maximum) and high-intensity interval training (approximately 91.6% of maximum) protocols before returning to baseline following three days of recovery (48, 61). Declines in countermovement jump height 24 hours after a soccer match are related to the number of hard changes in direction during match play, and values did not return to baseline within the 3-day period examined (41). Youth rugby players showed consistent declines in countermovement jump height (approximately 85.4% from reference values) over a 7-week competitive period demonstrating an accumulation of fatigue over the course of approximately 10 matches (45). These declines in countermovement jump height may indicate that the physical readiness of the athlete or client was compromised compared to typical, nonfatigued performance capabilities.

Exercise HR following a five-minute submaximal run has shown to differentiate between youth soccer athletes with higher (lower minute five HR) and lower (higher minute five HR) cardiorespiratory fitness, while HR recovery was significantly related to repeated sprint performance (11).

Submaximal Yo-Yo IR1 postexercise HR as a percentage of maximum has been shown to be related to high-intensity running during a soccer match, with lower values indicating the potential for greater distances covered at higher speeds (2). HR measured in soccer athletes after the submaximal Yo-Yo IR1 was 176 beats per minute during preseason and dropped to between 166 and 169 beats per minute throughout the regular season (38). This finding coincided with a decrease in postexercise HR as percentage of maximum from preseason (approximately 97%) to the beginning of the competitive period (approximately 87%), denoting improved cardiovascular fitness during the preparatory period (38).

Applied Examples

Following are five applied examples:

Scenario 1

Determine the percentage of maximum jump height for an athlete or client with a typical countermovement jump height of 82 centimeters and who jumps 78 centimeters during a preworkout countermovement jump assessment:

$$\text{\% of typical capacity} = \frac{78 \text{ cm (measured jump)}}{82 \text{ cm (typical jump)}} \times 100 = 95.0\%$$

In this scenario, the athlete or client jumped at 95 percent of his or her typical capacity, which could also be interpreted as being a 5-percent lower jump height than on a typical day.

Scenario 2

Determine the percentage of maximum sprint time for an athlete or client with a typical 30-meter sprint time of 4.5 seconds and who runs a preworkout 20-meter sprint in 4.8 seconds:

$$\text{\% of typical capacity} = \frac{4.5 \text{ sec (typical sprint)}}{4.8 \text{ sec (measured sprint)}} \times 100 = 93.8\%$$

In this scenario, the athlete's or client's 20-meter sprint speed is 93.8 percent of his or her typical capacity, which could also be interpreted as taking 6.2 percent longer to cover the desired distance.

Scenario 3

Determine the HR recovery and postexercise HR for an athlete with a known maximum HR of 202 beats per minute and who has a HR of 172 beats per minutes immediately following a 5-minute run at 9 km/hr (5.6 mph) and a HR of 118 beats per minute after 60 seconds of recovery:

$$\text{Absolute HR recovery} = 172 \text{ bpm (min 5 HR)} - 118 \text{ bpm (recovery HR)} = 54 \text{ bpm}$$

$$\text{Postexercise HR as \% of max} = \frac{172 \text{ bpm (min 5 HR)}}{202 \text{ bpm (maximum HR)}} = 85.1\%$$

Scenario 4

Determine the HR recovery and postexercise HR for an athlete with a known maximum HR of 198 beats per minute and who has a HR of 170 beats per minutes immediately following a 6-minute submaximal Yo-Yo IR1 and a HR of 105 beats per minute after 90 seconds of recovery:

$$\text{HR recovery \%} = \frac{170 \text{ bpm (min 6 HR)} - 105 \text{ bpm (recovery HR)}}{170 \text{ bpm (min 6 HR)}} \times 100 = 38.2\%$$

$$\text{Postexercise HR as \% of max} = \frac{147 \text{ bpm (recovery HR)}}{198 \text{ bpm (maximum 6 HR)}} \times 100 = 86.4\%$$

Scenario 5

Determine the HR recovery for an athlete who has a HR of 175 beats per minutes immediately following a 4-minute submaximal Yo-Yo IR2 and a HR of 110 beats per minute after 90 seconds of recovery:

$$\text{HR recovery \%} = \frac{175 \text{ bpm (min 4 HR)} - 110 \text{ bpm (recovery HR)}}{175 \text{ bpm (min 4 HR)}} \times 100 = 37.1\%$$

References

Chapter 1

1. Armstrong, LE, Maresh, CM, Castellani, JW, Bergeron, MF, Kenefick, RW, LaGasse, KE, and Riebe, D. Urinary indices of hydration status. *Int J Sport Nutr* 4:265-279, 1994.

2. Armstrong, LE, Soto, JA, Hacker, FT, Jr., Casa, DJ, Kavouras, SA, and Maresh, CM. Urinary indices during dehydration, exercise, and rehydration. *Int J Sport Nutr* 8:345-355, 1998.

3. Australian Institute of Sport. AIS Sports Draft searches for future champions. 2015. www.ausport.gov.au/news/ais_news/story_635185_ais_sports_draft_searches_for_future_champions. Accessed December 6, 2017.

4. Center for Community Health and Development. Assessing community needs and resources. Section 14. SWOT analysis: Strengths, weaknesses, opportunities, and threats. In *Community Tool Box*. Lawrence, KS: University of Kansas, 2017. http://ctb.ku.edu/en/table-of-contents/assessment/assessing-community-needs-and-resources/swot-analysis/main.

5. David, FR. *Strategic Management: Concepts and Cases*. 13th ed. Upper Saddle River, NJ: Prentice Hall, 2011.

6. Gonzalez-Badillo, JJ, and Sanchez-Medina, L. Movement velocity as a measure of loading intensity in resistance training. *Int J Sports Med* 31:347-352, 2010.

7. Hewett, TE, Ford, KR, Hoogenboom, BJ, and Myer, GD. Understanding and preventing ACL injuries: Current biomechanical and epidemiologic considerations—Update 2010. *N Am J Sports Phys Ther* 5:234-251, 2010.

8. Hewett, TE, Myer, GD, Ford, KR, Heidt, RS, Jr., Colosimo, AJ, McLean, SG, van den Bogert, AJ, Paterno, MV, and Succop, P. Biomechanical measures of neuromuscular control and valgus loading of the knee predict anterior cruciate ligament injury risk in female athletes: A prospective study. *Am J Sports Med* 33:492-501, 2005.

9. Johnson, CN. The benefits of PDCA: Use this cycle for continual process improvement. *Quality Progress* 35:120-120, 2002.

10. Lloyd, RS, and Oliver, JL. The youth physical development model: A new approach to long-term athletic development. *Strength Cond J* 34:61-72, 2012.

11. Lloyd, RS, and Oliver, JL. *Strength and Conditioning for Young Athletes: Science and Application*. New York: Routledge, 2013.

12. Lloyd, RS, Oliver, JL, Faigenbaum, AD, Howard, R, De Ste Croix, MB, Williams, CA, Best, TM, Alvar, BA, Micheli, LJ, Thomas, DP, Hatfield, DL, Cronin, JB, and Myer, GD. Long-term athletic development, part 1: A pathway for all youth. *J Strength Cond Res* 29:1439-1450, 2015.

13. Maughan, RJ, and Shirreffs, SM. Dehydration and rehydration in competative sport. *Scand J Med Sci Sports* 20 Suppl 3:40-47, 2010.

14. Meir, R, Diesel, W, and Archer, E. Developing a prehabilitation program in a collision sport: A model developed within English premiership rugby union football. *Strength Cond J* 29:50-62, 2007.

15. Meylan, C, and Cronin, JB. Talent identification. In *Strength and Conditioning for Young Athletes: Science and Application*. Lloyd, RS, Oliver, JL, eds. New York: Routledge, 19-32, 2013.

16. Newell, KM. Constraints on the development of coordination. In *Motor Development in Children: Aspects of Coordination and Control*. Wade, MG, Whiting, HTA, eds. Boston: Martinus Nijhoff, 341-361, 1986.

17. Philippaerts, RM, Vaeyens, R, Janssens, M, Van Renterghem, B, Matthys, D, Craen, R, Bourgois, J, Vrijens, J, Beunen, G, and Malina, RM. The relationship between peak height velocity and physical performance in youth soccer players. *Journal of Sports Sciences* 24:221-230, 2006.

18. Rampinini, E, Bishop, D, Marcora, SM, Ferrari Bravo, D, Sassi, R, and Impellizzeri, FM. Validity of simple field tests as indicators of match-related physical performance in top-level professional soccer players. *Int J Sports Med* 28:228-235, 2007.

19. Reilly, T, Williams, AM, Nevill, A, and Franks, A. A multidisciplinary approach to talent identification in soccer. *J Sports Sci* 18:695-702, 2000.

20. Rivera-Brown, AM, and De Felix-Davila, RA. Hydration status in adolescent judo athletes before and after training in the heat. *Int J Sports Physiol Perform* 7:39-46, 2012.

21. Stolberg, M, Sharp, A, Coutto, AS, Lloyd, RS, Oliver, JL, and Cronin, J. Triple and quintuple hops: Utility, reliability, asymmetry, and relationship to performance. *Strength Cond J* 38:18-25, 2016.

22. Suchomel, TJ, and Bailey, CA. Monitoring and managing fatigue in baseball players. *Strength Cond J* 36:39-45, 2014.

23. Vaeyens, R, Lenoir, M, Williams, AM, and Philippaerts, RM. Talent identification and development programmes in sport: Current models and future directions. *Sports Med* 38:703-714, 2008.

24. Wattie, N, Schorer, J, and Baker, J. The relative age effect in sport: A developmental systems model. *Sports Med* 45:83-94, 2015.

25. Weihrich, H. The tows matrix: A tool for situational analysis. *Long Range Planning* 15:54-66, 1982.

26. Wild, CY, Steele, JR, and Munro, BJ. Why do girls sustain more anterior cruciate ligament injuries than boys? A review of the changes in estrogen and musculoskeletal structure and function during puberty. *Sports Med* 42:733-749, 2012.

27. Williams, CA, Oliver, JL, and Lloyd, RS. Talent Development. In *Strength and Conditioning for Young Athletes: Science and Application*. Lloyd, RS, Oliver, JL, eds. New York: Routledge, 33-46, 2013.

Chapter 2

1. Brechue, WF. Structure-function relationships that determine sprint performance and running speed in sport. *Int J Appl Sports Sci* 23:313-350, 2011.

2. Coswig, VS, Machado Freitas, DF, Gentil, P, Fukuda, DH, and Del Vecchio, FB. Kinematics and kinetics of multiple sets using lifting straps during deadlift training. *J Strength Cond Res* 29:3399-3404, 2015.

3. Earp, JE, and Newton, RU. Advances in electronic timing systems: Considerations for selecting an appropriate timing system. *J Strength Cond Res* 26:1245-1248, 2012.

4. Fukuda, DH, Smith-Ryan, AE, Kendall, KL, Moon, JR, and Stout, JR. Simplified method of clinical phenotyping for older men and women using established field-based measures. *Exp Gerontol* 48:1479-1488, 2013.

5. Heyward, VH, and Wagner, DR. *Bioelectrical Impedance Analysis Method.* 2nd ed. Champaign, IL: Human Kinetics, 2004.

6. Hudy, A. Facility design, layout, and organization. In *Essentials of Strength Training and Conditioning.* 4th ed. Haff, G, Triplett, NT, eds. Champaign, IL: Human Kinetics, 623-639, 2016.

7. Kattan, MW, and Marasco, J. What is a real nomogram? *Seminars in Oncology* 37:23-26, 2010.

8. Kendall, KL, Fukuda, DH, Hyde, PN, Smith-Ryan, AE, Moon, JR, and Stout, JR. Estimating fat-free mass in elite-level male rowers: A four-compartment model validation of laboratory and field methods. *J Sports Sci* 35:624-633, 2017.

9. Malyszek, KK, Harmon, RA, Dunnick, DD, Costa, PB, Coburn, JW, and Brown, LE. Comparison of Olympic and hexagonal barbells with midthigh pull, deadlift, and countermovement jump. *J Strength Cond Res* 31:140-145, 2017.

10. McGuigan, M. Principles of test selection and administration. In *Essentials of Strength Training and Conditioning.* 4th ed. Haff, G, Triplett, NT, eds. Champaign, IL: Human Kinetics, 249-258, 2016.

11. Rana, S, and White, JB. Fitness assessment selection and administration. In *NSCA's Essentials of Personal Training.* 2nd ed. Coburn, JW, Malek, MH, eds. Champaign, IL: Human Kinetics, 179-200, 2012.

12. Renfro, GJ, and Ebben, WP. A review of the use of lifting belts. *Strength Cond J* 28:68-74, 2006.

13. Tanner, JM, Goldstein, H, and Whitehouse, RH. Standards for children's height at ages 2-9 years allowing for heights of parents. *Arch Dis Child* 45:755-762, 1970.

Chapter 3

1. Bredin, SS, Gledhill, N, Jamnik, VK, and Warburton, DE. PAR-Q+ and ePARmed-X+: New risk stratification and physical activity clearance strategy for physicians and patients alike. *Can Fam Physician* 59:273-277, 2013.

2. Center for Community Health and Development. Assessing community needs and resources. Section 14. SWOT analysis: Strengths, weaknesses, opportunities, and threats. In *Community Tool Box.* Lawrence, KS: University of Kansas, 2017. http://ctb.ku.edu/en/table-of-contents/assessment/assessing-community-needs-and-resources/swot-analysis/main.

3. Chiarlitti, NA, Delisle-Houde, P, Reid, RER, Kennedy, C, and Andersen, RE. The importance of body composition in the national hockey league combine physiologic assessments. *J Strength Cond Res*, 2017.

4. David, FR. *Strategic Management: Concepts and Cases.* 13th ed. Upper Saddle River, NJ: Prentice Hall, 2011.

5. Fernandez-Fernandez, J, Ulbricht, A, and Ferrauti, A. Fitness testing of tennis players: How valuable is it? *Br J Sports Med* 48 Suppl 1:i22-31, 2014.

6. Flanagan, SP. Putting it all together. In *Biomechanics: A Case-Based Approach.* 1st ed. Burlington, MA: Jones & Bartlett Learning, 327-354, 2014.

7. Hurley, WL, Denegar, CR, and Hertel, J. Validity and reliability. In *Research Methods: A Framework for Evidence-Based Clinical Practice.* 1st ed. Philadelphia: Wolters Kluwer/Lippincott Williams & Wilkins Health, 139-154, 2011.

8. Julio, UF, Panissa, VLG, Esteves, JV, Cury, RL, Agostinho, MF, and Franchini, E. Energy-system contributions to simulated judo matches. *Int J Sports Physiol Perform* 12:676-683, 2017.

9. Kondo, M, Abe, T, Ikegawa, S, Kawakami, Y, and Fukunaga, T. Upper limit of fat-free mass in humans: A study on Japanese sumo wrestlers. *Am J Hum Biol* 6:613-618, 1994.

10. Kovacs, MS. Tennis physiology: Training the competitive athlete. *Sports Med* 37:189-198, 2007.

11. Little, T, and Williams, AG. Effects of sprint duration and exercise: Rest ratio on repeated sprint performance and physiological responses in professional soccer players. *J Strength Cond Res* 21:646-648, 2007.

12. Mann, JB, Stoner, JD, and Mayhew, JL. NFL-225 test to predict 1RM bench press in NCAA Division I football players. *J Strength Cond Res* 26:2623-2631, 2012.

13. McBride, JM, Triplett-McBride, T, Davie, A, and Newton, RU. A comparison of strength and power characteristics between power lifters, Olympic lifters, and sprinters. *J Strength Cond Res* 13:58-66, 1999.

14. McGuigan, M. Administration, scoring, and interpretation of selected tests. In *Essentials of Strength Training and Conditioning.* 4th ed. Haff, G, Triplett, NT, eds. Champaign, IL: Human Kinetics, 259-316, 2016.

15. McGuigan, M. Principles of test selection and administration. In *Essentials of Strength Training and Conditioning.* 4th ed. Haff, G, Triplett, NT, eds. Champaign, IL: Human Kinetics, 249-258, 2016.

16. Newell, KM. Constraints on the development of coordination. In *Motor Development in Children: Aspects of Coordination and Control.* Wade, MG, Whiting, HTA, eds. Boston: Martinus Nijhoff, 341-361, 1986.

17. Perrin, P, Deviterne, D, Hugel, F, and Perrot, C. Judo, better than dance, develops sensorimotor adaptabilities involved in balance control. *Gait Posture* 15:187-194, 2002.

18. Rana, S, and White, JB. Fitness assessment selection and administration. In *NSCA's Essentials of Personal Training.* 2nd ed. Coburn, JW, Malek, MH, eds. Champaign, IL: Human Kinetics, 179-200, 2012.

19. Ryan, ED, and Cramer, JT. Fitness testing protocols and norms. In *NSCA's Essentials of Personal Training.* 2nd ed. Coburn, JW, Malek, MH, eds. Champaign, IL: Human Kinetics, 201-247, 2012.

20. Serpell, BG, Ford, M, and Young, WB. The development of a new test of agility for rugby league. *J Strength Cond Res* 24:3270-3277, 2010.

21. Wattie, N, Schorer, J, and Baker, J. The relative age effect in sport: A developmental systems model. *Sports Med* 45:83-94, 2015.

22. Weihrich, H. The tows matrix: A tool for situational analysis. *Long Range Planning* 15:54-66, 1982.

23. Wells, AJ, Hoffman, JR, Beyer, KS, Hoffman, MW, Jajtner, AR, Fukuda, DH, and Stout, JR. Regular- and postseason comparisons of playing time and measures of running performance in NCAA Division I women soccer players. *Appl Physiol Nutr Metab* 40:907-917, 2015.

24. Woolford, SM, Polglaze, T, Rowsell, G, and Spencer, M. Field testing principles and protocols. In *Physiological Tests for Elite Athletes*. 2nd ed. Tanner, RK, Gore, CJ, eds. Champaign, IL: Human Kinetics, 231-248, 2013.

25. Stratton, G. and J. L. Oliver (2013). The Impact of Growth and Maturation on Physical Performance. *Strength and Conditioning for Young Athletes: Science and Application*. R. S. Lloyd and J. L. Oliver. New York, Routledge: 3-18.

Chapter 4

1. Artioli, GG, Franchini, E, Nicastro, H, Sterkowicz, S, Solis, MY, and Lancha, AH, Jr. The need of a weight management control program in judo: A proposal based on the successful case of wrestling. *J Int Soc Sports Nutr* 7:15, 2010.

1. Baechle, TR, Earle, RW, eds. *Essentials of Strength Training and Conditioning*. 3rd ed. Champaign, IL: Human Kinetics, 2008.

2. Baun, WB, Baun, MR, and Raven, PB. A nomogram for the estimate of percent body fat from generalized equations. *Res Q Exerc Sport* 52:380-384, 1981.

3. Bray, GA. Definition, measurement, and classification of the syndromes of obesity. *Int J Obes* 2:99-112, 1978.

4. Bray, GA, and Gray, DS. Obesity: Part I—Pathogenesis. *West J Med* 149:429-441, 1988.

5. Douda, HT, Toubekis, AG, Avloniti, AA, and Tokmakidis, SP. Physiological and anthropometric determinants of rhythmic gymnastics performance. *Int J Sports Physiol Perform* 3:41-54, 2008.

6. Fryar, CD, Gu, Q, and Ogden, CL. Anthropometric reference data for children and adults: United States, 2007-2010. *Vital Health Stat 11*:1-48, 2012.

7. Haff, GG, and Triplett, NT, eds. *Essentials of Strength Training and Conditioning*. 4th ed. Champaign, IL: Human Kinetics, 2016.

8. Heyward, VH, and Gibson, AL. Assessing body composition. In *Advanced Fitness Assessment and Exercise Prescription*. 7th ed. Champaign, IL: Human Kinetics, 219-266, 2014.

9. Jackson, AS, and Pollock, ML. Generalized equations for predicting body density of men. *Br J Nutr* 40:497-504, 1978.

10. Jackson, AS, Pollock, ML, and Ward, A. Generalized equations for predicting body density of women. *Med Sci Sports Exerc* 12:175-181, 1980.

11. Marfell-Jones, MJ, Stewart, AD, and de Ridder, JH. *International Standards for Anthropometric Assessment*. Wellington, New Zealand: International Society for the Advancement of Kinanthropometry, 2012.

12. Moon, JR. Body composition in athletes and sports nutrition: An examination of the bioimpedance analysis technique. *Eur J Clin Nutr* 67 Suppl 1:S54-59, 2013.

13. Ratamess, NA. Body composition. In *NSCA's Guide to Tests and Assessments*. Miller, T, ed. Champaign, IL: Human Kinetics, 15-41, 2012.

14. Rossow, LM, Fukuda, DH, Fahs, CA, Loenneke, JP, and Stout, JR. Natural bodybuilding competition preparation and recovery: A 12-month case study. *Int J Sports Physiol Perform* 8:582-592, 2013.

15. Ryan, ED, and Cramer, JT. Fitness testing protocols and norms. In *NSCA's Essentials of Personal Training*. 2nd ed. Coburn, JW, Malek, MH, eds. Champaign, IL: Human Kinetics, 201-247, 2012.

16. Santos, DA, Dawson, JA, Matias, CN, Rocha, PM, Minderico, CS, Allison, DB, Sardinha, LB, and Silva, AM. Reference values for body composition and anthropometric measurements in athletes. *PLoS One* 9:e97846, 2014.

17. Sedeaud, A, Marc, A, Marck, A, Dor, F, Schipman, J, Dorsey, M, Haida, A, Berthelot, G, and Toussaint, JF. BMI, a performance parameter for speed improvement. *PLoS One* 9:e90183, 2014.

18. Slater, G, Woolford, SM, and Marfell-Jones, MJ. Assessment of physique. In *Physiological Tests for Elite Athletes*. 2nd ed. Tanner, RK, Gore, CJ, eds. Champaign, IL: Human Kinetics, 167-198, 2013.

19. W. H. O. Expert Consultation. Appropriate body-mass index for Asian populations and its implications for policy and intervention strategies. *Lancet* 363:157-163, 2004.

Chapter 5

1. SCAT3. *Br J Sports Med* 47:259, 2013. https://bjsm.bmj.com/content/47/5/259.long. 47.

2. Accvedo, EO, and Starks, MA. Evaluating flexibility. In *Exercise Testing and Prescription Lab Manual*. 2nd ed. Champaign, IL: Human Kinetics, 65-74, 2011.

3. Boguszewski, D, Adamczyk, JG, Buda, M, Kloda, M, and Bialoszewski, D. The use of functional tests to assess risk of injuries in judokas. *Arch Budo Sci Martial Arts Extrem Sports* 12:57-62, 2016.

4. Bressel, E, Yonker, JC, Kras, J, and Heath, EM. Comparison of static and dynamic balance in female collegiate soccer, basketball, and gymnastics athletes. *J Athl Train* 42:42-46, 2007.

5. Castro-Piñero, J, Girela-Rejón, MJ, González-Montesinos, JL, Mora, J, Conde-Caveda, J, Sjöström, M, and Ruiz, JR. Percentile values for flexibility tests in youths aged 6 to 17 years: Influence of weight status. *Eur J Sport Sci* 13:139-148, 2013.

5a. Cornell, DJ, Gnacinski, SL, Langford, MH, Mims, J, and Ebersole, KT. Backwards overhead medicine ball throw and countermovement jump performance among firefighter candidates. *J Trainol* 4: 11-14, 2015.

6. Davis, WJ, Wood, DT, Andrews, RG, Elkind, LM, and Davis, WB. Concurrent training enhances athletes' strength, muscle endurance, and other measures. *J Strength Cond Res* 22:1487-1502, 2008.

7. Dejanovic, A, Cambridge, ED, and McGill, S. Isometric torso muscle endurance profiles in adolescents aged

15-18: Normative values for age and gender differences. *Ann Hum Biol* 41:153-158, 2014.

8. Dejanovic, A, Harvey, EP, and McGill, SM. Changes in torso muscle endurance profiles in children aged 7 to 14 years: Reference values. *Arch Phys Med Rehabil* 93:2295-2301, 2012.

9. Duncan, PW, Weiner, DK, Chandler, J, and Studenski, S. Functional reach: A new clinical measure of balance. *J Gerontol* 45:M192-M197, 1990.

10. Durall, CJ, Udermann, BE, Johansen, DR, Gibson, B, Reineke, DM, and Reuteman, P. The effects of preseason trunk muscle training on low-back pain occurrence in women collegiate gymnasts. *J Strength Cond Res* 23:86-92, 2009.

11. Gorman, M, Hecht, S, Samborski, A, Lunos, S, Elias, S, and Stovitz, SD. SCAT3 assessment of non-head injured and head injured athletes competing in a large international youth soccer tournament. *Appl Neuropsychol Child* 6:364-368, 2017.

12. Haff, GG, and Dumke, C. Flexibility testing. In *Laboratory Manual for Exercise Physiology.* Champaign, IL: Human Kinetics, 79-114, 2012.

13. Hetu, FE, Christie, CA, and Faigenbaum, AD. Effects of conditioning on physical fitness and club head speed in mature golfers. *Percept Mot Skills* 86:811-815, 1998.

14. Heyward, VH, and Gibson, AL. Assessing flexibility. In *Advanced Fitness Assessment and Exercise Prescription.* 7th ed. Champaign, IL: Human Kinetics, 305-324, 2014.

15. Hoeger, WWK, Hoeger, SA, Hoeger, CI, and Fawson, AL. Muscular flexibility. In *Lifetime Physical Fitness and Wellness.* Stamford, CT: Cengage Learning, 302-330, 2018.

16. Hong, Y, Li, JX, and Robinson, PD. Balance control, flexibility, and cardiorespiratory fitness among older Tai Chi practitioners. *Br J Sports Med* 34:29-34, 2000.

17. Hutchinson, MR. Low back pain in elite rhythmic gymnasts. *Med Sci Sports Exerc* 31:1686-1688, 1999.

18. Isles, RC, Choy, NL, Steer, M, and Nitz, JC. Normal values of balance tests in women aged 20-80. *J Am Geriatr Soc* 52:1367-1372, 2004.

19. Iverson, GL, and Koehle, MS. Normative data for the balance error scoring system in adults. *Rehabil Res Pract* 2013:846418, 2013.

19a. Johnson, BL, Nelson, JK. *Practical Measurements for Evaluation in Physical Education.* Minneapolis, MN: Burgess Publishing Company, 1969.

20. Kjaer, IG, Torstveit, MK, Kolle, E, Hansen, BH, and Anderssen, SA. Normative values for musculoskeletal- and neuromotor fitness in apparently healthy Norwegian adults and the association with obesity: A cross-sectional study. *BMC Sports Sci Med Rehabil* 8:37, 2016.

21. McGill, SM, Childs, A, and Liebenson, C. Endurance times for low back stabilization exercises: Clinical targets for testing and training from a normal database. *Arch Phys Med Rehabil* 80:941-944, 1999.

22. McGuigan, M. Administration, scoring, and interpretation of selected tests. In *Essentials of Strength Training and Conditioning.* 4th ed. Haff, G, Triplett, NT, eds. Champaign, IL: Human Kinetics, 259-316, 2016.

23. McLeod, TC, Armstrong, T, Miller, M, and Sauers, JL. Balance improvements in female high school basketball players after a 6-week neuromuscular-training program. *J Sport Rehabil* 18:465-481, 2009.

24. Nieman, DC. Musculoskeletal Fitness. In *Exercise Testing and Prescription: A Health-Related Approach.* 7th ed. Boston: McGraw-Hill, 136-158, 2011.

25. Oldham, JR, DiFabio, MS, Kaminski, TW, DeWolf, RM, and Buckley, TA. Normative tandem gait in collegiate student-athletes: Implications for clinical concussion assessment. *Sports Health* 9:305-311, 2017.

26. Reiman, MP, and Manske, RC. Balance testing. In *Functional Testing in Human Performance.* Champaign, IL: Human Kinetics, 103-117, 2009.

27. Reiman, MP, and Manske, RC. Trunk testing. In *Functional Testing in Human Performance.* Champaign, IL: Human Kinetics, 211-240, 2009.

28. Ryan, ED, and Cramer, JT. Fitness testing protocols and norms. In *NSCA's Essentials of Personal Training.* 2nd ed. Coburn, JW, Malek, MH, eds. Champaign, IL: Human Kinetics, 201-247, 2012.

29. Santo, A, Lynall, RC, Guskiewicz, KM, and Mihalik, JP. Clinical utility of the Sport Concussion Assessment Tool 3 (SCAT3) tandem-gait test in high school athletes. *J Athl Train* 52:1096-1100, 2017.

30. Schneiders, AG, Sullivan, SJ, Gray, AR, Hammond-Tooke, GD, and McCrory, PR. Normative values for three clinical measures of motor performance used in the neurological assessment of sports concussion. *J Sci Med Sport* 13:196-201, 2010.

31. Schneiders, AG, Sullivan, SJ, Handcock, P, Gray, A, and McCrory, PR. Sports concussion assessment: The effect of exercise on dynamic and static balance. *Scand J Med Sci Sports* 22:85-90, 2012.

32. Sekendiz, B, Cug, M, and Korkusuz, F. Effects of Swiss-ball core strength training on strength, endurance, flexibility, and balance in sedentary women. *J Strength Cond Res* 24:3032-3040, 2010.

33. Stanziano, DC, Signorile, JF, Mow, S, Davidson, EE, Ouslander, JG, and Roos, BA. The modified total body rotation test: A rapid, reliable assessment of physical function in older adults. *J Am Geriatr Soc* 58:1965-1969, 2010.

34. Tomkinson, GR, Carver, KD, Atkinson, F, Daniell, ND, Lewis, LK, Fitzgerald, JS, Lang, JJ, and Ortega, FB. European normative values for physical fitness in children and adolescents aged 9-17 years: Results from 2 779 165 Eurofit performances representing 30 countries. *Br J Sports Med*, 2017.

35. Vescovi, JD, Murray, TM, and Vanheest, JL. Positional performance profiling of elite ice hockey players. *Int J Sports Physiol Perform* 1:84-94, 2006.

36. Warr, BJ, Heumann, KJ, Dodd, DJ, Swan, PD, and Alvar, BA. Injuries, changes in fitness, and medical demands in deployed National Guard soldiers. *Mil Med* 177:1136-1142, 2012.

Chapter 6

1. Beckett, JR, Schneiker, KT, Wallman, KE, Dawson, BT, and Guelfi, KJ. Effects of static stretching on repeated sprint and change of direction performance. *Med Sci Sports Exerc* 41:444-450, 2009.

2. Burgess, DJ, and Gabbett, TJ. Football (soccer) players. In *Physiological Tests for Elite Athletes.* 2nd ed.

Tanner, RK, Gore, CJ, eds. Champaign, IL: Human Kinetics, 323-330, 2013.

3. Castro-Pinero, J, Gonzalez-Montesinos, JL, Keating, XD, Mora, J, Sjostrom, M, and Ruiz, JR. Percentile values for running sprint field tests in children ages 6-17 years: Influence of weight status. *Res Q Exerc Sport* 81:143-151, 2010.

4. Gabbett, T, and Georgieff, B. Physiological and anthropometric characteristics of Australian junior national, state, and novice volleyball players. *J Strength Cond Res* 21:902-908, 2007.

5. Gabbett, TJ, Kelly, JN, and Sheppard, JM. Speed, change of direction speed, and reactive agility of rugby league players. *J Strength Cond Res* 22:174-181, 2008.

6. Gabbett, TJ, and Sheppard, JM. Testing and training agility. In *Physiological Tests for Elite Athletes*. 2nd ed. Tanner, RK, Gore, CJ, eds. Champaign, IL: Human Kinetics, 199-205, 2013.

7. Gillam, GM, and Marks, M. 300 yard shuttle run. *Strength Cond J* 5:46-46, 1983.

8. Grier, TL, Canham-Chervak, M, Bushman, TT, Anderson, MK, North, WJ, and Jones, BH. Evaluating injury risk and gender performance on health- and skill-related fitness assessments. *J Strength Cond Res* 31:971-980, 2017.

9. Haff, GG, and Dumke, C. Anaerobic fitness measurements. In *Laboratory Manual for Exercise Physiology*. Champaign, IL: Human Kinetics, 305-360, 2012.

10. Haugen, T, Tonnessen, E, Hisdal, J, and Seiler, S. The role and development of sprinting speed in soccer. *Int J Sports Physiol Perform* 9:432-441, 2014.

11. Herman, SL, and Smith, DT. Four-week dynamic stretching warm-up intervention elicits longer-term performance benefits. *J Strength Cond Res* 22:1286-1297, 2008.

12. Hoffman, J. Anaerobic power. In *Norms for Fitness, Performance, and Health*. Champaign, IL: Human Kinetics, 53-66, 2006.

13. Hoffman, J. Athletic performance testing and normative data. In *Physiological Aspects of Sport Training and Performance*. Second edition. ed. Champaign, IL: Human Kinetics, 237-267, 2014.

14. Langley, JG, and Chetlin, RD. Test re-test reliability of four versions of the 3-cone test in non-athletic men. *J Sports Sci Med* 16:44-52, 2017.

15. Lockie, RG, Jeffriess, MD, McGann, TS, Callaghan, SJ, and Schultz, AB. Planned and reactive agility performance in semiprofessional and amateur basketball players. *Int J Sports Physiol Perform* 9:766-771, 2014.

16. Mangine, GT, Hoffman, JR, Vazquez, J, Pichardo, N, Fragala, MS, and Stout, JR. Predictors of fielding performance in professional baseball players. *Int J Sports Physiol Perform* 8:510-516, 2013.

17. McGuigan, M. Administration, scoring, and interpretation of selected tests. In *Essentials of Strength Training and Conditioning*. 4th ed. Haff, G, Triplett, NT, eds. Champaign, IL: Human Kinetics, 259-316, 2016.

18. Nuzzo, JL. The National Football League scouting combine from 1999 to 2014: Normative reference values and an examination of body mass normalization techniques. *J Strength Cond Res* 29:279-289, 2015.

19. Paul, DJ, Gabbett, TJ, and Nassis, GP. Agility in team sports: Testing, training and factors affecting performance. *Sports Med* 46:421-442, 2016.

20. Pauole, K, Madole, K, Garhammer, J, Lacourse, M, and Rozenek, R. Reliability and validity of the T-test as a measure of agility, leg power, and leg speed in college-aged men and women. *J Strength Cond Res* 14:443-450, 2000.

21. Rampinini, E, Bishop, D, Marcora, SM, Ferrari Bravo, D, Sassi, R, and Impellizzeri, FM. Validity of simple field tests as indicators of match-related physical performance in top-level professional soccer players. *Int J Sports Med* 28:228-235, 2007.

22. Reiman, MP, and Manske, RC. Lower extremity anaerobic power testing. In *Functional Testing in Human Performance*. Champaign, IL: Human Kinetics, 263-274, 2009.

23. Reiman, MP, and Manske, RC. Speed, agility, and quickness testing. In *Functional Testing in Human Performance*. Champaign, IL: Human Kinetics, 191-208, 2009.

24. Reiman, MP, and Manske, RC. Strength and power testing. In *Functional Testing in Human Performance*. Champaign, IL: Human Kinetics, 131-190, 2009.

25. Robbins, DW, Goodale, TL, Kuzmits, FE, and Adams, AJ. Changes in the athletic profile of elite college American football players. *J Strength Cond Res* 27:861-874, 2013.

26. Seitz, LB, Reyes, A, Tran, TT, Saez de Villarreal, E, and Haff, GG. Increases in lower-body strength transfer positively to sprint performance: a systematic review with meta-analysis. *Sports Med* 44:1693-1702, 2014.

27. Sheppard, JM, Young, WB, Doyle, TL, Sheppard, TA, and Newton, RU. An evaluation of a new test of reactive agility and its relationship to sprint speed and change of direction speed. *J Sci Med Sport* 9:342-349, 2006.

28. Sierer, SP, Battaglini, CL, Mihalik, JP, Shields, EW, and Tomasini, NT. The National Football League Combine: performance differences between drafted and nondrafted players entering the 2004 and 2005 drafts. *J Strength Cond Res* 22:6-12, 2008.

29. Slater, LV, Vriner, M, Zapalo, P, Arbour, K, and Hart, JM. Difference in agility, strength, and flexibility in competitive figure skaters based on level of expertise and skating discipline. *J Strength Cond Res* 30:3321-3328, 2016.

30. Speirs, DE, Bennett, MA, Finn, CV, and Turner, AP. Unilateral vs. bilateral squat training for strength, sprints, and agility in academy rugby players. *J Strength Cond Res* 30:386-392, 2016.

31. Spiteri, T, Nimphius, S, Hart, NH, Specos, C, Sheppard, JM, and Newton, RU. Contribution of strength characteristics to change of direction and agility performance in female basketball athletes. *J Strength Cond Res* 28:2415-2423, 2014.

32. Triplett, NT. Speed and agility. In *NSCA's Guide to Tests and Assessments*. Miller, T, ed. Champaign, IL: Human Kinetics, 253-274, 2012.

33. Wong del, P, Chan, GS, and Smith, AW. Repeated-sprint and change-of-direction abilities in physically active individuals and soccer players: Training and testing implications. *J Strength Cond Res* 26:2324-2330, 2012.

34. Wong del, P, Hjelde, GH, Cheng, CF, and Ngo, JK. Use of the RSA/RCOD index to identify training priority in soccer players. *J Strength Cond Res* 29:2787-2793, 2015.

Chapter 7

1. Beckenholdt, SE, and Mayhew, JL. Specificity among anaerobic power tests in male athletes. *J Sports Med Phys Fitness* 23:326-332, 1983.

2. Chu, DA. Assessment. In *Explosive Power and Strength: Complex Training for Maximum Results*. Champaign, IL: Human Kinetics, 167-180, 1996.

3. Clayton, MA, Trudo, CE, Laubach, LL, Linderman, JK, De Marco, GM, and Barr, S. Relationships between isokinetic core strength and field based athletic performance tests in male collegiate baseball players. *J Exerc Physiol Online* 14, 2011.

4. Clemons, J, and Harrison, M. Validity and reliability of a new stair sprinting test of explosive power. *J Strength Cond Res* 22:1578-1583, 2008.

5. Clemons, JM, Campbell, B, and Jeansonne, C. Validity and reliability of a new test of upper body power. *J Strength Cond Res* 24:1559-1565, 2010.

5a. Cornell, DJ, Gnacinski, SL, Langford, MH Mims, J, and Ebersole, KT. Backwards overhead medicine ball throw and canter movement jump performance among firefighter candidates. *J Trainol* 4:11-14, 2015.

6. Davis, KL, Kang, M, Boswell, BB, DuBose, KD, Altman, SR, and Binkley, HM. Validity and reliability of the medicine ball throw for kindergarten children. *J Strength Cond Res* 22:1958-1963, 2008.

7. Dobbs, CW, Gill, ND, Smart, DJ, and McGuigan, MR. Relationship between vertical and horizontal jump variables and muscular performance in athletes. *J Strength Cond Res* 29:661-671, 2015.

8. Duncan, MJ, Al-Nakeeb, Y, and Nevill, AM. Influence of familiarization on a backward, overhead medicine ball explosive power test. *Res Sports Med* 13:345-352, 2005.

9. Ellenbecker, TS, and Roetert, EP. An isokinetic profile of trunk rotation strength in elite tennis players. *Med Sci Sports Exerc* 36:1959-1963, 2004.

10. Fernandez-Fernandez, J, Saez de Villarreal, E, Sanz-Rivas, D, and Moya, M. The effects of 8-week plyometric training on physical performance in young tennis players. *Pediatr Exerc Sci* 28:77-86, 2016.

11. Freeston, JL, Carter, T, Whitaker, G, Nicholls, O, and Rooney, KB. Strength and power correlates of throwing velocity on subelite male cricket players. *J Strength Cond Res* 30:1646-1651, 2016.

12. Haff, GG, and Dumke, C. Anaerobic fitness measurements. In *Laboratory Manual for Exercise Physiology*. Champaign, IL: Human Kinetics, 305-360, 2012.

13. Hamilton, RT, Shultz, SJ, Schmitz, RJ, and Perrin, DH. Triple-hop distance as a valid predictor of lower limb strength and power. *J Athl Train* 43:144-151, 2008.

14. Harris, C, Wattles, AP, DeBeliso, M, Sevene-Adams, PG, Berning, JM, and Adams, KJ. The seated medicine ball throw as a test of upper body power in older adults. *J Strength Cond Res* 25:2344-2348, 2011.

15. Hetzler, RK, Vogelpohl, RE, Stickley, CD, Kuramoto, AN, Delaura, MR, and Kimura, IF. Development of a modified Margaria-Kalamen anaerobic power test for American football athletes. *J Strength Cond Res* 24:978-984, 2010.

16. Hoffman, J. Athletic performance testing and normative data. In *Physiological Aspects of Sport Training and Performance*. 2nd ed. Champaign, IL: Human Kinetics, 237-267, 2014.

17. Hoffman, JR, Ratamess, NA, Klatt, M, Faigenbaum, AD, Ross, RE, Tranchina, NM, McCurley, RC, Kang, J, and Kraemer, WJ. Comparison between different off-season resistance training programs in Division III American college football players. *J Strength Cond Res* 23:11-19, 2009.

18. Hoog, P, Warren, M, Smith, CA, and Chimera, NJ. Functional hop tests and tuck jump assessment scores between female Division I collegiate athletes participating in high versus low ACL injury prone sports: A cross sectional analysis. *Int J Sports Phys Ther* 11:945-953, 2016.

19. Housh, TJ, Cramer, JT, Weir, JP, Beck, TW, and Johnson, GO. Muscular power. In *Physical Fitness Laboratories on a Budget*. Scottsdale, AZ: Holcomb Hathaway, 127-162, 2009.

20. Ikeda, Y, Kijima, K, Kawabata, K, Fuchimoto, T, and Ito, A. Relationship between side medicine-ball throw performance and physical ability for male and female athletes. *Eur J Appl Physiol* 99:47-55, 2007.

21. Izquierdo-Gabarren, M, Exposito, RG, de Villarreal, ES, and Izquierdo, M. Physiological factors to predict on traditional rowing performance. *Eur J Appl Physiol* 108:83-92, 2010.

22. Kellis, SE, Tsitskaris, GK, Nikopoulou, MD, and Mousikou, KC. The evaluation of jumping ability of male and female basketball players according to their chronological age and major leagues. *J Strength Cond Res* 13:40-46, 1999.

23. Kendall, KL, and Fukuda, DH. Rowing ergometer training for combat sports. *Strength Cond J* 33:80-85, 2011.

24. Lawton, TW, Cronin, JB, and McGuigan, MR. Strength, power, and muscular endurance exercise and elite rowing ergometer performance. *J Strength Cond Res* 27:1928-1935, 2013.

25. Lockie, RG, Stage, AA, Stokes, JJ, Orjalo, AJ, Davis, DL, Giuliano, DV, Moreno, MR, Risso, FG, Lazar, A, Birmingham-Babauta, SA, and Tomita, TM. Relationships and predictive capabilities of jump assessments to soccer-specific field test performance in Division I collegiate players. *Sports* 4, 2016.

26. Loturco, I, Pereira, LA, Cal Abad, CC, D'Angelo, RA, Fernandes, V, Kitamura, K, Kobal, R, and Nakamura, FY. Vertical and horizontal jump tests are strongly associated with competitive performance in 100-m dash events. *J Strength Cond Res* 29:1966-1971, 2015.

27. Marques, MC, Izquierdo, M, Gabbett, TJ, Travassos, B, Branquinho, L, and van den Tillaar, R. Physical fitness profile of competitive young soccer players: Determination of positional differences. *Int J Sports Sci Coa* 11:693-701, 2016.

28. Marques, MC, Tillaar, R, Vescovi, JD, and Gonzalez-Badillo, JJ. Changes in strength and power performance in elite senior female professional volleyball players

during the in-season: A case study. *J Strength Cond Res* 22:1147-1155, 2008.

29. Marques, MC, van den Tillaar, R, Gabbett, TJ, Reis, VM, and Gonzalez-Badillo, JJ. Physical fitness qualities of professional volleyball players: Determination of positional differences. *J Strength Cond Res* 23:1106-1111, 2009.

30. Mayhew, JL, Bemben, MG, Rohrs, DM, and Bemben, DA. Specificity among anaerobic power tests in college female athletes. *J Strength Cond Res* 8:43-47, 1994.

31. Mayhew, JL, Bird, M, Cole, ML, Koch, AJ, Jacques, JA, Ware, JS, Buford, BN, and Fletcher, KM. Comparison of the backward overhead medicine ball throw to power production in college football players. *J Strength Cond Res* 19:514-518, 2005.

32. Mayhew, JL, Piper, FC, Etheridge, GL, Schwegler, TM, Beckenholdt, SE, and Thomas, MA. The Margaria-Kalamen anaerobic power test: Norms and correlates. *J Hum Movement Stud* 18:141-150, 1991.

33. McGuigan, MR, Doyle, TL, Newton, M, Edwards, DJ, Nimphius, S, and Newton, RU. Eccentric utilization ratio: Effect of sport and phase of training. *J Strength Cond Res* 20:992-995, 2006.

34. Metikos, B, Mikulic, P, Sarabon, N, and Markovic, G. Peak power output test on a rowing ergometer: A methodological study. *J Strength Cond Res* 29:2919-2925, 2015.

35. Moran, JJ, Sandercock, GR, Ramirez-Campillo, R, Meylan, CM, Collison, JA, and Parry, DA. Age-related variation in male youth athletes' countermovement jump after plyometric training: A meta-analysis of controlled trials. *J Strength Cond Res* 31:552-565, 2017.

36. Myers, BA, Jenkins, WL, Killian, C, and Rundquist, P. Normative data for hop tests in high school and collegiate basketball and soccer players. *Int J Sports Phys Ther* 9:596-603, 2014.

37. Noyes, FR, Barber, SD, and Mangine, RE. Abnormal lower limb symmetry determined by function hop tests after anterior cruciate ligament rupture. *Am J Sports Med* 19:513-518, 1991.

38. Nuzzo, JL. The National Football League scouting combine from 1999 to 2014: Normative reference values and an examination of body mass normalization techniques. *J Strength Cond Res* 29:279-289, 2015.

39. Palozola, MV, Koch, AJ, and Mayhew, JL. Relationship of backward overhead medicine ball throw with Olympic weightlifting performances. *J Strength Cond Res* 24:1, 2010.

40. Patterson, DD, and Peterson, DF. Vertical jump and leg power norms for young adults. *Meas Phys Educ Exerc Sci* 8:33-41, 2004.

41. Peterson, MD. Power. In *NSCA's Guide to Tests and Assessments*. Miller, T, ed. Champaign, IL: Human Kinetics, 217-252, 2012.

42. Power, A, Faught, BE, Przysucha, E, McPherson, M, and Montelpare, W. Establishing the test–retest reliability & concurrent validity for the Repeat Ice Skating Test (RIST) in adolescent male ice hockey players. *Meas Phys Educ Exerc Sci* 16:69-80, 2012.

43. Read, PJ, Lloyd, RS, De Ste Croix, M, and Oliver, JL. Relationships between field-based measures of strength and power and golf club head speed. *J Strength Cond Res* 27:2708-2713, 2013.

44. Reiman, MP, and Manske, RC. *Functional Testing in Human Performance*. Champaign, IL: Human Kinetics, 2009.

45. Reiman, MP, and Manske, RC. Strength and power testing. In *Functional Testing in Human Performance*. Champaign, IL: Human Kinetics, 131-190, 2009.

46. Reiman, MP, and Manske, RC. Upper extremity testing. In *Functional Testing in Human Performance*. Champaign, IL: Human Kinetics, 241-262, 2009.

47. Salonia, MA, Chu, DA, Cheifetz, PM, and Freidhoff, GC. Upper-body power as measured by medicine-ball throw distance and its relationship to class level among 10- and 11-year-old female participants in club gymnastics. *J Strength Cond Res* 18:695-702, 2004.

48. Sayers, SP, Harackiewicz, DV, Harman, EA, Frykman, PN, and Rosenstein, MT. Cross-validation of three jump power equations. *Med Sci Sports Exerc* 31:572-577, 1999.

49. Seiler, S, Taylor, M, Diana, R, Layes, J, Newton, P, and Brown, B. Assessing anaerobic power in collegiate football players. *J Strength Cond Res* 4:9-15, 1990.

50. Stockbrugger, BA, and Haennel, RG. Validity and reliability of a medicine ball explosive power test. *J Strength Cond Res* 15:431-438, 2001.

51. Stockbrugger, BA, and Haennel, RG. Contributing factors to performance of a medicine ball explosive power test: a comparison between jump and nonjump athletes. *J Strength Cond Res* 17:768-774, 2003.

52. Stoggl, R, Muller, E, and Stoggl, T. Motor abilities and anthropometrics in youth cross-country skiing. *Scand J Med Sci Sports* 25:e70-81, 2015.

53. Stojanovic, E, Ristic, V, McMaster, DT, and Milanovic, Z. Effect of plyometric training on vertical jump performance in female athletes: A systematic review and meta-analysis. *Sports Med* 47:975-986, 2017.

54. Stolberg, M, Sharp, A, Comtois, AS, Lloyd, RS, Oliver, JL, and Cronin, J. Triple and quintuple hops: Utility, reliability, asymmetry, and relationship to performance. *Strength Cond J* 38:18-25, 2016.

55. Suchomel, TJ, Sole, CJ, and Stone, MH. Comparison of methods that assess lower-body stretch-shortening cycle utilization. *J Strength Cond Res* 30:547-554, 2016.

56. Szymanski, DJ, Szymanski, JM, Schade, RL, Bradford, TJ, McIntyre, JS, DeRenne, C, and Madsen, NH. The relation between anthropometric and physiological variables and bat velocity of high-school baseball players before and after 12 weeks of training. *J Strength Cond Res* 24:2933-2943, 2010.

57. Tomkinson, GR, Carver, KD, Atkinson, F, Daniell, ND, Lewis, LK, Fitzgerald, JS, Lang, JJ, and Ortega, FB. European normative values for physical fitness in children and adolescents aged 9-17 years: Results from 2 779 165 Eurofit performances representing 30 countries. *Br J Sports Med*, 2017.

58. Ulbricht, A, Fernandez-Fernandez, J, and Ferrauti, A. Conception for fitness testing and individualized training programs in the German Tennis Federation. *Sport Orthop Traumatol* 29:180-192, 2013.

59. Wagner, DR, and Kocak, MS. A multivariate approach to assessing anaerobic power following a plyometric training program. *J Strength Cond Res* 11:251-255, 1997.

60. Zwolski, C, Schmitt, LC, Thomas, S, Hewett, TE, and Paterno, MV. The utility of limb symmetry indices in return-to-sport assessment in patients with bilateral anterior cruciate ligament reconstruction. *Am J Sports Med* 44:2030-2038, 2016.

Chapter 8

1. American College of Sports Medicine. Health-related physical fitness testing and interpretation. In *ACSM's Guidelines for Exercise Testing and Prescription*. 9th ed. Pescatello, LS, Arena, R, Riebe, D, Thompson, PD, eds. Philadelphia: Wolters Kluwer/Lippincott Williams & Wilkins Health, 60-113, 2014.

2. Baker, DG, and Newton, RU. Discriminative analyses of various upper body tests in professional rugby-league players. *Int J Sports Physiol Perform* 1:347-360, 2006.

3. Baláš, J, Pecha, O, Martin, AJ, and Cochrane, D. Hand–arm strength and endurance as predictors of climbing performance. *Eur J Sport Sci* 12:16-25, 2012.

4. Bianco, A, Lupo, C, Alesi, M, Spina, S, Raccuglia, M, Thomas, E, Paoli, A, and Palma, A. The sit up test to exhaustion as a test for muscular endurance evaluation. *Springerplus* 4:309, 2015.

5. Bohannon, RW, Steffl, M, Glenney, SS, Green, M, Cashwell, L, Prajerova, K, and Bunn, J. The prone bridge test: Performance, validity, and reliability among older and younger adults. *J Bodyw Mov Ther*, 22:385-389, 2018.

6. Brzycki, M. Strength testing—predicting a one-rep max from reps-to-fatigue. *J Phys Health Educ Recreat Dance* 64:88-90, 1993.

7. Caulfield, S, and Berninger, D. Exercise technique for free weight and machine training. In *Essentials of Strength Training and Conditioning*. 4th ed. Haff, G, Triplett, NT, eds. Champaign, IL: Human Kinetics, 351-408, 2016.

8. Centers for Disease Control and Prevention. *National Health and Nutrition Examination Survey (NHANES): Muscle Strength Procedures Manual*. Atlanta: Centers for Disease Control and Prevention, 2011.

9. Cronin, J, Lawton, T, Harris, N, Kilding, A, and McMaster, DT. A brief review of handgrip strength and sport performance. *J Strength Cond Res* 31:3187-3217, 2017.

10. Haff, GG, Berninger, D, and Caulfield, S. Exercise technique for alternative modes and nontraditional implement training. In *Essentials of Strength Training and Conditioning*. 4th ed. Haff, G, Triplett, NT, eds. Champaign, IL: Human Kinetics, 409-438, 2016.

11. Heyward, VH, and Gibson, AL. Assessing muscular fitness. In *Advanced Fitness Assessment and Exercise Prescription*. 7th ed. Champaign, IL: Human Kinetics, 153-180, 2014.

12. Hodgdon, JA. A history of the US Navy physical readiness program from 1976 to 1999. San Diego, CA: Naval Health Research Center, 1999.

13. Hoffman, J. Muscular endurance. In *Norms for Fitness, Performance, and Health*. Champaign, IL: Human Kinetics, 41-52, 2006.

14. Hoffman, J. Muscular strength. In *Norms for Fitness, Performance, and Health*. Champaign, IL: Human Kinetics, 27-40, 2006.

15. Jurimae, T, Perez-Turpin, JA, Cortell-Tormo, JM, Chinchilla-Mira, IJ, Cejuela-Anta, R, Maestu, J, Purge, P, and Jurimae, J. Relationship between rowing ergometer performance and physiological responses to upper and lower body exercises in rowers. *J Sci Med Sport* 13:434-437, 2010.

16. Kayihan, G. Comparison of physical fitness levels of adolescents according to sports participation: Martial arts, team sports and non-sports. *Arch Budo* 10:227-232, 2014.

17. Kim, PS, Mayhew, JL, and Peterson, DF. A modified YMCA bench press test as a predictor of 1 repetition maximum bench press strength. *J Strength Cond Res* 16:440-445, 2002.

18. Kramer, JF, Leger, A, Paterson, DH, and Morrow, A. Rowing performance and selected descriptive, field, and laboratory variables. *Can J Appl Physiol* 19:174-184, 1994.

19. Kyrolainen, H, Hakkinen, K, Kautiainen, H, Santtila, M, Pihlainen, K, and Hakkinen, A. Physical fitness, BMI and sickness absence in male military personnel. *Occup Med (Lond)* 58:251-256, 2008.

20. Leyk, D, Witzki, A, Willi, G, Rohde, U, and Ruther, T. Even one is too much: Sole presence of one of the risk factors overweight, lack of exercise, and smoking reduces physical fitness of young soldiers. *J Strength Cond Res* 29 Suppl 11:S199-S203, 2015.

21. McGuigan, M. Administration, scoring, and interpretation of selected tests. In *Essentials of Strength Training and Conditioning*. 4th ed. Haff, G, Triplett, NT, eds. Champaign, IL: Human Kinetics, 259-316, 2016.

22. McIntosh, G, Wilson, L, Affieck, M, and Hall, H. Trunk and lower extremity muscle endurance: Normative data for adults. *J Rehabil Outcome Meas* 2:20-39, 1998.

23. Moir, GL. Muscular endurance. In *NSCA's Guide to Tests and Assessments*. Miller, T, ed. Champaign, IL: Human Kinetics, 193-216, 2012.

24. Nieman, DC. Physical fitness norms. In *Exercise Testing and Prescription: A Health-Related Approach*. 7th ed. Boston: McGraw-Hill, 582-622, 2011.

25. Pearson, SN, Cronin, JB, Hume, PA, and Slyfield, D. Kinematics and kinetics of the bench-press and bench-pull exercises in a strength-trained sporting population. *Sports Biomech* 8:245-254, 2009.

26. Peterson, MD, and Krishnan, C. Growth charts for muscular strength capacity with quantile regression. *Am J Prev Med* 49:935-938, 2015.

27. Phillips, M, Petersen, A, Abbiss, CR, Netto, K, Payne, W, Nichols, D, and Aisbett, B. Pack hike test finishing time for Australian firefighters: Pass rates and correlates of performance. *Appl Ergon* 42:411-418, 2011.

28. Reiman, MP, and Manske, RC. Trunk testing. In *Functional Testing in Human Performance*. Champaign, IL: Human Kinetics, 211-240, 2009.

29. Reiman, MP, and Manske, RC. Upper extremity testing. In *Functional Testing in Human Performance*. Champaign, IL: Human Kinetics, 241-262, 2009.

30. Reynolds, JM, Gordon, TJ, and Robergs, RA. Prediction of one repetition maximum strength from multiple repetition maximum testing and anthropometry. *J Strength Cond Res* 20:584-592, 2006.

31. Ryman Augustsson, S, and Ageberg, E. Weaker lower extremity muscle strength predicts traumatic knee injury in youth female but not male athletes. *BMJ Open Sport Exerc Medi* 3:e000222, 2017.

32. Sanchez-Medina, L, Gonzalez-Badillo, JJ, Perez, CE, and Pallares, JG. Velocity- and power-load relationships of the bench pull vs. bench press exercises. *Int J Sports Med* 35:209-216, 2014.

33. Schram, B, Hing, W, and Climstein, M. Profiling the sport of stand-up paddle boarding. *J Sports Sci* 34:937-944, 2016.

34. Sheppard, JM, and Triplett, NT. Program design for resistance training. In *Essentials of Strength Training and Conditioning*. 4th ed. Haff, G, Triplett, NT, eds. Champaign, IL: Human Kinetics, 439-470, 2016.

35. Speranza, MJ, Gabbett, TJ, Johnston, RD, and Sheppard, JM. Muscular strength and power correlates of tackling ability in semiprofessional rugby league players. *J Strength Cond Res* 29:2071-2078, 2015.

36. Speranza, MJ, Gabbett, TJ, Johnston, RD, and Sheppard, JM. Effect of strength and power training on tackling ability in semiprofessional rugby league players. *J Strength Cond Res* 30:336-343, 2016.

37. Stoggl, T, Muller, E, Ainegren, M, and Holmberg, HC. General strength and kinetics: Fundamental to sprinting faster in cross country skiing? *Scand J Med Sci Sports* 21:791-803, 2011.

37a. Strand, SL, Hjelm, J, Shoepe, TC, and Fajardo, MA. Norms for an Isometric Muscle Endurance Test. *J Hum Kinet* 40:93-102, 2014.

38. Tanner, RK, Gore, CJ, and Australian Institute of Sport. *Physiological Tests for Elite Athletes*. 2nd ed. Champaign, IL: Human Kinetics, 2013.

39. Tomkinson, GR, Carver, KD, Atkinson, F, Daniell, ND, Lewis, LK, Fitzgerald, JS, Lang, JJ, and Ortega, FB. European normative values for physical fitness in children and adolescents aged 9-17 years: Results from 2 779 165 Eurofit performances representing 30 countries. *Br J Sports Med*, 2017.

40. Tong, RJ, and Wood, GL. A comparison of upper body strength in collegiate rugby players. In *Science and Football III: Proceedings of the Third World Congress of Science and Football, Cardiff, Wales, 9-13 April, 1995*. Bangsbo, J, Reilly, T, Hughes, M, eds. London: Taylor & Francis, 16-20, 1997.

41. Vaara, JP, Kyrolainen, H, Niemi, J, Ohrankammen, O, Hakkinen, A, Kocay, S, and Hakkinen, K. Associations of maximal strength and muscular endurance test scores with cardiorespiratory fitness and body composition. *J Strength Cond Res* 26:2078-2086, 2012.

42. Wathen, D. Load selection. In *Essentials of Strength and Conditioning*. 1st ed. Baechle, TR, ed. Champaign, IL: Human Kinetics, 435-436, 1994.

43. Wilkerson, GB, Giles, JL, and Seibel, DK. Prediction of core and lower extremity strains and sprains in collegiate football players: A preliminary study. *J Athl Train* 47:264-272, 2012.

44. Wind, AE, Takken, T, Helders, PJ, and Engelbert, RH. Is grip strength a predictor for total muscle strength in healthy children, adolescents, and young adults? *Eur J Pediatr* 169:281-287, 2010.

45. Zourladani, A, Zafrakas, M, Chatzigiannis, B, Papasozomenou, P, Vavilis, D, and Matziari, C. The effect of physical exercise on postpartum fitness, hormone and lipid levels: A randomized controlled trial in primiparous, lactating women. *Arch Gynecol Obstet* 291:525-530, 2015.

Chapter 9

1. *Army Physical Readiness Training, Training Circular 3-22.20*. Washington, DC: Headquarters, Department of the Army, 2010.

2. Adams, GM, and Beam, WC. Aerobic stepping. In *Exercise Physiology Laboratory Manual*. 7th ed. New York: McGraw-Hill, 135-144, 2014.

3. Almansba, R, Sterkowicz, S, Belkacem, R, Sterkowicz-Przybycien, K, and Mahdad, D. Anthropometrical and physiological profiles of the Algerian Olympic judoists. *Arch Budo* 6:185-193, 2010.

4. American College of Sports Medicine. Health-related physical fitness testing and interpretation. In *ACSM's Guidelines for Exercise Testing and Prescription*. 9th ed. Pescatello, LS, Arena, R, Riebe, D, Thompson, PD, eds. Philadelphia: Wolters Kluwer/Lippincott Williams & Wilkins Health, 60-113, 2014.

5. Asaka, M, and Higuchi, M. Rowing: A favorable tool to promote elderly health which offers both aerobic and resistance exercise. In *Physical Activity, Exercise, Sedentary Behavior and Health*. Kanosue, K, Oshima, S, Cao, Z-B, Oka, K, eds. Tokyo: Springer Japan, 307-318, 2015.

6. Bangsbo, J, Iaia, FM, and Krustrup, P. The Yo-Yo intermittent recovery test: A useful tool for evaluation of physical performance in intermittent sports. *Sports Med* 38:37-51, 2008.

7. Bendiksen, M, Ahler, T, Clausen, H, Wedderkopp, N, and Krustrup, P. The use of Yo-Yo intermittent recovery level 1 and Andersen testing for fitness and maximal heart rate assessments of 6- to 10-year-old school children. *J Strength Cond Res* 27:1583-1590, 2013.

8. Bennett, H, Parfitt, G, Davison, K, and Eston, R. Validity of submaximal step tests to estimate maximal oxygen uptake in healthy adults. *Sports Med* 46:737-750, 2016.

9. Bohannon, RW, Bubela, DJ, Wang, YC, Magasi, SS, and Gershon, RC. Six-minute walk test vs. three-minute step test for measuring functional endurance. *J Strength Cond Res* 29:3240-3244, 2015.

10. Bradley, PS, Bendiksen, M, Dellal, A, Mohr, M, Wilkie, A, Datson, N, Orntoft, C, Zebis, M, Gomez-Diaz, A, Bangsbo, J, and Krustrup, P. The application of the Yo-Yo intermittent endurance level 2 test to elite female soccer populations. *Scand J Med Sci Sports* 24:43-54, 2014.

11. Castagna, C, Impellizzeri, FM, Belardinelli, R, Abt, G, Coutts, A, Chamari, K, and D'Ottavio, S. Cardiorespiratory responses to Yo-Yo intermittent endurance test in nonelite youth soccer players. *J Strength Cond Res* 20:326-330, 2006.

12. Castagna, C, Impellizzeri, FM, Rampinini, E, D'Ottavio, S, and Manzi, V. The Yo-Yo intermittent recovery test in basketball players. *J Sci Med Sport* 11:202-208, 2008.

13. Cooper, KH. A means of assessing maximal oxygen intake: Correlation between field and treadmill testing. *J Amer Med Assoc* 203:201-&, 1968.

14. Cureton, KJ, Sloniger, MA, O'Bannon, JP, Black, DM, and McCormack, WP. A generalized equation for prediction of VO2peak from 1-mile run/walk performance. *Med Sci Sports Exerc* 27:445-451, 1995.

15. Fanchini, M, Castagna, C, Coutts, AJ, Schena, F, McCall, A, and Impellizzeri, FM. Are the Yo-Yo intermittent recovery test levels 1 and 2 both useful? Reliability, responsiveness and interchangeability in young soccer players. *J Sports Sci* 32:1950-1957, 2014.

16. George, JD, Vehrs, PR, Allsen, PE, Fellingham, GW, and Fisher, AG. VO2max estimation from a submaximal 1-mile track jog for fit college-age individuals. *Med Sci Sports Exerc* 25:401-406, 1993.

17. Gorski, T, Rosser, T, Hoppeler, H, and Vogt, M. An anthropometric and physical profile of young Swiss alpine skiers between 2004 and 2011. *Int J Sports Physiol Perform* 9:108-116, 2014.

18. Gorski, T, Rosser, T, Hoppeler, H, and Vogt, M. Relative age effect in young Swiss Alpine skiers from 2004 to 2011. *Int J Sports Physiol Perform* 11:455-463, 2016.

19. Haff, GG, and Dumke, C. Aerobic power field assessments. In *Laboratory Manual for Exercise Physiology*. Champaign, IL: Human Kinetics, 187-208, 2012.

20. Haff, GG, and Dumke, C. Submaximal exercise testing. In *Laboratory Manual for Exercise Physiology*. Champaign, IL: Human Kinetics, 165-186, 2012.

21. Heyward, VH, and Gibson, AL. Assessing cardiorespiratory fitness. In *Advanced Fitness Assessment and Exercise Prescription*. 7th ed. Champaign, IL: Human Kinetics, 79-120, 2014.

22. Hoffman, J. Aerobic power and endurance. In *Norms for Fitness, Performance, and Health*. Champaign, IL: Human Kinetics, 67-80, 2006.

23. Ingebrigtsen, J, Bendiksen, M, Randers, MB, Castagna, C, Krustrup, P, and Holtermann, A. Yo-Yo IR2 testing of elite and sub-elite soccer players: Performance, heart rate response and correlations to other interval tests. *J Sports Sci* 30:1337-1345, 2012.

24. Johnston, RD, Gabbett, TJ, Jenkins, DG, and Hulin, BT. Influence of physical qualities on post-match fatigue in rugby league players. *J Sci Med Sport* 18:209-213, 2015.

25. Kendall, KL, and Fukuda, DH. Rowing ergometer training for combat sports. *Strength Cond J* 33:80-85, 2011.

26. Krustrup, P, and Bangsbo, J. Physiological demands of top-class soccer refereeing in relation to physical capacity: Effect of intense intermittent exercise training. *J Sports Sci* 19:881-891, 2001.

27. Krustrup, P, and Mohr, M. Physical demands in competitive Ultimate Frisbee. *J Strength Cond Res* 29:3386-3391, 2015.

28. Krustrup, P, Mohr, M, Nybo, L, Jensen, JM, Nielsen, JJ, and Bangsbo, J. The Yo-Yo IR2 test: Physiological response, reliability, and application to elite soccer. *Med Sci Sports Exerc* 38:1666-1673, 2006.

29. Lakomy, HK, and Lakomy, J. Estimation of maximum oxygen uptake from submaximal exercise on a Concept II rowing ergometer. *J Sports Sci* 11:227-232, 1993.

30. Latour, AW, Peterson, DD, Rittenhouse, MA, and Riner, DD. Comparing alternate aerobic tests for United States Navy physical readiness test. *Int J Kinesiol High Educ* 1:89-99, 2017.

31. Leger, LA, Mercier, D, Gadoury, C, and Lambert, J. The multistage 20 metre shuttle run test for aerobic fitness. *J Sports Sci* 6:93-101, 1988.

32. Lockie, RG, Moreno, MR, Lazar, A, Orjalo, AJ, Giuliano, DV, Risso, FG, Davis, DL, Crelling, JB, Lockwood, JR, and Jalilvand, F. The physical and athletic performance characteristics of Division I collegiate female soccer players by position. *J Strength Cond Res* 32:334-343, 2018.

33. Mara, JK, Thompson, KG, Pumpa, KL, and Ball, NB. Periodization and physical performance in elite female soccer players. *Int J Sports Physiol Perform* 10:664-669, 2015.

34. Mayorga-Vega, D, Aguilar-Soto, P, and Viciana, J. Criterion-related validity of the 20-m shuttle run test for estimating cardiorespiratory fitness: A meta-analysis. *J Sports Sci Med* 14:536-547, 2015.

35. Mayorga-Vega, D, Bocanegra-Parrilla, R, Ornelas, M, and Viciana, J. Criterion-related validity of the distance- and time-based walk/run field tests for estimating cardiorespiratory fitness: A systematic review and meta-analysis. *PLoS One* 11:e0151671, 2016.

36. McArdle, WD, Katch, FI, and Katch, VL. Measuring and evaluating human-generating capacities during exercise. In *Essentials of Exercise Physiology*. 3rd ed. Baltimore, MD: Lippincott Williams & Wilkins, 223-259, 2006.

37. McClain, JJ, and Welk, GJ. Comparison of two versions of the PACER aerobic fitness test. *Med Sci Sports Exerc* 36:S5-S5, 2004.

38. McGuigan, M. Administration, scoring, and interpretation of selected tests. In *Essentials of Strength Training and Conditioning*. 4th ed. Haff, G, Triplett, NT, eds. Champaign, IL: Human Kinetics, 259-316, 2016.

39. Mello, RP, Murphy, MM, and Vogel, JA. Relationship between a two mile run for time and maximal oxygen uptake. *J Strength Cond Res* 2:9-12, 1988.

40. Mohr, M, and Krustrup, P. Yo-Yo intermittent recovery test performances within an entire football league during a full season. *J Sports Sci* 32:315-327, 2014.

40a. Morrow, JR, Jackson, A, Disch, J, and Mood, D. Measurement and evaluation in human performance. 3E. Champaign, IL: Human Kinetics, 2005.

41. Mujika, I, Santisteban, J, Impellizzeri, FM, and Castagna, C. Fitness determinants of success in men's and women's football. *J Sports Sci* 27:107-114, 2009.

42. Owen, C, Jones, P, and Comfort, P. The reliability of the submaximal version of the Yo-Yo intermittent recovery test in elite youth soccer. *J Trainol* 6:31-34, 2017.

43. Perroni, F, Guidetti, L, Cignitti, L, and Baldari, C. Absolute vs. weight-related maximum oxygen uptake in firefighters: Fitness evaluation with and without protective clothing and self-contained breathing apparatus among age group. *PLoS One* 10:e0119757, 2015.

44. Piquet, L, Dalmay, F, Ayoub, J, Vandroux, JC, Menier, R, Antonini, MT, and Pourcelot, L. Study of blood flow

parameters measured in femoral artery after exercise: Correlation with maximum oxygen uptake. *Ultrasound Med Biol* 26:1001-1007, 2000.

45. Purkhus, E, Krustrup, P, and Mohr, M. High-intensity training improves exercise performance in elite women volleyball players during a competitive season. *J Strength Cond Res* 30:3066-3072, 2016.

46. Reiman, MP, and Manske, RC. Aerobic testing. In *Functional Testing in Human Performance.* Champaign, IL: Human Kinetics, 119-130, 2009.

47. Rikli, RE, and Jones, CJ. *Senior fitness test manual.* 2nd ed. Champaign, IL: Human Kinetics, 2013.

48. Roberts, CK, Freed, B, and McCarthy, WJ. Low aerobic fitness and obesity are associated with lower standardized test scores in children. *J Pediatr* 156:711-718, 718 e711, 2010.

49. Rospo, G, Valsecchi, V, Bonomi, AG, Thomassen, IW, van Dantzig, S, La Torre, A, and Sartor, F. Cardiorespiratory improvements achieved by American College of Sports Medicine's exercise prescription implemented on a mobile app. *JMIR Mhealth Uhealth* 4:e77, 2016.

50. Santana, CCA, Azevedo, LB, Cattuzzo, MT, Hill, JO, Andrade, LP, and Prado, WL. Physical fitness and academic performance in youth: A systematic review. *Scand J Med Sci Sports* 27:579-603, 2017.

51. Sartor, F, Bonato, M, Papini, G, Rosio, A, Mohammed, RA, Bonomi, AG, Moore, JP, Mcrati, G, La Torre, A, and Kubis, HP. A 45-second self-test for cardiorespiratory fitness: Heart rate-based estimation in healthy individuals. *PLoS One* 11:e0168154, 2016.

52. Silva, G, Aires, L, Mota, J, Oliveira, J, and Ribeiro, JC. Normative and criterion related standards for shuttle run performance in youth. *Pediatr Exerc Sci* 24:157-169, 2012.

53. Tachibana, K, Yashiro, K, Miyazaki, J, Ikegami, Y, and Higuchi, M. Muscle cross-sectional areas and performance power of limbs and trunk in the rowing motion. *Sports Biomech* 6:44-58, 2007.

54. Tomkinson, GR, Lang, JJ, Tremblay, MS, Dalc, M, LeBlanc, AG, Belanger, K, Ortega, FB, and Leger, L. International normative 20 m shuttle run values from 1 142 026 children and youth representing 50 countries. *Br J Sports Med* 51:1545-1554, 2017.

55. Tomkinson, GR, Leger, LA, Olds, TS, and Cazorla, G. Secular trends in the performance of children and adolescents (1980-2000): An analysis of 55 studies of the 20m shuttle run test in 11 countries. *Sports Med* 33:285-300, 2003.

56. Vernillo, G, Silvestri, A, and La Torre, A. The Yo-Yo intermittent recovery test in junior basketball players according to performance level and age group. *J Strength Cond Res* 26:2490-2494, 2012.

57. Veugelers, KR, Naughton, GA, Duncan, CS, Burgess, DJ, and Graham, SR. Validity and reliability of a submaximal intermittent running test in elite Australian football players. *J Strength Cond Res* 30:3347-3353, 2016.

58. Wong, PL, Chaouachi, A, Castagna, C, Lau, PWC, Chamari, K, and Wisloff, U. Validity of the Yo-Yo intermittent endurance test in young soccer players. *Eur Sport Sci* 11:309-315, 2011.

59. Woolford, SM, Polglaze, T, Rowsell, G, and Spencer, M. Field testing principles and protocols. In *Physiological Tests for Elite Athletes.* 2nd ed. Tanner, RK, Gore, CJ, eds. Champaign, IL: Human Kinetics, 231-248, 2013.

60. YMCA of the USA. *YMCA Fitness Testing and Assessment Manual.* 4th ed. Champaign, IL: Human Kinetics, 2000.

61. Thomas, A, Dawson, B, and Goodman, C. The yo-yo-test: reliability and association with a 20-m shuttle run and VO(2max). *Int J Sports Physiol Perform* 1:137-149, 2006.

Chapter 10

1. Armstrong, LE. Assessing hydration status: The elusive gold standard. *J Am Coll Nutr* 26:575S-584S, 2007.

1a. Baker, LB, Barnes, KA, Anderson, ML, Passe, DH, and Stofan, JR. Normative data for regional sweat sodium concentration and whole-body sweating rate in athletes. *J Sports Sci* 34: 358-368, 2016.

2. Bangsbo, J, Iaia, FM, and Krustrup, P. The Yo-Yo intermittent recovery test: A useful tool for evaluation of physical performance in intermittent sports. *Sports Med* 38:37-51, 2008.

3. Bartolomei, S, Sadres, E, Church, DD, Arroyo, E, Gordon, JA, III, Varanoske, AN, Wang, R, Beyer, KS, Oliveira, LP, Stout, JR, and Hoffman, JR. Comparison of the recovery response from high-intensity and high-volume resistance exercise in trained men. *Eur J Appl Physiol* 117:1287-1298, 2017.

4. Bellenger, CR, Fuller, JT, Thomson, RL, Davison, K, Robertson, EY, and Buckley, JD. Monitoring athletic training status through autonomic heart rate regulation: A systematic review and meta-analysis. *Sports Med* 46:1461-1486, 2016.

5. Borg, E, and Borg, G. A comparison of AME and CR100 for scaling perceived exertion. *Acta Psychol (Amst)* 109:157-175, 2002.

6. Borg, GA. Perceived exertion. *Exerc Sport Sci Rev* 2:131-153, 1974.

7. Bosquet, L, Merkari, S, Arvisais, D, and Aubert, AE. Is heart rate a convenient tool to monitor over-reaching? A systematic review of the literature. *Br J Sports Med* 42:709-714, 2008.

8. Buchheit, M. Monitoring training status with HR measures: Do all roads lead to Rome? *Front Physiol* 5:73, 2014.

9. Buchheit, M, Mendez-Villanueva, A, Quod, MJ, Poulos, N, and Bourdon, P. Determinants of the variability of heart rate measures during a competitive period in young soccer players. *Eur J Appl Physiol* 109:869-878, 2010.

10. Buchheit, M, Simpson, BM, Garvican-Lewis, LA, Hammond, K, Kley, M, Schmidt, WF, Aughey, RJ, Soria, R, Sargent, C, Roach, GD, Claros, JCJ, Wachsmuth, N, Gore, CJ, and Bourdon, PC. Wellness, fatigue and physical performance acclimatisation to a 2-week soccer camp at 3600 m (ISA3600). *Br J Sports Med* 47:i100-i106, 2013.

11. Buchheit, M, Simpson, MB, Al Haddad, H, Bourdon, PC, and Mendez-Villanueva, A. Monitoring changes in

physical performance with heart rate measures in young soccer players. *Eur J Appl Physiol* 112:711-723, 2012.

12. Cheuvront, SN, Carter, R, 3rd, Montain, SJ, and Sawka, MN. Daily body mass variability and stability in active men undergoing exercise-heat stress. *Int J Sport Nutr Exerc Metab* 14:532-540, 2004.

13. Claudino, JG, Cronin, J, Mezencio, B, McMaster, DT, McGuigan, M, Tricoli, V, Amadio, AC, and Serrao, JC. The countermovement jump to monitor neuromuscular status: A meta-analysis. *J Sci Med Sport* 20:397-402, 2017.

14. Daanen, HA, Lamberts, RP, Kallen, VL, Jin, A, and Van Meeteren, NL. A systematic review on heart-rate recovery to monitor changes in training status in athletes. *Int J Sports Physiol Perform* 7:251-260, 2012.

15. Edwards, AM, Bentley, MB, Mann, ME, and Seaholme, TS. Self-pacing in interval training: A teleoanticipatory approach. *Psychophysiology* 48:136-141, 2011.

16. Eston, R. Use of ratings of perceived exertion in sports. *Int J Sports Physiol Perform* 7:175-182, 2012.

17. Fernandez-Elias, VE, Martinez-Abellan, A, Lopez-Gullon, JM, Moran-Navarro, R, Pallares, JG, De la Cruz-Sanchez, E, and Mora-Rodriguez, R. Validity of hydration non-invasive indices during the weightcutting and official weigh-in for Olympic combat sports. *PLoS One* 9:e95336, 2014.

18. Foster, C, Florhaug, JA, Franklin, J, Gottschall, L, Hrovatin, LA, Parker, S, Doleshal, P, and Dodge, C. A new approach to monitoring exercise training. *J Strength Cond Res* 15:109-115, 2001.

19. Franchini, E, Brito, CJ, and Artioli, GG. Weight loss in combat sports: Physiological, psychological and performance effects. *J Int Soc Sports Nutr* 9:52, 2012.

20. Fullagar, HH, Skorski, S, Duffield, R, Julian, R, Bartlett, J, and Meyer, T. Impaired sleep and recovery after night matches in elite football players. *J Sports Sci* 34:1333-1339, 2016.

21. Gabbett, TJ, Nassis, GP, Oetter, E, Pretorius, J, Johnston, N, Medina, D, Rodas, G, Myslinski, T, Howells, D, Beard, A, and Ryan, A. The athlete monitoring cycle: A practical guide to interpreting and applying training monitoring data. *Br J Sports Med* 51:1451-1452, 2017.

22. Gathercole, RJ, Sporer, BC, Stellingwerff, T, and Sleivert, GG. Comparison of the capacity of different jump and sprint field tests to detect neuromuscular fatigue. *J Strength Cond Res* 29:2522-2531, 2015.

23. Gibson, JC, Stuart-Hill, LA, Pethick, W, and Gaul, CA. Hydration status and fluid and sodium balance in elite Canadian junior women's soccer players in a cool environment. *Appl Physiol Nutr Metab* 37:931-937, 2012.

24. Haddad, M, Stylianides, G, Djaoui, L, Dellal, A, and Chamari, K. Session-RPE method for training load monitoring: Validity, ecological usefulness, and influencing factors. *Front Neurosci* 11:612, 2017.

25. Hagerman, P. Aerobic endurance training program design. In *NSCA's Essentials of Personal Training*. 2nd ed. Coburn, JW, Malek, MH, eds. Champaign, IL: Human Kinetics, 389-410, 2012.

26. Heyward, VH, and Gibson, AL. Preliminary health screening and risk classification. In *Advanced Fitness Assessment and Exercise Prescription*. 7th ed. Champaign, IL: Human Kinetics, 23-46, 2014.

27. Hooper, SL, Mackinnon, LT, Howard, A, Gordon, RD, and Bachmann, AW. Markers for monitoring overtraining and recovery. *Med Sci Sports Exerc* 27:106-112, 1995.

28. Kavouras, SA, Johnson, EC, Bougatsas, D, Arnaoutis, G, Panagiotakos, DB, Perrier, E, and Klein, A. Validation of a urine color scale for assessment of urine osmolality in healthy children. *Eur J Nutr* 55:907-915, 2016.

29. Lau, WY, Blazevich, AJ, Newton, MJ, Wu, SS, and Nosaka, K. Assessment of muscle pain induced by elbow-flexor eccentric exercise. *J Athl Train* 50:1140-1148, 2015.

30. Laurent, CM, Fullenkamp, AM, Morgan, AL, and Fischer, DA. Power, fatigue, and recovery changes in national collegiate athletic association Division I hockey players across a competitive season. *J Strength Cond Res* 28:3338-3345, 2014.

31. Laurent, CM, Green, JM, Bishop, PA, Sjokvist, J, Schumacker, RE, Richardson, MT, and Curtner-Smith, M. A practical approach to monitoring recovery: Development of a perceived recovery status scale. *J Strength Cond Res* 25:620-628, 2011.

32. Lieberman, HR. Hydration and cognition: A critical review and recommendations for future research. *J Am Coll Nutr* 26:555S-561S, 2007.

33. Malone, S, Owen, A, Newton, M, Mendes, B, Tiernan, L, Hughes, B, and Collins, K. Wellbeing perception and the impact on external training output among elite soccer players. *J Sci Med Sport* 21:29-34, 2018.

34. Marston, KJ, Peiffer, JJ, Newton, MJ, and Scott, BR. A comparison of traditional and novel metrics to quantify resistance training. *Sci Rep* 7:5606, 2017.

35. McBride, JM, McCaulley, GO, Cormie, P, Nuzzo, JL, Cavill, MJ, and Triplett, NT. Comparison of methods to quantify volume during resistance exercise. *J Strength Cond Res* 23:106-110, 2009.

36. McDermott, BP, Anderson, SA, Armstrong, LE, Casa, DJ, Cheuvront, SN, Cooper, L, Kenney, WL, O'Connor, FG, and Roberts, WO. National Athletic Trainers' Association position statement: Fluid replacement for the physically active. *J Athl Train* 52:877-895, 2017.

37. McGuigan, M. Quantifying training stress. In *Monitoring Training and Performance in Athletes*. Champaign, IL: Human Kinetics, 69-102, 2017.

38. Mohr, M, and Krustrup, P. Yo-Yo intermittent recovery test performances within an entire football league during a full season. *J Sports Sci* 32:315-327, 2014.

39. Murray, B. Hydration and physical performance. *J Am Coll Nutr* 26:542S-548S, 2007.

40. Nagahara, R, Morin, JB, and Koido, M. Impairment of sprint mechanical properties in an actual soccer match: A pilot study. *Int J Sports Physiol Perform* 11:893-898, 2016.

41. Nedelec, M, McCall, A, Carling, C, Legall, F, Berthoin, S, and Dupont, G. The influence of soccer playing actions on the recovery kinetics after a soccer match. *J Strength Cond Res* 28:1517-1523, 2014.

42. Nilsson, J, Csergo, S, Gullstrand, L, Tveit, P, and Refsnes, PE. Work-time profile, blood lactate concentration and rating of perceived exertion in the 1998

Greco-Roman Wrestling World Championship. *J Sports Sci* 20:939-945, 2002.

43. Nuccio, RP, Barnes, KA, Carter, JM, and Baker, LB. Fluid balance in team sport athletes and the effect of hypohydration on cognitive, technical, and physical performance. *Sports Med* 47:1951-1982, 2017.

44. Ohnhaus, EE, and Adler, R. Methodological problems in the measurement of pain: A comparison between the verbal rating scale and the visual analogue scale. *Pain* 1:379-384, 1975.

45. Oliver, JL, Lloyd, RS, and Whitney, A. Monitoring of in-season neuromuscular and perceptual fatigue in youth rugby players. *Eur J Sport Sci* 15:514-522, 2015.

46. Owen, C, Jones, P, and Comfort, P. The reliability of the submaximal version of the Yo-Yo intermittent recovery test in elite youth soccer. *J Trainol* 6:31-34, 2017.

47. Peterson, MD, Pistilli, E, Haff, GG, Hoffman, EP, and Gordon, PM. Progression of volume load and muscular adaptation during resistance exercise. *Eur J Appl Physiol* 111:1063-1071, 2011.

48. Raeder, C, Wiewelhove, T, Simola, RA, Kellmann, M, Meyer, T, Pfeiffer, M, and Ferrauti, A. Assessment of fatigue and recovery in male and female athletes after 6 days of intensified strength training. *J Strength Cond Res* 30:3412-3427, 2016.

49. Rauch, JT, Ugrinowitsch, C, Barakat, CI, Alvarez, MR, Brummert, DL, Aube, DW, Barsuhn, AS, Hayes, D, Tricoli, V, and De Souza, EO. Auto-regulated exercise selection training regimen produces small increases in lean body mass and maximal strength adaptations in strength-trained individuals. *J Strength Cond Res*, 2017.

50. Rivera Brown, AM, and De Felix Davila, RA. Hydration status in adolescent judo athletes before and after training in the heat. *Int J Sports Physiol Perform* 7:39-46, 2012.

51. Santos, L, Fernandez-Rio, J, Winge, K, Barragán-Pérez, B, Rodríguez-Pérez, V, González-Díez, V, Blanco-Traba, M, Suman, OE, Philip Gabel, C, and Rodríguez-Gómez, J. Effects of supervised slackline training on postural instability, freezing of gait, and falls efficacy in people with Parkinson's disease. *Disabil Rehabil* 39:1573-1580, 2017.

52. Saw, AE, Main, LC, and Gastin, PB. Monitoring the athlete training response: Subjective self-reported measures trump commonly used objective measures: A systematic review. *Br J Sports Med* 50:281-291, 2016.

53. Sikorski, EM, Wilson, JM, Lowery, RP, Joy, JM, Laurent, CM, Wilson, SM, Hesson, D, Naimo, MA, Averbuch, B, and Gilchrist, P. Changes in perceived recovery status scale following high-volume muscle damaging resistance exercise. *J Strength Cond Res* 27:2079-2085, 2013.

54. Slimani, M, Davis, P, Franchini, E, and Moalla, W. Rating of perceived exertion for quantification of training and combat loads during combat sport-specific activities: A short review. *J Strength Cond Res* 31:2889-2902, 2017.

55. Smith, MF, Newell, AJ, and Baker, MR. Effect of acute mild dehydration on cognitive-motor performance in golf. *J Strength Cond Res* 26:3075-3080, 2012.

56. Stone, MH, O'Bryant, HS, Schilling, BK, Johnson, RL, Pierce, KC, Haff, GG, and Koch, AJ. Periodization: Effects of manipulating volume and intensity. Part 1. *Strength Cond J* 21:56, 1999.

56a. Tanaka, H, Monahan, KD, and Seals, DR. Age-predicted maximal heart rate revisited. *J Am Coll Cardiol* 37:153-6, 2001.

57. Thorpe, RT, Strudwick, AJ, Buchheit, M, Atkinson, G, Drust, B, and Gregson, W. Tracking morning fatigue status across in-season training weeks in elite soccer players. *Int J Sports Physiol Perform* 11:947-952, 2016.

58. Thorpe, RT, Strudwick, AJ, Buchheit, M, Atkinson, G, Drust, B, and Gregson, W. The influence of changes in acute training load on daily sensitivity of morning-measured fatigue variables in elite soccer players. *Int J Sports Physiol Perform* 12:S2107-S2113, 2017.

59. Turner, AN, Buttigieg, C, Marshall, G, Noto, A, Phillips, J, and Kilduff, L. Ecological validity of the session rating of perceived exertion for quantifying internal training load in fencing. *Int J Sports Physiol Perform* 12:124-128, 2017.

60. Veugelers, KR, Naughton, GA, Duncan, CS, Burgess, DJ, and Graham, SR. Validity and reliability of a submaximal intermittent running test in elite Australian football players. *J Strength Cond Res* 30:3347-3353, 2016.

61. Wiewelhove, T, Raeder, C, Meyer, T, Kellmann, M, Pfeiffer, M, and Ferrauti, A. Markers for routine assessment of fatigue and recovery in male and female team sport athletes during high-intensity interval training. *PLoS One* 10:e0139801, 2015.

Index

Note: The italicized *f* and *t* following page numbers refer to figures and tables, respectively.

About the Author

David Fukuda, PhD, CSCS,*D, CISSN, is an associate professor and head of the division of kinesiology at the University of Central Florida. He was previously an assistant professor at Creighton University and a research assistant at the University of Oklahoma, where he earned his doctorate in exercise physiology. His research interests include the development of performance-based testing methodologies, the analysis of physiological profiles in athletes, and the assessment of adaptations to exercise training and nutritional interventions for various populations.

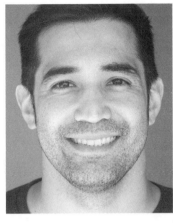

Courtesy of Randall Aarestad

Fukuda is certified as a strength and conditioning specialist with distinction through the National Strength and Conditioning Association and is certified as a sports nutritionist through the International Society of Sports Nutrition. He was awarded the Terry J. Housh Outstanding Young Investigator Award in 2016 by the National Strength and Conditioning Association. Fukuda is a fourth-degree black belt in judo and for the past 20 years has been involved in the sport as a competitor, instructor, coach, and referee.

You read the book—now complete an exam to earn continuing education credit!

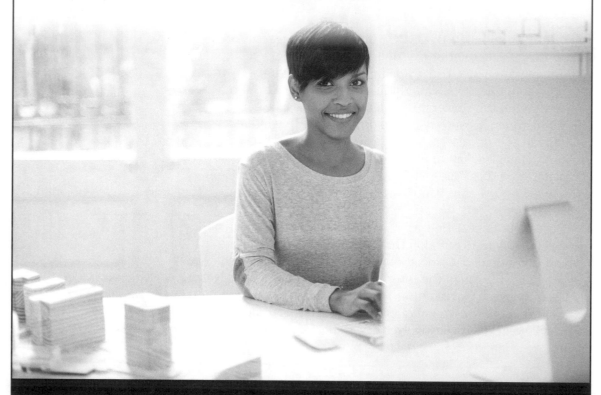

Congratulations on successfully preparing for this continuing education exam!

If you would like to earn CE credit, please visit

www.HumanKinetics.com/CE-Exam-Access

for complete instructions on how to access your exam.
Take advantage of a discounted rate by entering
promo code **ASAP2019** when prompted.

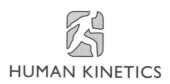

HUMAN KINETICS